As a doctor on the front lines of the current obesity epidemic, I have become increasingly alarmed that people simply are unaware of how to eat, or what the food they put into their mouths is doing to them. People no longer know what or how to eat. Food choices are based on what's fast and what big business and big agriculture tells us is correct. We are dealing with a country of obese people who are chronically malnourished. Drs. Pottingers and Price showed us decades ago what was to come of tainting our food supply, yet we failed to heed their warnings. This book has again introduced us to concepts that we should have listened to decades ago. Perhaps this generation will pay attention! We will continue to die of obesity related chronic illnesses until people begin to reclaim their health by understanding what and how to eat again. This book lays it out for us.

—Tyna Moore, ND, DC

This is an excellent book illustrating the current plight facing our Western culture, warning us of the perils of a poor diet as predicted by Dr. Pottenger in his book Pottenger's Cats, published in 1946. After giving an intriguing explanation of the new science of epigenetics, and how that profoundly influences our health, the authors then provide us all with timely, healthy, well-reasoned, scientifically-sound nutritional strategies to fetch us back from the brink of nutritional melt-down. Bravo!

—John A. Walck, MD

POTTENGER'S
PROPHECY

Deborah Kesten is the author of:
The Enlightened Diet
The Healing Secrets of Food
Feeding the Body, Nourishing the Soul

Larry Scherwitz is co-author of:
The Enlightened Diet

Gray Graham is the founder of the
Nutritional Therapy Association (NTA)

Pottenger's Prophecy

How Food Resets Genes for Wellness or Illness

GRAY GRAHAM, B.A., N.T.P.

DEBORAH KESTEN, M.P.H.

LARRY SCHERWITZ, PH.D.

White River Press
Amherst, Massachusetts

White River Press
PO Box 3561
Amherst, MA 01004
www.whiteriverpress.com

Printed in the United States of America
ISBN: 978-1-935052-33-3

Book design: Rebecca S. Neimark, Twenty-Six Letters

Library of Congress Cataloging-in-Publication Data

Graham, Gray, 1950–
Pottenger's prophecy : how food resets genes for wellness or illness / by Gray Graham, Deborah Kesten, Larry Scherwitz.
        p.   cm.
    Includes bibliographical references and index.
    ISBN 978-1-935052-33-3 (pbk. : alk. paper)
1. Nutrition—Genetic aspects. 2. Epigenesis. I. Kesten, Deborah, 1948– II. Scherwitz, Larry, 1946–. III. Title. IV. Title: Pottenger's prophecy.
    QP144.G45G73 2010
    613.2—dc22
                            2010029393

This publication contains the opinions and ideas of its authors. It is intended to provide helpful and informative material on the subjects addressed in the publication. It is sold with the understanding that the authors and publisher are not engaged in rendering medical, health, or any other kind of personal professional services in the book. The reader should consult his or health practitioner before adopting any of the suggestions in the book or drawing inferences from it.

The authors and publisher specifically disclaim all responsibility for any liability, loss, or risk, personal or otherwise, which is incurred as a consequence, directly or indirectly, of the use and application of any of the contents of the book.

This book is dedicated to the memory of
Weston A. Price, D.D.S. and
Frances M. Pottenger Jr., M.D.,
whose nutritional wisdom guides us to this day.

Acknowledgments

This book is possible only because of the landmark and ground-breaking research of individuals who preceded it. With this in mind, we extend gratitude to Gregor Johann Mendel for his discovery in the mid-1800s of how individual traits are passed on through generations; the pioneering work in the 1930s of innovators Francis M. Pottenger, Jr., M.D., and Weston A. Price, D.D.S., who made the link between diet, genes, and health-through-generations, well before the concept existed. We also owe thanks to British geneticists James D. Watson and Francis Crick, who identified the structure of DNA in the early 1950s; and the relatively recent discoveries by Swedish epidemiologist Lars Olov Bygren, Ph.D., and British geneticist Marcus Pembrey, Ph.D., who not only revealed that diet affects genes and whether they express through wellness or illness, but also that gene expression can be passed on to the next generation. Clearly, these foundational discoveries, which show that *food and nutrition are far more important than we previously realized*, provide the thesis of this book. In this regard, we also want to acknowledge the Price-Pottenger Nutrition Foundation in Lemon Grove, California, whose work is exceedingly relevant to this book.

Each health professional and research scientist interviewed for this book is continuing to contribute to the rich repository of wisdom about food, nutrition, genetics, and epigenetics that has evolved over the decades.

To Robert T. Pottenger, Jr., M.D., who generously shared memories about his uncle, Francis M. Pottenger, Jr., and his before-their-time feeding experiments in the 1930s with cats—which provided early clues about the food-gene-health link.

To educator, doctor, researcher, and a leading authority on natural medicine, Joseph Pizzorno, N.D. Founder of Bastyr University, who discussed his knowledge about genetic testing and genes as they relate to health and healing and the future of medicine.

To Lara Pizzorno, M.A.(Div), M.A.(Lit), L.M.T., and Senior Medical Editor, who generously shared both her medical expertise and personal gene-nutrient health odyssey.

To Pamela Snider, N.D., a brilliant, beautiful friend who is Founding Executive Director of the Academic Consortium for Complementary and Alternative Health Care (ACCAHC), and Executive Editor, Foundations of Naturopathic Medicine Project. Heartfelt thanks for providing pearls of wisdom about epigenetics and natural medicine.

To Dana Dolinoy, M.P.H., Ph.D., for insights about her research on genistein and its ability to alter coat color and protect avy mice offspring from obesity by modifyng the fetal epigenome; thank you, too, for giving us permission to print a photo about your research in our book.

To David Granatstein, a sustainable agriculture specialist from Wenatchee, Washington, who provided invaluable insights into the full spectrum of organic and conventional farming practices; for providing his excellent chart on this topic; and for his broad-spectrum wisdom about soil and food quality.

To Malea Balmuth, her husband, Edward, and their children Eliza and Jake, for sharing their "food pioneer" experience about the sustainable and organic farm they created for the nourishment of the family.

To Preston Andrews, Ph.D., Associate Professor of Horticulture, Department of Horticulture & Landscape Architecture, Washington State University at Pullman, who shared his knowledge about living soil, food quality . . . and more.

To John P. Reganold, Ph.D., director and founder of Washington State University's organic farming major. His novel and pioneering farming systems research has shown that organic, biodynamic, and integrated farming practices are sustainable, and can mitigate some of the hazardous effects of conventional agriculture on the environment.

To Matthew Anway, Ph.D., for his time and in-depth insights into both his own innovative research on epigenetics, and also for providing an "arc overview" of this emerging new science.

To Linda Roghaar, for her ongoing support, enthusiasm, and publishing expertise extraordinaire.

To Joanne McCall, for applying her finely honed public relations skills to get the word out about our book. We appreciate the coverage she achieved in top-tier print, broadcast, and online media, and her ability to help create a "spot on" platform that effectively communicates our work.

To book designer Rebecca Neimark, of Twenty-Six Letters, whose brilliant work superbly reflects the quality of the contents.

To Joy Graham, for her ongoing support, and for sprinkling her intelligence and "sparkling" personality on our many meetings; and, wow, what a cook!

And to all those who continue to research and eat the "green-gene" way that resets genes for wellness . . . thank you for contributing to the stream of wisdom about optimal eating—for yourself, your children, and future generations.

CONTENTS

POTTENGER'S PROPHECY

In the 1930s, in a small town in southern California, pediatrician and research scientist Dr. Francis M. Pottenger, Jr., made two discoveries that were nothing less than prophetic. His first discovery revealed that mother cats fed a *poor* diet passed their health problems onto their kittens *over three generations*. Pottenger's second discovery was as revolutionary, for he found that it took at least four generations of a *healthy* diet for kittens to recover from—meaning, to turn around—the health-robbing effects of the poor diet fed to the first generation. Is it really possible to pass on health problems to unborn generations? Is diet-related health status—*over generations*—relevant to human beings? Conversely, can consuming a healthful diet reverse the trend and turn illness to wellness for ourselves and our offspring? An emerging new state-of-the-art science called *epigenetics* is offering early answers to questions raised by Pottenger and his prophecy of diet-based wellness or illness decades ago. And recent research is doing even more, for it is providing a crystal ball into the future of food and our health, indeed, into the role diet plays in our survival as a species.

I

The city of Monrovia lies in the foothills of the San Gabriel Mountains of Los Angeles County, California. Originally a residential community of orange ranches, all that changed when the Santa Fe railroad forged its way through Monrovia in the late 1800s, bringing new people looking for homes and work and business opportunities.[1] One such settler was Francis Marion Pottenger, a physician from Ohio who came to Monrovia in 1895 to open a medical facility—called a sanatorium at the time—to treat people with the often deadly disease tuberculosis, or TB, and related respiratory chest ailments. Founded by Pottenger and his two brothers, the Pottenger Sanatorium and Clinic opened its doors in 1903.

Pottenger had a special, personal interest in helping those with the ailment because his first wife had died from it. When he married his second wife, Adelaide (Kitty), in 1900, they lived in the family home on the property's many acres. Called The Oaks, the facility included a working farm and a first-of-its-kind government-accredited dairy whose cows were certified to be TB-free. Not only did the farm provide fresh food and milk for the sanatorium's TB patients, but fresh fare and farming know-how became the norm for the Pottengers and their three children, Francis Marion Jr., Robert Thomas, and Adelaide Marie.[2]

Early on, the Pottengers' first-born son, Francis, born in 1901, showed a strong inclination toward combining his innovative inventions with farm-fresh food, so that he could be of help to others. If you visited The Oaks when he was a teenager in the second decade of the 1900s, you might have observed a tractor-drawn cart he designed so that he could deliver hot meals prepared in the kitchen of the sanatorium to patients in outlying cottages on the grounds.[3] Pottenger was exceptionally smart; however, such inventions also may have been motivated by the health problems he had experienced throughout his childhood. They had been so severe that by the time he began college, he had spent almost three years bedridden. Was it possible that Pottenger had turned such suffering into care and compassion for others? His career choice might offer a clue.

Though he was attracted to engineering for his life's work, Pottenger honored his father's wishes and, like his father, became a physician. Throughout his medical education, he continued to care deeply about how heath and healing could be achieved, and how children in particular might maintain wellness and not suffer as he had. "He lived from the heart," his nephew, Dr. Robert Thomas Pottenger, Jr., would say years later in an interview. "My uncle wanted to figure out how to make sick people better—and to understand why they got better."[4]

In medical school, Pottenger had specialized in pediatric allergies. After graduating, Pottenger knew he could put his passion for high-quality patient care into action if he were to return to the sanatorium to live, practice medicine, and conduct research studies that would help those with respiratory conditions. What he didn't know was that the first research project he initiated not only would change the course of his life but would lead to a dynamic and new understanding of food and nutrition, and in turn, of the pivotal role that they play in medicine, health and healing—in life itself.

2

In 1931, when Pottenger began his work at the Pottenger Sanatorium and Clinic, it had evolved into a well-known, well-respected institution, with a reputation for paying careful attention to patients' physical and emotional well-being, as well as to the disease itself. In this way, it was a good fit for Pottenger's caring values, as well as for his new wife, Teresa Elizabeth, and ultimately for their four children.[5] As a dynamic young doctor, he would wear various hats—from serving as a vice president and associate medical director to beginning a private practice in a separate building on the grounds of the sanatorium.

At the same time, he would launch a first-of-its-kind research project, motivated by his father's theory that TB was linked to deficiencies in the adrenal gland.[3] To put his plan into action, Pottenger and his father administered fresh adrenal extract—taken from cattle on the family farm—to their TB patients. What they discovered was encouraging, for the health of most TB patients who received the extract improved. The next step would be to discover the *exact dosage* needed to bring optimal benefits. To proceed, Pottenger removed the adrenals (called an *adrenalectomy*) of cats, so that they no longer produced adrenal extract; he then gave the cats various doses of adrenal extract from cattle to determine how much the cats would need to survive and recover. His thinking was that if he could identify the dosage that could help cats heal, he could use this information to work out the optimal dosage needed to treat TB patients (or for those with other respiratory ailments, such as asthma or emphysema).

Given today's scientific sensibilities, such a study may seem unusual, but in the 1930s and '40s, it was common for scientists to use animals such as mice or guinea pigs for the purpose of standardizing hormonal extracts that could be used therapeutically. "In those days, there was no way of measuring the biological effect [called *pharmacokinetics*], so it was done by feed," that is, experimenting with dosage levels in animals, Pottenger's nephew Robert said. "He would feed the extracts to the cats to find out how much was needed to keep the cats alive. This was his standardization method."[4]

To begin his investigation, Pottenger turned to cats who were donated especially for the study. After surgically removing their adrenal glands, he would give them various doses of his newly created adrenal extract. Then, to determine the effectiveness of each batch, he would observe the cats' responses. In this way, "he was able to determine the strength of each batch of extract and to obtain the necessary uniformity in potency," states a biography.[2]

Throughout his adrenal studies, Pottenger kept careful notes on the food he fed the cats, which consisted of cooked meat scraps from the kitchen in the sanatorium, raw milk from cows raised on the property's dairy, and cod liver oil.[6] At the time, such a diet was believed to be healthful and nutritious for cats. Even so, Pottenger noted that many of the cats didn't survive the surgery or died soon after the operation. He also began to realize he had more donated cats than food to feed them. And if he didn't have enough food, he couldn't move forward with his work. In response, he turned to the local meat packing plant, from which he ordered scraps of *raw* meat, as well as organs and bone.[4]

It seemed simple enough: to proceed, Pottenger would feed one group of cats the *raw* meat scraps from the meat packing plant, while the second group would continue to eat the *cooked* meat diet from the sanatorium. At the time, Pottenger didn't consider that the way in which the meat was prepared (meaning, cooked versus raw) would matter. This was the 1930s, and we knew a lot less about nutrition then than now. Not only would it be years before researchers discovered the existence of more vitamins and minerals, they hadn't yet made a strong link between the food we eat, how it is prepared, and health status.

It was during this time that Pottenger made an unexpected observation: the cats receiving the new diet of raw meat appeared to be healthier than the cats fed the cooked meat scraps. Not only did cats receiving the raw meat seem to be in better shape, he observed that more of them were surviving the surgical removal of their adrenal glands compared to the cats who were consuming the cooked meat. "Within a very short time the cats in the pens [fed raw meat] survived the operations, the unoperated cats appeared to be in better health, and the kittens born were vigorous," he would later write. "The contrast in apparent health between the cats in the pens fed on raw-meat scraps and those fed on the cooked-meat scraps was . . . startling."[7] Such unexpected serendipitous insights piqued Pottenger's interest—so much so that he decided to investigate further.

The question he posed was this: what is the effect, if any, of heat-processed foods and pasteurized vitamin D milk on the dentofacial and other anatomical structures of experimental animals? Put another way, does the cooking process somehow render food nutritionally different and deficient, causing eventual physiological degeneration?[2] Ultimately, his intention was to discover more about the nutrient quality—or difference, if any—of raw versus cooked meat, as well as raw versus pasteurized milk. And he wanted to know if meat and milk, when modified by high heat, had an impact on growth and development. To find out, he would do a controlled scientific study to see what impact the differently prepared meat and milk had on the cats' and kittens' teeth and related structures such as gums and jaw structure.[6]

The year was 1932. Pottenger's adrenal-based discoveries happened more than 75 years ago. [6, 8–10] At the time, he didn't know he was about to launch a study that would lead to an exceptional discovery. Nor did he know that his future pioneering breakthrough would be of such magnitude that it would plant a seed for a new science and medicine that would emerge in the latter part of the twentieth century, poised to take flight at the start of the 21st century.

3

Back to the 1930s and Pottenger's first-of-its-kind project. "To begin the study, a population of animals was selected, which Pottenger aptly dubbed 'run of the pen cats,'" states a documentary on his work. "His major concern was that his cats represent the normal sampling of animals," meaning, to be selected for the study, they needed to be disease-free.[11] The cats were then weighed, numbered, and described, and kept in open-air pens with a partially covered roof and bedding on the floor for comfort. With such thorough preparation, Pottenger was poised to launch the first series of his meat and milk experiments, unaware that it would turn into a series of experiments that would continue for ten years.

During the ten years, "approximately nine hundred cats were studied," he would later write in a research paper that summarized his work, for "six hundred of whom we have completed records."[8] Pottenger kept such a thorough account, and continued his experiments for such a long period of time, because not only did he want to see the short-term impact the different cooking methods had on the health of the cats, but he had the great foresight to study the influence the cats' diet and health status would have on their kittens over three generations. In other words, starting with the first generation of cats, Pottenger carefully documented the link between diet and health for a total of four generations.

The first series of studies, which focused on meat, was fairly simple and straightforward: one group of cats was fed a diet of two-thirds *raw* meat, one-third raw milk, and cod-liver oil, and cats in the second group consumed a diet of two-thirds *cooked* meat, one-third raw milk, and cod-liver oil.[6] The results were both innovative and intriguing. When the cats ate a raw meat, raw milk diet, they and their kittens over three generations exhibited similar traits: pregnancies were carried to full term; litters averaged five, and the mother cats nursed their young with no difficulty. These cats also had strong immune systems that effectively warded off infections. In other words, "their organic development was complete and functioned normally," reported Pottenger.[8]

In contrast, the cats and kittens born to cats that had been fed cooked meat experienced a variety of health problems. For instance, instead of being similar, the skeletal structure of each kitten differed; and many cats, unable to carry their young to term, experienced naturally occurring abortions. "Deliveries were in general difficult," observed Pottenger, with "many cats dying in labor." And "mortality rates of the kittens were high, frequently due to the failure of the mother to lactate," but also because "kittens were often too frail to nurse."[12]

For some reason, still unknown to Pottenger, these cats and their offspring also had a plethora of other problems. The mothers' health often worsened after giving birth, subsequent pregnancies were difficult, and they were irritable and some tended to bite their keeper; males, on the other hand, presented as passive. The cats were more prone to other problems ranging from skin lesions, allergies, and pneumonia, to cardiac lesions, thyroid disease, and arthritis—the kinds of conditions with which many human beings still struggle today.[8]

Perhaps as telling was the wide range of dental conditions. From generation to generation, those on the raw meat diet continued to maintain a balanced, broad face with normal arches and regular teeth, and membranes remained firm, pink, and virtually infection-free. But the generations of cats fed the diet that included scraps of *cooked* meat fared less well. Within three to six months of being put on the cooked-meat diet, the first generation of adult cats developed infections in their mouth and lost teeth. When these cats had kittens, their newborns exhibited similar dental problems that worsened through generations.

Pottenger faced similar challenges and results with his second series of studies, this time, with milk as the variable. To find out more about the health impact, if any, on cats fed raw milk compared to various types of heated milk, he fed the cats a diet that included one-third raw meat, while two-thirds of their diet consisted of one of the following: raw, pasteurized, evaporated, sweetened condensed, or raw vitamin D-added milk. "Roughly, our results corresponded with those of the previous experiments," Pottenger wrote in his in-depth research paper on his meat and milk studies.[2] In other words, although there were two different studies—one focusing on meat and the other targeting milk—the results of both studies were nearly identical: a diet of raw meat or milk, compared to heated, cooked versions, seemed to make a difference in the health and well-being of cats fed the different diets. And the impact was so powerful that not only did it influence the health of the cats, but for better or worse the cats' diet-induced health status carried over to the kittens they produced for the next three generations.

4

The implications of Pottenger's studies are quite remarkable. Actually, they're stunning. Is it really possible that a seemingly simple modification in diet—in this case, consuming raw meat and raw milk versus heated and cooked meat and milk—can affect cats' health over four generations? Pottenger's experimental studies suggest this is so.

We can draw two conclusions from his studies that are nothing short of life-changing. The first is that they raised the possibility—for the first time—that *physical degeneration caused by a poor diet in the mother is inherited in the offspring and passed on through the third generation.* Pottenger also discovered that the converse also seems true: *when a mother's diet is nutritious, not only does she benefit with good health, so, too, do her offspring . . . and their offspring, and so on.*

If he were not so meticulous, intelligent, and caring, he may have stopped with these groundbreaking findings. But he didn't. Instead, the second interesting thing is that Pottenger focused his intellectual curiosity on a series of studies on what he called "regeneration," meaning, reversing health problems. The question he posed is this: if a cooked meat and processed milk diet caused poor health across four generations of cats, could a diet based on seemingly more nutritious raw meat and raw milk reverse negative health effects that had been inherited, and, in turn, produce healthy cats?

To find out, Pottenger turned to a third generation of cats from his prior studies, all of whom appeared to have health problems linked to the *cooked* food their mothers and grandmothers had been fed. To find out if it were possible—and what it would take—to turn around their poor health, for six months Pottenger fed these cats the *raw* meat and milk diet, plus cod liver oil, which seemed to produce healthier cats. Over time, what he noticed with the first generation of cats—as well with the three successive generations of litters they produced—was that each ensuing litter was healthier than the prior litter.

For instance, he observed that the third generation of cats who had been fed a good diet resisted disease more effectively than their second-generation parents. But with allergic reactions that persisted, their health still wasn't optimal. Not only did this mean that the fourth generation of cats were the healthiest, it told Pottenger that it takes four generations of normal, raw-food feeding for the cats to return to the positive health status of the first generation of healthy cats. In other words, Pottenger discovered that poor health could, indeed, be reversed; that what was inherited from parents didn't necessarily determine health destiny; rather, the quality of the cats' diet seemed to hold the power to harm or heal—regardless of what was passed down to them from their parents. As powerful was the discovery that while dietary damage could be quick, recovery was slower. But it did appear to be possible.

And there's yet another revealing piece of the diet-and-health-destiny puzzle to consider: when Pottenger tried to do a similar series of experiments with cats over four generations—cats to whom he would feed *cooked* meat and milk, he couldn't continue the series. Why? These cats were so unhealthy that they did not survive beyond the third generation, because they were unable to produce live offspring. The question that lingers is this: does diet impact not only fertility but lifespan?

A meticulously careful thinker and researcher, Pottenger stated that "While no attempt will be made to correlate the changes in the animals studied with malformations found in humans, the similarity is so obvious that parallel pictures will suggest themselves."[3] Indeed, more—much more—than "parallel pictures" suggest themselves, because, since Pottenger started his studies in the 1930s, American scientists have been keeping statistics on health trends in human beings, beginning in the 1930s. And these statistical trends tell us a lot. From them emerge powerfully profound questions that go to the core of life, health and healing.

In relationship to Pottenger's work, the statistics raise the question: is it possible that mothers and fathers who ate a poor diet of predominantly processed and fast foods in the 1970s, '80s, and '90s, passed on the probability of illness to their children? More specifically, might a poor parental diet be a major contributing cause to today's alarming increase in childhood allergies; the fast rise in obesity since the 1980s; the onset of adolescent Type II diabetes that is occurring earlier and earlier in children; the increase in depression, autism, and Attention Deficit Disorder (ADD) in infants and children; and the increase in fertility problems?[13–19] In other words, is it possible that the generation of parents who consumed a predominantly denatured, fast- and processed-food diet, passed on "weakened genes" to their children, making them more prone to today's chronic conditions? And if so—as with Pottenger's studies with cats—will it take generations of optimal eating to restore good health; indeed, is "regeneration" at all possible?

Pottenger didn't wait for further research to answer questions like this; rather, the pediatrician decided to apply what seemed obvious to him to children struggling with various ailments. "My uncle applied what he learned [about nutritious, fresh food] to his patients," Pottenger's nephew Robert recalled during an interview. "He would take kids with allergies, or those with bone problems, and he would feed them and exercise them. He had the best playground where the kids could play. It had a real train with a track that went around the hills that you had to pump for it to work. And he would turn their health around." Continuing, his nephew said that "he didn't know what he was doing when he started his studies. Now we know that he was giving people a way of life that included regular exercise, getting a good night's sleep, and eating fresh food. His patients would feel good for the first time in their lives. So they could stay that way, he gave them lifestyle skills and natural sources of vitamins (through food)." With a smile in his voice, Robert added, "We're finally catching up with him."[4]

5

What we're catching up with is not only that a poor diet leads to poor health within one's lifetime. Pottenger realized this throughout his studies, as we do now. What we're catching up with is his landmark discovery that *when either a mother or father is in poor health because of an unhealthy diet, they pass on their health problems both to their children and to future generations.*[20–25] Today, more and more, there is still more emerging scientific support for Pottenger's pioneering findings. For instance, we know that a diet of mostly denatured fast- and processed-food products can threaten health and lead to life-threatening conditions, such as obesity, heart disease, and diabetes. We know from the field of developmental biology that children inherit health problems caused by their parents' poor diet. We also know that the way we prepare food—such as baking, boiling, barbequing, or frying—affects its nutrient content, and in turn, health and healing. And we also know what it takes to achieve what Pottenger called "regeneration," meaning, what and how to eat to reverse poor health in both ourselves and our children, so that we may all fulfill our health potential. Yes, we are indeed catching up with Pottenger's prophecy of wellness or illness over generations through the food we eat and how we live our lives.

As riveting, we're on the precipice of unraveling the reasons behind what Pottenger learned more than 70 years ago: *the food we eat each day has a cascading effect. It influences illness or wellness, not only in ourselves, but in our children, grandchildren, even our great-grandchildren, born or unborn.* This is Pottenger's prophecy, his prediction for what researchers are now beginning to unravel, and many more are starting to understand and apply to their own lives, today. Such is the legacy he has left science, medicine, and humankind.

Empowered by today's scientific and medical advances, Pottenger's ideas provide enormous implications that are pregnant with promise and potential for re-creating our health destiny. For it suggests that many health conditions can be reversed, that what we think we inherited from our parents is changeable, and that what is passed down from generation to generation isn't necessarily fixed. In other words, DNA isn't destiny, something else is. And that "something else" tells us that even devastating and often life-threatening ailments can be reversed; that both *de*generation and *re*generation—for both ourselves and our progeny—may be possible through the quality of food and lifestyle choices we make each day. In other words, we believe from recent evidence in transgenerational studies that Pottenger got it right:[20–25] *the food we eat each day is a strong determinant of our health, which, in turn, reflects the health of the genes we pass on to our children.*

In the childhood fairy tale "Hansel and Gretel," siblings sprinkled breadcrumbs on the dense and dark forest floor to create a path that would enable them to find their way home to safety. But birds ate the crumbs and the children were lost—until a duck appeared to take them across an expanse of water, which in turn, led to their safe return home. In the same way, as we travel further and further away from our evolutionary food and nutrition roots, we are losing our direction and our way home to health and healing.

As in "Hansel and Gretel," *Pottenger's Prophecy* travels a previously untrodden path, full of unexpected scientific twists, turns, and vistas. However, like the duck who led the children toward safety, we lead you "home" to a way of eating that can reset your genes—including those you pass on to your children—so that that you create health for yourself and generations to come. The next chapters begin where Pottenger's prophecy ends, by revealing the discovery of the genetic underpinnings of why and how food has the power to re-create our health destiny. You'll discover the emerging discoveries and new medicine that validate Pottenger's work and his prophecy of wellness or illness through your daily diet. At the same time, you'll discover a lexicon of emerging gene-diet specialties that didn't exist a decade ago, such as epigenetics, nutritional genetics, and nutritional genomics.

To further the discovery process, you will meet pioneering doctors and scientists who are putting their newly acquired gene-diet medicine and scientific discoveries into action. Through their evidence-based work, you will be given the practical insights you need to eat to reset illness and to maintain wellness. With a private visit to their offices and research laboratories, you will discover how they are using their scientifically sound revelations to replace a genetic tendency you may have toward certain ailments with a positive health destiny. You will also get a firsthand look at their groundbreaking studies, which are shedding light on the power that food has to reset genes and in turn influence the chronic conditions with which many of us struggle today: obesity, heart disease, diabetes, metabolic syndrome, and cancer. And you will meet patients who have applied such breakthrough medicine and science to make a difference in their own health destiny. Along the way, you will get a close-up look at how a change in your food choices—a shift in what you eat each day—holds the timeless genetic secret not only to your own health status and that of your children, but also to your unborn children, regardless of their "starter" genes. And we will show you how you can enhance and use other aspects of your lifestyle, from stress and exercise to social support and sleep, to reset your genes and maintain wellness for a lifetime.

If you want to know how to eat to increase the odds of resetting your genes (and your children's' genes) for wellness, we'll also give you the practical guidelines you need with our new, innovative, and *scientifically sound* way of eating. To give still more substance to your new way of eating, we will reveal research about the diets on which our ancestors thrived for millennia, and, as a contrast, how the diet most of us typically eat each day enables our genes either to "express" or "suppress" illness or wellness. To make it easy for you to put our insights into action, we created four "putting-it-all-together" chapters. The first introduces you to food pioneers, people who are already practicing the principles of eating to re-create their food destiny: farmers, through the food they grow; ranchers, by raising free-range cattle; individuals like you and families like yours, through the food choices they make, for example an award-winning restaurateur who serves grass-fed meat and organic vegetables. We further empower you with our "10 Green-Gene Food Guidelines" chapter, which gives you sound nutrition guidelines and ways to make modifications to meals based on your personal food preferences.

The final chapter is a call to action, asking the question "If not now, when?" Filled with practical steps you can take to turn "green-gene dining" into your everyday way of eating, it also looks at a larger picture, offering suggestions on how, together, we can start to change our food culture into one that is not only healthier for each mother, father, child, family, community, and nation, but to a way of eating and living that is more enjoyable, environmentally friendly—even more economical.

By illuminating the links among diet, genetic expression, and health destiny, *Pottenger's Prophecy* gives you the insights and understanding you need to redefine the role of food and eating in your life. In the same light, it also offers a re-visioning of what it means to eat healthfully and optimally. In this way, *Pottenger's Prophecy* is a genuine alternative to the eating-by-number, rigid and restricted, reductionist, diet and "food product" mentality to which many of us have become accustomed and which contributes to the plague of obesity and other food-related health conditions, from heart disease and diabetes to certain cancers, and more. With *Pottenger's Prophecy*, we give you the skills, tools, insights, and guidelines you need to proceed with confidence, to do a dietary U-turn and to take a direction other than the unsatisfying, unhealthful, self-defeating relationship to food for which many of us have settled.

Ultimately, we wrote *Pottenger's Prophecy* to introduce you to a new nutritional concept: that as much as 95 percent of today's chronic conditions may be due to the nutritional environment of cells and not to defective genes. This means that most of us have the power to create and re-create our health destiny through the foods we eat each day. But there is a caveat: It is not easy. While we provide evidence-based inspiration, information, suggestions, and specific guidelines, success depends on *your* dedication and commitment to take action. Then the solution lies in your applying the scientifically sound insights in this book, and the personalized optimal eating guidelines, to ignite the epigenetic mechanisms that lead to health and healing. In this way, our book aims at healing the split between today's state-of-the-art nutritional science and food's timeless place in the evolution of humankind and its powerful role in health and healing.

Pottenger's Prophecy does even more: it gives you and later generations the chance to choose the same careful and caring dietary care that Pottenger provided for his cats. In this way, it empowers you and your descendents to benefit from Pottenger's prophecy of wellness or illness through food choices. After all, when you consider what's important in life, isn't good health the most precious thing you can give yourself, and pass on to your children and to your future family members for generations to come?

Chapter 1

THE GENE-HEALTH PROMISE

In the mid-1800s, Gregor Johann Mendel made the groundbreaking discovery that individual traits are passed on through generations. Since then, a steady stream of Nobel-winning geneticists have built on Mendel's work by answering such questions as: What are genes? Where are they located in our cells? What do they do and of what are they made? And how are our genes put together to create the human genome? This succession of genetic discoveries led to the *gene-health promise*: solving the mystery of hereditary disorders through genetic testing, and creating wellness with genetic engineering. Can such an ambitious promise be fulfilled?

I

Medical journalist and mother Lara Pizzorno went through menopause with no symptoms whatsoever—no hot flashes, no fatigue, and no forgetfulness. That she breezed through the cessation of her menses was not surprising. "Lara lives a lifestyle that's as healthy as anyone I know," her husband, Dr. Joseph E. Pizzorno, Jr., a naturopathic physician who specializes in gene-based health solutions,[1] said in a recent interview.[2,3] What, exactly, was Lara's "everything right" lifestyle? For years, she had pursued a regular exercise regimen that included bone-building strength training and aerobic exercise; and her most-of-the-time way of eating included lots of fresh organic food. Aware that adequate vitamin D consumption is linked with bone health, Lara had added even more bone-building ammunition to her lifestyle by taking a multiple vitamin that included 400 IUs of vitamin D; add the 200 IUs in her daily dose of cod liver oil, and she typically took in 600 IUs each day.

Given her excellent lifestyle, several years *prior* to menopause, something unexpected happened: Lara developed osteopenia (a precursor to osteoporosis)—as had her mother, grandmother, and aunt on their way to osteoporosis; indeed, virtually all the females in Lara's family had developed brittle, porous bones that are prone to breaking or cracking, although none had manifested the dreaded dowager's hump, bent-over posture that occurs in advanced osteoporosis due to weakened and fractured spinal vertebrae.[4] Both Joe and Lara were surprised she was losing bone—mostly because of her bone-building lifestyle, which included vitamin D—but also because many "women think they do not lose much bone until menopause, but this is incorrect," clarifies Lara. Adds Pizzorno: "We knew her bone mass wasn't building up because when Lara had a bone mineral density [DEXA] test,[5] it was clear the problem was continuing; that her bone-health was worsening. She was on her way to full-blown osteoporosis."[6]

At the time of Lara's diagnosis, conventional medical wisdom held that a nutrient-dense diet, regular weight resistance exercise, and adequate supplementation with the DRI (daily recommended amount) of calcium and vitamin D, were the best strategies for achieving bone-building results.[7] Why wasn't it working for Lara? Even more unsettling was the uncertainty about "next steps." After all, if Lara's state-of-the-art lifestyle wasn't bringing the hoped-for results, what would?

Lara got her answer a year or so after being diagnosed with osteopenia with a pioneering and new scientific breakthrough: genetic testing. This new specialty was—and still is—pregnant with promise because it has the potential to reveal defective or missing genes, and in turn, whether you have inherited—or your children are vulnerable to inheriting—a particular condition.[8] Geneticists tell us this is especially powerful knowledge to have because if you can pinpoint the genetic cause of a disease, you may be able to use this information to prevent or treat the condition—both for yourself or your children. In other words, if tests reveal you have a *single-gene* disease or variation, your doctor may be able to create a treatment plan for you, personally, to prevent or reverse the condition.[9] Might this be the "next step" the Pizzornos were seeking? Would the new option of genetic testing enable them to

Osteoporosis is a disorder whereby the bones become increasingly porous, brittle, and subject to fracture, because of a loss of calcium and other mineral components. **Osteopenia** is a condition where bone mineral density (BMD) is lower than normal peak BMD but not low enough to be considered osteoporosis. **Bone mineral density** is a measurement of the level of minerals in the bones, which indicates how dense and strong they are. If your BMD is low compared to normal peak BMD, you are said to have osteopenia.

develop a scientifically sound treatment for Lara's osteopenia that, so far, had eluded them?

It was natural for Lara to link genetic testing to her osteopenia because the quick mental scan she did of close female relatives reminded her they all had osteoporosis. She had thought her healthier lifestyle would help her avoid the same fate, but it obviously was not going to be enough. Now, however, with the advent of genetic testing, she knew she could do more. Not only might she be able to use this newly emerging specialty to solve her genetic puzzle, the Pizzornos might be able to apply what they would learn to treat and reverse Lara's condition.

To start the process, Dr. Pizzorno needed to submit a sample of Lara's tissue—blood, hair, or skin—to a genetics laboratory; in turn, the lab would use the sample to perform genetic tests targeting Lara's risks for osteoporosis. Deciding on a *buccal smear*, Pizzorno used a cotton swab to collect a sample of cells from the inside surface of Lara's cheek. Then he sent the sample to a genomics laboratory (one of a handful in the country) for an analysis of core genetic components of cells, such as DNA chromosomes, RNA, and proteins and enzymes. In turn, the lab would use its findings to make genetic discoveries about what Lara might have inherited that made her vulnerable to osteoporosis.[10]

The answer that emerged was unequivocal: Lara had what is called a *VDR* (vitamin D receptor) *genetic variation*, called a *single nucleotide polymorphism* or SNP, which about 10 percent of women have. This meant she had less effective binding of vitamin D to her cell receptors—and therefore, poor vitamin D absorption—in other words, it meant it was especially difficult for the circulating vitamin D in her body to do its job. Such a discovery was especially significant because by helping calcium do its job in the formation of bones and teeth, and proper functioning of heart, muscles, and nerves, vitamin D plays a pivotal role in the proper development of bones. But because of the genetic variation Lara inherited from both parents, her cells were unable to utilize most of her circulating vitamin D, and in turn, bring calcium into her bones. Clearly, Pizzorno realized Lara's low absorption levels meant she would need more vitamin D than is typically recommended to reap its bone-health benefits. But how much more? In other words, what exact dosage would it take—if at all—for vitamin D to work its wonders on Lara? The Pizzornos were committed to finding out. Here is the clinical odyssey they took after realizing Lara's VDR genetic variation meant it was difficult for her body to use vitamin D. We're quoting Pizzorno at length to emphasize the challenge they faced before getting results:

At the time of the diagnosis, we weren't really as aware as we are today of the way in which genetics can influence vitamin D's absorption. After the diagnosis, to get her bone mass up, we gave her higher amounts of vitamin D, starting at 1500 IUs a day; 1500 mg. of calcium; and carefully monitored bio-identical hormone replacement therapy [HRT], prepared by a compounding pharmacist, in order to meet Lara's individual estrogen needs. Even so, it just kept continuing to go down. We followed this regimen for three years, but the bone mineral density tests showed it wasn't working. It was at this point that we did the genetic test; afterward, it took several years of trial and error to determine just how much vitamin D she needed.[11, 12, 13] We next went to 4000 IUs daily, and even at this dosage, her vitamin D levels didn't budge. So we kept upping it and upping it until we got to 10,000 IUs a day. Then we discovered that 25,000 IUs of vitamin D3 twice a week, and 4,000 IUs on the other days, was what it took for her vitamin D levels to increase to normal, and for her bones to start re-calcifying over the next two years. At first, Lara's bone mass leveled out. The last BMD test showed she had some osteopenia, but she also began to get some bone mass back. Without genetic testing, I would not have been aware of her inability to absorb vitamin D, nor would I have been comfortable giving her such a large dosage, which is far above the RDI [recommended daily intake] for vitamin D. Without the genetic insights derived from the tests, health professionals—including myself—would have considered that level to be possibly toxic. Now I know it is simply what her body needs.[2]

It is hard to look at this evidence of genetic testing and how the Pizzornos used it to turn around a potentially debilitating disease, and not appreciate the contribution that genetics, cell biology, biotechnology, and nutritional science have made to medicine, health and healing. Prior to such genetic testing, Lara would likely have perceived her osteopenia as an inherited disease that would worsen. Yet with the breakthrough of gene- and nutrition-based testing, not only did they discover the *singular* genetic polymorphism causing the problem, they also were able to target the optimal dosage of vitamin D that would bring the desired results; in Lara's case, this meant more than halting the progression of bone loss, it also included reversing the process and actually building up her bones. And it is the marriage of genetic testing and "smart" supplementation that made it possible. Clearly, Lara benefited from the science behind the gene-health promise that emerged in the twentieth century: identify the genetic defect and treat it.

2

It seems so simple: find the problem-causing gene, then take a supplement to "fix" it. But it is not so simple. Rather, the scientific path that brought health benefits for Lara took many decades of scientific discovery and a multitude of twists and turns in untraveled genetic territory. Imagine: first, the concept of the gene itself had to be discovered. Geneticists needed to tease out genes' location and how they function and develop an understanding of normal versus abnormal genes. Questions about which diagnostic tests could locate the problem gene had to be answered. Finally, for Lara, vitamin D biochemistry also entered the picture. Viewed from this vantage point, Lara benefited from a culmination of a century and a half of scientific discoveries about genes. It is Gregor Johann Mendel whom we have to thank for creating the foundation that launched humankind on its genetic journey.

On July 22, 1822, when Mendel was born to farmers of German heritage in Hyncice, Moravia (now the Czech Republic), the word "gene" had not been coined and the gene's role in heredity had not been discovered yet. The ruling belief about the basis of life—now considered folk wisdom—was based on environmental theories of Mendel's predecessor, zoologist Jean-Baptiste Lamarck: that *environmental* forces somehow influence traits in plants and in their offspring.[14] It was this theory that Mendel would put to the test when he had the opportunity as an adult interested in evolution.

Having grown up on a farm, Mendel had a strong interest in nature—especially in plants with unusual, atypical features. One day, during one of his walks around the monastery where he lived as a monk and taught physics to high school students, his eyes lit on an ornamental plant with foliage that differed from other plants of the same species in the garden. Given his natural curiosity, he decided to transplant the unusual plant next to more typical varieties of the same species to test the environmental theory of the time. To do this, the question he posed is this: If two related plants with different foliage were planted side by side, would the proximity of one plant influence or change the foliage of the next generation?

To find out, Mendel transplanted the unusual varietal he had found next to the more common version; when each plant produced seeds, he planted the seeds from each varietal in close proximity. Then he waited and observed the offspring. Would the characteristics of the more unusual plant be influenced by the proximity of the typical plant? And would the traits from the typical plant be transferred to the unusual varietal? After the offspring matured, the answer was clear, categorical, and unequivocal: no, proximity did not play a role. The next generation of plants retained the original traits of their parents.[15] Such a milestone observation became a turning point that shifted Mendel's perspective and determined his next research focus: what was *inside* the plant somehow determines traits of the offspring. What he didn't know at the time was that his new research focus would lead to the science of genetics as we know it today.

Inspired by his associates at the monastery, Mendel was well into his middle years when he turned his attention to this question: if environment did not lead to changes in a plant's characteristics, what was the mechanism that led to variations? How were traits inherited and passed from one generation to the next? To find out, he would patiently and slowly tease out the answer over seven years. Between 1856 and 1863, Mendel cultivated and conducted studies on about 29,000 pea plants (*Pisum sativum*), across four to six generations, with a special focus on tracing the peas' characteristics: the shape and color of the peas and pea pods; length of the stems; and the position and color of the flowers. But he did more than passively observe the generations; rather, he created *hybrids* by crossing pea plants with distinctly different characteristics, because this would allow him to study the distinct features each "parent" passed on to their offspring.

After meticulously recording each generation's distinct characteristics, what emerged were two basic laws that were to form the basis of modern genetics. Mendel's first Law of Segregation stated that parents passed on discrete traits to their offspring. Prior to this understanding, botanists believed that traits inherited by children happened in the same way that one might mix two colors of paint; that a trait was a *mixture* of the parents' characteristics, rather than being the specific, individual trait that a parent passed on. Examples of such individual traits might be the length of the plant stem and the shape of the seed kernel. Mendel's second Law of Independent Assortment told us that individual traits are inherited independently of one another; in other words, the size that the pea pod inherited was independent of, say, the length of the stem that had been passed on to it.[16,17]

At the time, Mendel did not know that the patterns of inheritance he had defined also applied to other plants as well as to human beings. Nor did he know that he had discovered the foundation on which genetics would build in the next century. As a matter of fact, even though Mendel published his findings in 1866,[18] his work remained obscure until well after his death 18 years later. It would be the early 1900s before two German botanists would replicate Mendel's work and launch the rediscovery of what came to be called Mendelian inheritance; it would be 1911 before Danish geneticist Wilhelm L. Johannsen would coin the word "gene" to describe the basic physical unit of heredity;[19] and it would be 1915 before Mendel's discoveries would find their "home"—both literally and figuratively—when American geneticist and embryologist Thomas Hunt Morgan demonstrated that genes and the genetic information they hold are housed in chromosomes in the nucleus of the cell.[20, 21]

Between 1900 and 1915, Mendel's laws were *verified*, they were *named* (as genes), and they were *located* in the chromosome. The next intriguing question loomed on the genetic horizon: how, exactly, did genes work?

3

It's 1915, and geneticists are wondering whether genes are pivotal to creating proteins—the building blocks in our body that sustain life. Did genes do more than pass on traits? Did genes somehow direct our biochemistry by playing a role in the creation of naturally occurring chemical substances that our bodies produce? And if so, did this mean that genes also influenced our body's chemical activities, such as the way in which we metabolize various substances?

By this time, genetic science had advanced enough that geneticists were exploring the role genes play in the creation of functional proteins called *enzymes*, which catalyze chemical reactions in the body and in turn, our life processes, from digestion to reproduction. They also knew enzymes form chemical precursors for other enzymes to perform biochemical reactions, such as digestion, creating new cells, repairing tissue, developing antibodies that fight disease, and more. But they still didn't know the relationship between genes and enzymes. If they knew this, they could shed light on the riddle of the role genes play in inherited human diseases—what, in 1909, British physician Archibald Garrod called "inborn errors of metabolism."[22]

Fast-forward to 1941, when two American geneticists, George Beadle and Edward Tatum of Stanford University, set out to tackle the connection, if any, between specific genes and specific enzymes. Was there in fact a relationship? And if so, might this mean that "dysfunctional" genes, such as Lara's genetic variation on her vitamin D receptor sites, played a role in "inborn errors of metabolism" and in turn some types of illness? Beadle and Tatum posed these questions: Is there a one-to-one relationship between specific genes and specific enzymes? And if so, would *in*activating specific genes stop the production of specific enzymes?

To test their theory, Beadle and Tatum performed a series of experiments with a single-spore orange bread mold, a fungus called *Neurospora*. After growing it in test tubes, the geneticists exposed spores of *Neurospora* to x-rays (UV radiation) in order to change (*mutate*) specific genes so they could no longer function. Their next step: give the impaired mold food that was deficient in specific vitamins, then observe the growth of the mold, if any.

The first-of-their-kind results were quite illuminating. The normal mold that had not received x-rays needed only one B vitamin (biotin) to grow, while x-rayed molds needed other nutrients such as thiamine, choline, or amino acids to live. The specific needed nutrient depended on which gene had been altered. In other words, the mutant molds needed special nutrients to grow and thrive. The reason for these life-and-death dietary differences became clearer when Beadle and Tatum took a closer look. Not only did the mutants differ from their normal counterparts in just one gene; they also lacked various enzymes. This seemingly minor change was really quite major, for without the enzyme, the metabolic pathway the mold needed to produce the amino acid *arginine* was blocked. And without arginine, the mold couldn't grow.

Three insights surfaced from this study that were so powerful that not only did Beadle and Tatum garner a Nobel Prize in Physiology or Medicine in 1958, but their findings influenced the direction of genetics well into the 21st century. By creating a series of mutant genes, each of which produced a different non-functional enzyme, Beadle and Tatum pieced together the sequence of steps mold needed to produce arginine, essential for growth.

Armed with an understanding of the enzymatic pathway of proteins and where each gene fit in the picture, Beadle and Tatum's second theory surfaced: the function of each gene is to produce a specific enzyme. Merged together, their findings led to what has come to be called the one gene/one enzyme hypothesis: that the purpose of each gene is to direct the building of a single, specific enzyme.[23-25] Viewed from a larger vantage point, this meant that each gene coding for a specific enzyme produces a catalyst for one step in a specific biochemical pathway, such as digestion or reproduction. If a mutation altered that structure, the enzyme might be knocked out of action.

The third insight provided the basis for the concept that intervention with specific vitamins could compensate for genes that were no longer able to create nutrients needed for life processes. In other words, when x-rays impaired specific genes in *Neurospora*, the mold could get the nutrients it needed from its diet. Not only did this discovery evolve into supplementation as a therapy, it led to the realization that food can compensate for certain deficiencies in genes that could potentially lead to health problems. This is exactly what happened when Lara Pizzorno realized she had a defective gene that led to osteoporosis. But she was able to compensate with mega doses of vitamin D.

With these discoveries, not only was Beadle and Tatum's one gene/ one protein hypothesis born, so, too, was its twin, the *gene-health promise*, which implied that if you can identify the problematic gene, you might be able prevent, treat, or cure its related ailment. For instance, in Lara's case, the one gene-one protein theory opened the door for geneticists to discover that it was her singular defective vitamin D receptor gene that made it difficult for her body to metabolize one nutrient, vitamin D, and in turn, prevent osteoporosis. But first, before the one gene-one protein hypothesis could help women like Lara and others struggling with single-gene disorders, science needed to climb yet another steep scientific slope. And the first step would entail identifying the architecture of a gene. What did a normal gene look like? What was it made of? If researchers knew this, they could shed light on the specific part of the gene that needed "fixing."

By the mid-1940s, scientists had discovered that genes were composed of DNA (*deoxyribonucleic acid*), which relies on four nitrogen-containing molecules, cytosine, adenosine, tyrosine, and guanine. Now, if they knew how structure of DNA was actually put together, medicine might be able to repair specific aspects of the defective gene and, hopefully, restore health. Identifying the structure was exactly what British geneticists James D. Watson and Francis Crick set out to accomplish in the early 1950s. Based upon previously accumulated scientific evidence, and using a special x-ray technique developed by chemists Roslyn Franklin and Maurice Wilkins, Watson and Crick were able to map the three-dimensional structure of the DNA molecule, which was comprised of two threadlike strands of a double helix or spiral that run in opposite directions.[26] The helical strands, composed of a phosphate-sugar "backbone," are linked to each other by bonds between pairs of nitrogen-containing bases: adenosine which links with *thymine* and *cytosine* which pairs up with *guanine*. The bonds that hold the bases to the sugar background are chemical and strong, but the bonds that link the base-pairs are weaker. Change one of these bases and the gene may produce a protein with a different structure from the normal one, and depending how serious the damage is, that structure may not be able to carry out its job.

Unraveling the structure of an individual gene was such an exceptional breakthrough that Watson and Crick were awarded the Nobel Prize in Physiology or Medicine in 1962. Still, it was but one piece of the overall human genome puzzle. The Nobel Prize winners said they had "found the secret of life."[27] But what they had found was a piece of it in the individual gene. In actuality, we have *many* genes that work together to create the mechanisms of life. This meant that to truly get a glimpse of how our genes work, scientists still needed to connect and combine *all* of our genes to complete the puzzle. With the big picture in place, they might be able to identify causes of diseases and create therapies that could alter health outcomes. To do this, scientists needed to identify all the components of human genetics, summed up in the *human genome*. This ambition relied on a major research push: the Human Genome Project.

4

When the international Human Genome Project was launched in the United States on October 1, 1990, its aim was to discover the whole of our genetic complement. It needed to discover what genes reside in each cell in our body, identify their sequence, meaning, learn how genes are pieced together, and map their location within the chromosomes themselves.

As the genome project evolved, many scientists did, indeed, expect miracles. Believers anticipated that the project would provide insights into how genes determine many diseases; that it would give the medical community the ability to diagnose the genetic cause of ailments; and that new treatments could be developed that would treat defective or missing genes. And why not expect such miracles? At first, it all seemed so simple: fix the gene, cure the disease. After 13 years of unrelenting, intensive work, in 2003, scientists completed the Project. And what they discovered was totally unexpected.

How many genes are there in the nucleus of each cell is probably the most common question asked about the human genome. When the project started, biochemists already had identified approximately 100,000 different proteins in the human body. Based on Beadle and Tatum's one gene-one protein theory and ensuing work, scientists on the Genome Project expected to find about 100,000 genes; in other words, one gene to match each protein.

But as the genome project continued toward its finish, members of the international team began to realize the awesome complexity of our genetic makeup. For starters, they discovered that instead of having one gene for each of the 100,000 proteins in the human body, we have only 25,000 or so genes! This caused a significant change in the one gene-one protein idea, because it meant that each gene is probably involved in creating, copying, and modifying more than one protein. And because each gene plays more than one role, if it is modified by, say, a drug created to prevent or treat one health problem to which a gene is linked, it is quite possible that the drug would alter the gene's other functions and cause unforeseen health problems.

Another compelling implication: it appears that genes "team up" with other genes to carry out various cellular processes. This means that if you change one gene, not only will it change the team chemistry, it could affect the efficacy of the whole "gene team." Clearly, what we are facing is an awesome complexity, a dynamic wherein changing one part of the web of interconnected genes could create unwelcome and unexpected changes in other parts of the gene team. This means that if (say) a specific drug is designed to affect one gene or part of a gene, any change made to the gene will likely affect the entire web, or organism. Until we understand more about the *whole* genome, turning to gene therapy as a "cure" is entering into risky territory.

Here's another way of looking at the conundrums that emerged. Let's change images. Imagine a large, intricate, delicate but complex spider web; then imagine that each intersection of all the major and minor strands is a single gene. With this image, it's easy to understand that if you disturb one intersection (gene) in the web, it will influence and modify all other aspects of the web in unimagined ways. For instance, not only could one or more intersections (for our purposes, various genes) be weakened, torn, broken, or impaired, so, too, might one or more strands that are connecting the intersections.

The gene-health promise was that the Genome Project would enable doctors to identify the genetic causes of many diseases and then treat these diseases by "repairing" the wayward gene. And "gene therapy" is the term created to describe this new medicine. But now, it had become clear that the one-gene-one protein simple solution was not feasible because human genes likely create more than one protein, individually or as a team. Where did this leave the one gene-one cure health promise?

5

What was promised and *is* being fulfilled is the ability to identify problematic *single* genes and then compensate for their weakness by one or more nutritional or other conservative approaches. And *genetic testing* is the diagnostic tool that enables doctors to do this. Undoubtedly, the most significant contribution of the genome project was the improved technology that led to genetic testing, which enabled medicine to identify genes linked with disease.

It was 2003 when the Pizzornos used a *diagnostic test* both to rule out or identify the specific single-gene genetic condition that made Lara prone to osteoporosis; armed with such knowledge, they created an effective treatment strategy of large doses of vitamin D. Five years later, by mid-2008, more than 1200 genetic tests would be available for clinical assessment by specialists such as medical geneticists, genetic counselors, or knowledgeable primary-care physicians. As a matter of fact, genetic testing helps in many ways unimaginable even a decade ago. For example, if you're part of a couple who is planning to have a child, and one or both of you have a close relative with an inherited illness, you may opt to take advantage of *carrier testing*, designed to identify a gene mutation that can cause a genetic disorder you could pass on to your child.[28] And genetic testing is being used in still other ways that are becoming integral to health care. Did you know that all states in America conduct *newborn screening* by testing millions of babies each year for genetic disorders such as Prader Willi (decreased motor skills, cognitive impairment, early death) or congenital hypothyroidism (a disorder of the thyroid gland), both of which can be treated early on? Or that many women already count on *prenatal testing* to identify genetic or chromosomal changes in a fetus prior to birth? And there are other tests that are part of the mix, such as *forensic* and *research testing.*[29]

Of all possible tests, it is *predictive* and *presymptomatic* assessments that are perhaps the most promising and potent options, because they can reveal the likelihood of your developing a particular disorder that may manifest later in life. For example, these tests could be especially useful for breast cancer, one of the most feared diagnoses by women. Consider, for example, the landmark Shanghai Breast Cancer Study (SBCS), a major research project that illuminates the benefits of genetic testing and the role of nutrition in lowering the odds of breast cancer.[30] Conducted by a team of geneticists, cell biologists, and epidemiologists from China and the United States, beginning in 1996, the question the researchers wanted to answer was this: Is there a relationship between the consumption of a particular group of vegetables, called cruciferous (*Brassicaceae*) vegetables, and a risky gene linked with breast cancer called GSTP1 val/val? Part of the mustard family, cruciferous vegetables include broccoli, radish, turnip, and arugula, and greens such as collard, kale, mustard, and China's bok choy.

If you've ever tasted any of these greens, especially (for instance) mustard greens, it is likely you noticed they had an especially pungent aroma and flavor. What you are smelling and tasting are the powerful sulfur-containing compounds called *glucosinolates* in these vegetables. When you chop or chew these greens, you are combining the naturally occurring enzyme in the vegetable, called *myrosinate*, with pungent glucosinolates, which in turn, produce *isothiocynates*, a powerful antioxidant that can prevent cancer. If your genes produce the right enzymes you can use the potent antioxidant properties of isothiocynates to reduce, suppress, or eliminate cancer-causing agents (called *carcinogens*) before they can damage your DNA; in this way, these powerful antioxidants can even prevent normal cells from being transformed into cancerous cells.[31, 32]

Scientists have known for decades that these compounds in cruciferous vegetables work together (that is, synergistically) to help prevent some cancers such as lung and colorectal cancer.[33] However, more and more evidence has recently surfaced revealing that each woman's genetic differences or tendencies play a significant role in whether her body can take full advantage of isothiocynates' potential to protect against breast cancer. In other words, some women have *genotypes*—inherited genetic make-up, or qualities, which determine a specific trait—that speed the elimination of isothiocynates from their bodies, making it difficult, if not impossible, for the isothiocynates to protect against carcinogens. On the other hand, others have genes that help the body retain isothiocynates, and it is these women who are less prone to breast cancer.[30]

At the time of the Shanghai study, completed in 2004, cancer research and genetics had advanced enough for scientists to know that three variations of the genotype GSTP1 might play a role in the development of breast cancer. They were able to determine this on the basis of animal studies, which had revealed that this family of genes can detoxify, or neutralize, carcinogens such as those created in over-cooked meat or in cigarette smoke. But if one of the three family members—the GSTP1 val/val genotype—is underactive and unable to create enzymes that detoxify carcinogens, its ability to use certain nutrients in food to fight cancer is weakened, which in turn, increases the risk for breast cancer. They also knew that the consumption of cruciferous vegetables was linked with a lower risk of various cancers. But scientists hadn't yet discovered if there was a link among cruciferous vegetable intake, the role of the three GSTP1 genotypes, and breast cancer. Making this connection could be important because of what it could tell us about protecting women against carcinogens that put them at risk for breast cancer.

Given these factors, what the scientists overseeing the Shanghai Breast Cancer Study specifically wanted to find out was this: is there a relationship among the GSTP1 genotype, cruciferous vegetable intake, and the phenotype, or "trait," of breast cancer? If so, what was the relationship? And might women benefit by knowing if they had this particular genotype, and in turn, whether consuming cruciferous vegetables could reduce their risk of breast cancer? The answers would be challenging to tease out, especially since similar studies had revealed contradictory findings: some had associated the presence of GSTP1 with greater risk of breast cancer whereas other studies revealed weak or no links.[30]

To find out more, the researchers created the largest and most comprehensive study of its kind. Called a population (epidemiological) case-control study, the three-year project included women between 20 and 70 years of age living in Shanghai, China. One group of 3035 women already had been diagnosed with breast cancer, while the second group of 3037 randomly selected women were cancer-free. At the start of the study, all women were given an extensive in-person interview about their medical, family, and lifestyle histories. They were asked to contribute samples of genomic DNA with buccal (cheek) cells the researchers would use for genotyping (genetic analysis)—as Lara Pizzorno had done for her genetic tests for osteoporosis. Finally, they were asked to provide details about their intake of cruciferous vegetables via a food-frequency questionnaire.

The two key results of the study are exceptional and groundbreaking because they provide insight, hope, and proactive dietary possibilities for the much-feared diagnosis of breast cancer. The first finding is that the scientists identified one of the genes that put women at risk for breast cancer; called the GSTP1 val/val genotype variation, it is one of the three variations in the GSTP1 genotype. The second key finding is that women with the val/val genotype who also have a low intake of cruciferous vegetables have a 1.7-fold increased risk for breast cancer. Women with the same genotype who consume a diet high in cruciferous vegetables lower their odds of breast cancer, because nutrients in these particular vegetables seem to lessen the potential cancer-causing effects of the val/val genotype.[30]

Ultimately, the key take-away message from the Shanghai Breast Cancer Study is this: if you have the GSTP1 val/val allele (the genetic variation that makes you vulnerable to breast cancer) certain phytonutrients in cruciferous vegetables can compensate for the breast-cancer gene you inherited and in turn, lower your risk for breast cancer.

6

Can current diet-gene science be of use to most of us, now? Can it help the millions of us, today, who struggle not only with osteoporosis and breast cancer, but also with weight concerns, heart disease, diabetes, cancer, and other ailments that have become a common part of many Americans' health landscape? Experts in the know believe that such medicine is just around the corner. Dr. Francis S. Collins, the "rock star" leader of the Human Genome Project, sees the evolution of genomic medicine this way:

> All physicians will soon need to understand the concept of genetic variability, its interaction with the environment, and its implications for patient care . . . The practice of medicine has now entered an era in which the individual patient's genome will help determine the optimal approach to care, whether it is preventive, diagnostic, or therapeutic. Genomics . . . is poised to take center stage in clinical medicine. . . .[34]

For the millions who suffer from single-gene and diet-related diseases, it does indeed seem that the emerging field of genomics can play a key role in medical care. After all, haven't we just seen two ailments that benefit from genetic testing and nutritional science, so much so that these conditions turned out to be more than treatable: osteoporosis was reversed, while the risk for breast cancer can be reduced? Clearly, this is the promise of genetics, nutrition, and medicine in action. Or is it? In other words, is it possible that our hope for genetic miracles, combined with ignorance about the immense biological complexity of our genes, led to an overstated promise about what is really feasible?

About the same time geneticists realized our human genome is comprised of a complicated and integrated web of 25,000 genes—not the anticipated 100,000—another key limitation surfaced that dampened expectations about how far-reaching genomic medicine could go: scientists also discovered that *fewer than 10 percent of diseases are caused by a single gene.* We saw this earlier in the chapter, for instance, when Lara Pizzorno was diagnosed with a VDR genetic variation on her vitamin D receptor cites, which about 10 percent of women have. (Actually, there are a number of VDR SNPs in addition to Lara's. If you add them together, between 45–50 percent of women will have one.) This single gene defect made it difficult for her body to absorb vitamin D, which in turn, meant it didn't have the tools it needed to absorb enough bone-building calcium to prevent osteoporosis. We saw a similar single-gene dynamic in the study on 3035 women from Shanghai who had been diagnosed with breast cancer. Of this group, only 5 percent had an underactive GSTP1 val/val genotype that was unable to create enzymes that detoxify carcinogens; because of this, the women with this gene had a higher risk for breast cancer. And it was this 5 percent of women who benefited by consuming lots of cruciferous vegetables, because of the powerful antioxidants they contain.

When researchers and media released the results of the genome project in 2003, some scientists believed it "will revolutionize biology and medicine" as we know it today. How so? The scientific community thought that not only will pharmaceuticals grow from 500 new drugs in 2000 to at least 3000 by 2020, but by then, your doctor would be able to match your individual genetic profile with a panel of drugs that will bring health-enhancing benefits. Other scientists predicted that "gene therapy for single-gene diseases will be routine and successful," and, through new techniques, that "certain aberrant disease-associated genes will be replaced with normally functioning versions, and several hundred diseases will be curable." What's more, because scientists will know "the timing of expression of most, perhaps all, of the human gene set, some of the mysteries of embryonic development will be solved."[35] This was the gene-health promise, the expectation that gene engineering would help cure most disease.

Such enthusiasm and the hope that our new understanding of genes will help to combat illness is understandable. Not only did the discovery of the human genome shed light on the previously hidden role of genes in health and healing, it also sparked new visions and speculation about how *genomic medicine* might be practiced. Here is the vision Dr. Francis S. Collins had for moving genomic medicine from the laboratory into your doctor's office: "For the promise of the Human Genome Project to be realized, the wealth of discoveries from our new-found genomic knowledge must be converted into diagnostic tests, prevention strategies and new medical treatments that can be used in the doctor's office. [We want to] steer a course that delivers on the promise of personalized medicine."[36]

When Collins uses the phrase "personalized medicine," he is referring to the leading-edge medicine that is emerging from genetic testing, and how the findings that are gleaned from genetic-based diagnostic tests can be used to create a personalized, individualized plan to treat or prevent gene-related ailments. Viewed from this vantage point, Collins's vision of the new medicine is nothing less than revolutionary, because it promises to change the way medicine is practiced today. Rather than solely treating symptoms, Collins suggests that health conditions—buoyed by genetic insights—can be treated or prevented by understanding, and then targeting, the underlying genetic source of the problem.

7

Given how complex the workings of our bodies are, it is humbling to stand before the unanswered questions raised by the Human Genome Project. Was it presumptuous of us to think the gene-health answer would be so simple; that finding a one-gene-one protein cure would be easy? Lara's success story in reversing her osteoporosis gives us clues, because she was able to reap the rewards of genetic testing, and learn she had VDR genetic variation, the single-gene defect that was causing her osteoporosis to continue, regardless of an optimal lifestyle. And then she was able to treat it by upping her dosage of vitamin D. What's pivotal to Lara's success story is realizing that *her weak genetic variation linked to osteoporosis never changed; rather, the vitamin D supplementation enabled her to work around her genetic limitations.* In other words, she was able to work around the problem, but not replace her weak genetic link. This is a significant difference, because the concept of a single-gene defect is key to taking advantage of genetic testing. The challenge comes when more than one gene is responsible for a particular ailment, for it isn't so easy to identify a family of two or more—perhaps hundreds—of genes, and then discover the nutrients or pharmaceuticals needed to compensate for many genetic weaknesses; indeed, it may not even be possible.

Clearly, fulfilling the gene-health promise made at the turn of the 21st century will require considerable commitment and resources before it can realized. Though we cannot turn to genetic engineering, by itself, to prevent or cure our chronic conditions, is it possible to benefit from wisdom derived from the genome project? Absolutely. But perhaps not in the way geneticists initially envisioned.

Surely, for the 10 percent or fewer of us who have a single-gene disease (indeed, some scientists say this applies to less than 2 percent of the population), genetic testing has the potential to offer evidence-based help by identifying the problematic gene, then using that knowledge to compensate for the weak gene. But what can the majority of us *without* a single-gene condition do to prevent or reverse health problems? Is there a genetic approach from which we, too, can benefit? Absolutely. Marry genetics with other state-of-the-art specialties, and you have the emergence of a new gene-health solution for all of us. But first you need to know what it is.

Chapter 2

EPIGENETICS:
A FAMILY AFFAIR . . . AND FARE

A revolution is taking place in biology. For decades, scientists believed DNA determined health destiny for both ourselves and what we pass on to our children. But the newly emerging science of *epigenetics* is rewriting the rules of heredity and health. For it tells us that while you might be born with a genetic predisposition to a particular ailment—say, obesity or diabetes—the tendency comes not only from genes you inherited from parents, it may also be due to your parents' *diet*—even your grandparents' diet. In other words, research on epigenetics tells us that the food choices we make each day, as well as other aspects of our lifestyle and environment, have the power to "override" the health tendency coded in your genes. This means that your daily diet may have a powerful impact on your health and the "health status" you pass on to your children. With this in mind, the potential of epigenetics is full of promise. Indeed, it may change medicine as it is practiced tomorrow and provide a new nutrition-health paradigm for the 21st century.

I

Six thousand years ago, the first settlers arrived in a remote area of Northern Sweden, now called Överkalix. Located in the far-north regions of Sweden's Lapland near the Arctic Circle, Överkalix is surrounded by dramatic mountains, lush coniferous forests, thousands of lakes, and even today, virgin wilderness. Two vigorous rivers run through this idyllic town: Torne äiv, which creates a border between Sweden and Finland, and Kalix äiv, renowned for its salmon fishing. Both rivers flow into an enchanting archipelago, resplendent with hundreds of island and islets.[1,2]

For centuries, the farmers of Överkalix complemented their access to fish with crops such as potatoes and grains, and farm animals, such as pigs, which provided ham, bacon, pork chops, and sausage. For centuries, forestry was the vocational mainstay of the area, but since the 1960s, the service industry replaced logging as work for many of the 946 people who live there today. If you wandered up and down the streets of Överkalix, you would still hear the distinctive dialect (*Överka-lixmäl*) of the inhabitants, as well as three other languages—Swedish, Lappish, and Finnish—due largely to the proximity of Överkalix to Finland. With its geographic isolation, Överkalix might have remained unknown had a particularly unique aspect of the tiny town not caught the attention of Dr. Lars Olov Bygren of the University of Umeå. A Swedish epidemiologist, his interest is studying causes of disease in different populations, ranging from entire nations and cities to towns and small parishes like Överkalix.

In the 1990s, Bygren developed a special interest in Överkalix because of its remoteness, combined with its sparse population. In particular, though, his fascination was with its centuries-old registry, meticulously recording births, marriages, deaths, and harvest records. What he wanted to learn from these data was whether the nutritional environment—in this case, the effects of famine and food scarcity—experienced by a generation of locals around the turn of the 20th century could affect their health. It seemed like a simple enough study: relate food availability to health. But while scanning the well-kept registry for clues, he stumbled on something curious that changed his focus: It appeared that *a famine affected the health of grandchildren born two generations after their grandparents had suffered a food shortage*—even though the grandchildren themselves hadn't experienced food scarcity. And the impact was so far-reaching, it seemed to be linked not only to an increased risk of diabetes, heart disease, and cancer in the grandchildren, but also to a much-shortened lifespan.

How could this be possible? To explore the seeming phenomenon, Bygren turned to the extensive database at the University library. Had anyone else ever written about what seemed impossible: that the food supply available to a generation of grandparents could leapfrog over the parent generation and affect the health of the grandchildren? After many hours, Bygren found a singular possibility in the work of clinical geneticist Marcus Pembrey, who had published a theory paper on the topic in an obscure medical journal in May 1996, four years earlier.[3] In his article, Pembrey speculated about if—and why—genes might carry a "memory" from one generation to the next. What evolutionary purpose could it possibly serve? And he wondered if some kind of "imprinting" in a generation of grandchildren could be linked to diet and other environmental influences experienced by their parents or earlier ancestors. And if so, might such imprinting lead to unexplained health problems in grandchildren? As incredible as it seemed, Pembrey thought this could be possible. Here is how the geneticist explains some of his "out-of-the-box" transgenerational thinking at the time:

> Something that always puzzled me ... was, What stops the baby's head from jamming up in the birth canal? The baby, of course, is growing in one generation, but the mother's pelvis was grown in the previous generation. If the mother was starving when she was growing—so she had a small pelvis—maybe her eggs had captured that information. And so they were instructing the growth of the genes of future babies to not work so much, or the baby not to grow so much ... so as not to jam up the birth canal.[4]

Clearly, Pembrey's professional imagination suggested some sort of not-yet-understood genetic communication between generations. But there was no evidence for this ... yet. Might the intriguing transgenerational theory Bygren had found in Pembrey's paper provide, for the first time, a scientific piece of the puzzle? Or might the mystery in Överkalix do even more, and reveal submerged pieces of the puzzle that connect past and future generations in previously unimagined ways?

2

· The concept itself was amazing. What Bygren and Pembrey wanted to know was whether the effects of the nutritional environment—in this case, food availability, experienced by one generation who lived in Överkalix around the turn of the 20th century—could be passed down through generations. To find out, they focused on this question: If grandparents under-eat at critical times in their lives due to famine, would this somehow affect the life expectancy of their grandchildren? If this proved to be so, it would be the first evidence that the genetic effects of a person's diet (nutritional environment) could be passed down and inherited by grandchildren.

By any measure, the question the scientists were posing was far beyond any prior research on the topic. At the time, as a geneticist, Pembrey was likely familiar with the work of British developmental biologist Conrad H. Waddington, who, in the mid-1900s, coined the word *epigenetics* (from the Greek prefix *epi*, which means "on," "over," or "above the genome") to provide a model for how cells differentiate or develop to assume their roles as nerves, muscle cells, and so on.[5, 6] Waddington knew that something *outside* the original DNA *genotype*, or blueprint, was directing cell development, but he didn't know the mechanisms.

Since Waddington's work six decades ago, our understanding of epigenetics has grown to such a degree, we now know more about the mechanisms that operate *on top of* or *outside* our genes and DNA; in other words, the mechanisms that eluded Waddington. With this understanding, the definition of epigenetics has come to mean the study of how the "instructions" we give our genes through our environment (such as the food we eat, stressful experiences, and other lifestyle factors) affect our biology and health. Think of it this way: If you were building a house, the architect would provide the blueprint (the *genotype*); and the builder would work with building materials from the *environment* (the epigenetic mechanism) to create the house. In turn, the finished house would be the *phenotype, the end result*. Though the concept of epigenetics—with its focus on the *interaction* among genotype, phenotype, and environment—was familiar to Pembrey, at the turn of the 21st century, its impact, if any, on and through generations was unknown territory.

What researchers *did* know at the time was based on previously done studies about the effects of parental nutrition on the long-term health of their children. Because of such studies, we've known for a long time that parents' poor nutrition could increase the odds of adult-onset ailments such as obesity, diabetes, or high blood pressure, in their children.[7-9] Surely, it's not surprising to find that a mother's nutrition could directly affect the health of her offspring. After all, mother and child share the same nutritional environment before the baby is born. But to show that access to food by both the grandmothers *and* grandfathers not only could influence the health of their children but also that of their grandchildren would mean that the quality of the diet of grandparents was passed on genetically; that genes had some kind of "memory" that could actually "remember" the effects of diet consumed two generations before. Would science be able to provide an actual explanation for Pembrey's seemingly fanciful speculation that health effects due to the diet consumed by parents could be passed on to their *grand*children?

Armed with such insights, Bygren and Pembrey set out to find out more. They were particularly excited about Överkalix because its registry had recorded crop failures as well as births and causes of death over centuries. This meant that the scientists could take a close look at food availability for specific people during specific periods of time. To proceed, they chose three sets of grandparents, the first born in 1890, the second in 1905, and the third in 1920. The Swedish scientists were particularly interested in these three generations because registry records revealed crop failures throughout the lifetimes of these generations, as well as moderate and good food availability for these three *cohorts*, the scientific word used to describe distinct groups of people that are followed over time.[10-13]

To the modern sensibility, the concept of "poor crops" sounds as if it should be straightforward. Today, when most of us think of crop failure, we think that less availability of a particular food means it will cost more in the supermarket. But a century ago, in isolated Överkalix, a crop failure meant less food—a lot less—to eat. And relief food from other communities wasn't an option, because during the winter, both rivers and the Baltic Sea were solidly frozen, making it impossible for ships or boats to reach the townspeople with food. Nor was there a railroad; indeed, roads adjoining communities hadn't been built yet. Truly, food was "less available."

In 1890, 1905, and 1920, the number of births for each of the cohorts comprised 108, 99, and 113 babies respectively. Pembrey and Bygren took a close look at the food for each group when the boys were between the ages of 9 and 12 and the girls were between 8 and 11. They were particularly interested in this pre-teen age range for both the boys and girls, because the years prior to puberty are considered to be a "slow growth period." The researchers wondered if this might have special significance for the study. Might it mean that the age in which a person experiences abundant versus limited food availability influences health outcomes *of* future generations? Such speculation prompted the researchers to pose this question: Would abundant-, moderate-, or low-food consumption during the slow-growth period of the three cohorts be linked to the health of their future grandchildren in some way? Given the limited information about birth and death dates and crop yields over two centuries in the registry records, what they would focus on was longevity. Would there be a difference in the grandchildren's lifespan, based on fluctuation in their grandparents' food supply?

The results were quite unexpected and surprising, in part, because they were sex specific. When the grandparents had an abundance of food, you would expect their offspring to live long lives and be healthy. But this isn't what happened. Rather, the archives revealed that the grandsons whose grandfathers had an abundance of food lived *31 years less* than grandsons of grandfathers who had had poor food availability. Not only did death certificates reveal their lifespan was significantly shorter, *they died early from heart disease and diabetes.* A similar shortened lifespan and tendency toward disease occurred with the granddaughters whose grandmothers had abundant food availability. Clearly, the food supply of the grandfathers affected their grandsons only, while the food supply of grandmothers affected the lifespan of granddaughters only. Why was this so? Is there a genetic *dietary* effect that is somehow passed on through two generations? Indeed, is this biologically possible? As intriguing, what was the genetic mechanism that seemed to enable sex-specific patterns of inheritance?

Traditional genetic theory of inheritance would tend to explain the phenomenon that occurred in Överkalix through a genetic mutation in the grandparents; a change that somehow occurred in the DNA of the gene that was passed on to the grandchildren. But since mutation is relatively rare, it is highly unlikely that it caused the shortened lifespan and chronic illnesses that occurred in not just a handful, but in scores of grandchildren. Could the diet-based transgenerational effect that occurred in Överkalix be similar to the same dynamic that happened with Pottenger's cats, which we discussed in the introduction chapter, "Pottenger's Prophecy?" Recall that when Pottenger fed a poor diet to a generation of cats, as with the Överkalix grandchildren, the "grand-kittens" also had a shortened lifespan and various illnesses. The "inheritance puzzle" gets even more confusing when we consider that genes pass on certain *fixed* traits or health conditions, but genes *don't* pass on health problems that manifest from the *food* we eat. Or so we thought. Which leaves us with this question: If genes aren't responsible for creating such diet-based serious health problems and shortened lifespans that were passed on to both grandkittens as well as the generation of grandchildren born in the 20th century in Överkalix what, then, is?

3

Reflecting on the diet-transgenerational dynamic that was emerging in Överkalix, Pembrey said, "Up to now, geneticists thought inheritance is just in the genes, the DNA sequence. I suspect that we're going to be able to demonstrate that inheritance is more than that."[14] The "that" to which Pembrey is referring is the cornerstone on which conventional genetics rests, which for more than six decades has held that our genetic inheritance is fixed and unchanging from the moment we're conceived. In chapter 1, we discussed this basic tenet of classic genetics, which tells us that our ancestors, grandparents, and parents pass on their genes to us. And throughout our life, the genes we inherit stay static and stone-like, locked away in every cell of our body. Protected by their chromosomal packaging, they remain incapable (except by accidental mutations) of inheriting the biological, environmental, or emotional influences our parents or grandparents accumulated throughout their life. Generation after generation, they are untouched both by the way we live as well as by what our ancestors did during their lifetime.

It was in the 1990s when Pembrey and Bygren began to speculate that our DNA does *not* carry all our heritable information, and that, instead, an individual's *life experiences* (such as diet, stress, starvation, etc.) are somehow passed on to their children and future generations. What made the timing of their new genetic theories so seemingly heretical was that they were surfacing while the hope and expectation of the Human Genome Project was at its pinnacle. With its focus on creating a "bible"—a clear set of instructions of humankind's genetic blueprint—the Project was the culmination of a century of work on genes and genetics. And the international scientific community working on it expected to identify the code of human biology at a molecular level, and in turn, use it to find the genetic cause and cure to an endless list of ailments. "We believed, naively, that we would be able to find the genetic components of common diseases," Prof. Jonathan Seckl of Edinburgh University said in an interview. "And that's proven to be very difficult. The idea of a one gene-one disease doesn't explain it all."[15] Indeed, when geneticists discovered 25,000 or so genes—instead of the 100,000 they expected—it was clear that human genetics was quite complex and that there was a missing piece to the puzzle.

Marcus Pembrey got his first clue about the missing part when he headed the Clinical Genetics Department at Great Ormond Street Hospital for Children in London, England. What he was observing was especially incredible, because not only did it go against everything the geneticist had learned, but it came hard up against a century of orthodoxy about the rules of inheritance. It was even more amazing, because what he was seeing were conditions that seemed to defy traditional genetics: "We were constantly coming across families that didn't fit the rules; that didn't fit any of the patterns that genetics was supposed to fit," Pembrey said. He was referring to children with Angelman syndrome, a neurogenetic disorder characterized by a happy demeanor with frequent laughter and smiling, no speech, and jerky movements;[16] and its sister disorder, Prader-Willi syndrome, which typically manifests with "floppyness" at birth, followed by an insatiable appetite that typically leads to obesity.[17]

What riveted Pembrey's attention was the similar *cause* of the ailments; that both syndromes are due to the same missing link in the DNA sequence of chromosome 15. To Pembrey, this was a paradox that made no sense. "We had a bizarre situation, really," he said. "How could we propose that the same deletion [on the DNA] could cause a different syndrome?" In other words, how could the same, exact, single, genetic fault cause two different diseases? When Pembrey looked beyond the genetic defect that caused the conditions and, instead, focused his attention on the *source* of the inheritance pattern, he got his answer: "What really mattered was the *origin* [emphasis added] of chromosome 15 at the deletion," he discovered. "If the deletion was on the chromosome 15 that the child had inherited from the *father* [emphasis added], then you had Prader-Willi syndrome, whereas if the deletion was inherited from the *mother* [emphasis added], you had the Angelman syndrome." Pembrey's discovery was both groundbreaking and remarkable: though both Angelman and Prader-Willi syndromes are due to the same missing sequence on the same chromosome, Angelman is *maternally* inherited, while Prader-Willi is *paternally* inherited.[18, 19]

To Pembrey, it was becoming clearer and clearer that DNA wasn't the only vehicle that could move between generations and influence development and health. Some other dynamic seemed to have the ability to influence genes and how they expressed themselves. Pembrey's work with Angelman and Prader-Willi syndromes had revealed this "something else" by showing that not only can genetic information be inherited, but it can be *modified* depending on whether it is passed to the child through the egg (via the mother) or the sperm (by the father).

With this new genetic mother-father-health link, Pembrey was another step closer to teasing out the scientific mechanism that made the transgenerational phenomenon in Överkalix possible. But huge questions needed to be resolved: Is it possible that if the infant genome can "remember" which parent gave it specific genes, can it also recall the quality of the diet and lifestyle of each parent? If so, this would give us the ability to anticipate, and to prepare for, the environment to which we'll be born, and in turn, better survive. But what was that mechanism—the hidden "non-DNA" dynamic that seemed to have the power to control how our children's and grandchildren's genes function?

In the esoteric article Pembrey published in an obscure science journal—the one that inspired Olov Bygren to contact him about the phenomenon he was observing in Överkalix—Pembrey speculated about if—and why—genes might carry a "memory" from one generation to the next. What evolutionary purpose could it possibly serve? And he wondered if some kind of "imprinting" in a generation of grandchildren could be linked to diet and other environmental influences experienced by their parents or earlier ancestors. And if so, might such imprinting lead to unexplained health problems in grandchildren? As incredible as it seemed, Pembrey thought this could be possible.

When it was completed in 2003, the Human Genome Project revealed the sequencing of the human genome—and it quickly became apparent that our genetic story is more—much more—complex than initially expected. For decades, conventional genetic wisdom had told us that when DNA is transcribed onto messenger RNA—a close "cousin" of DNA—the RNA creates proteins. In turn, these proteins are responsible for just about every process in our body, from eye color to how well our immune system works to ward off illness.

Recall that in chapter 1, we revealed the one gene-one protein promise: solve the mystery of illness by identifying the health-robbing gene, then "fix" the gene and create wellness with genetic engineering. But when the "project of the century" revealed the human genome contains only about 25,000 genes, it became obvious there isn't a one gene-one protein relationship. Indeed, only 2 percent of our DNA actually codes directly for proteins![20] Clearly, this meant that our genes, in collaboration with RNA, must create more than one protein to keep life processes going. Some other dynamic was at play. But what was that "something else," the biological mechanism that makes inheritance possible—not through the DNA we inherit, but through diet and other aspects of our parents' lifestyle and environment? By the 21st century, Bygren's work in Överkalix and Pembrey's findings about Angelman and Prader-Willi syndromes—which suggested that genetic information can be inherited based on the *gender* of the child's parents—had left some clues. Still, the *mechanism* wasn't clear ... until other independent scientists turned their attention to the challenge.

4

Stephanie Mullins and her husband were trying to conceive, but becoming pregnant wasn't easy. Filled with desperation and despair, their doctor recommended they try *in vitro fertilization* (IVF), a treatment for infertility. In England, where Stephanie and her husband live, about 8000 babies are conceived annually with assisted reproduction techniques such as IVF.[21] The process involves removing ova (eggs) from the woman's ovaries and letting sperm fertilize them in a fluid medium *outside* the uterus where the process would normally take place. Cultivating the embryo in this way typically takes place within a glass (in vitro) tube or petri dish. The fertilized egg is then transferred to the woman's uterus in the hope of establishing a successful pregnancy.[22]

After the third attempt, Stephanie became pregnant. "At the time, [the doctors] didn't really highlight any risk for us," recalls Stephanie, "and then we went for our routine scan, which was taking an awfully long time." She soon found out why: the doctors suspected her son, Claran, had Beckwith-Wiedemann syndrome (BWS), a relatively rare condition that causes oversized tongues and other symptoms, including a high risk for cancer.[23] When Claran was born, the doctors confirmed what they suspected: he had BWS. In response, a few hours after his birth, the baby had surgery to reduce the BWS symptoms with which he was born.[24]

It was around this time that BWS caught the attention of Professor Wolf Reik, a developmental geneticist at the Babraham Institute in Cambridge, England. He was interested in BWS, in part, because it was believed to be congenital and genetic, linked with a defect in chromosome number 11. But Reik was also interested in it because of the work he'd been doing with what is now called "genetic imprinting," the term that describes the mechanism that turns off the influence of a gene inherited from either the mother or father, allowing one or the other to have full expression.[25-27] As a matter of fact, genetic imprinting explains the phenomenon that Pembrey observed on the chromosome 15 gene that caused Angelman syndrome to be a maternal inheritance, and Prader-Willi syndrome to be paternally inherited.

Genetic imprinting is also used to describe genes that are imprinted from the allele inherited from the mother (such as *H19* or *CDKN1C*), or in other instances, from the allele inherited from the father (such as *IGF2*). The word allele, short for *allelomorph*, describes slight variations of specific genes. The concept of epigenetics would be of special interest to Pembrey in his search for the mechanism behind the Överkalix phenomenon because it is a process that is *independent* of classical Mendelian genetics, which holds the conventional view that DNA carries all developmental instructions within its genetic code, called the *genotype*. On the other hand, imprinting—the result of the way in which genes "express" or "reset" themselves based on the interaction between genotype and the environment—not only can originate from either your mother's or father's genes, *it can also be influenced by environmental factors* (such as diet) *and pos-*

sible interactions between the two. In 1911, Wilhelm Johannsen proposed that the difference between genotype and phenotype was *heredity* versus *what that heredity produces*; in other words, physical expression.[28,29] In other words, might genetics not be the reason Claran developed BWS? Instead, might the simple act of removing an embryo from its natural environment within its mother and placing it in a culture dish trigger heritable, non-DNA-based changes that led to the syndrome? Reik intended to find out.

Reik was poised to explore this phenomenon because he had already spent years studying the invisible layers of how genes "express" themselves—meaning, turn on or off—beyond the DNA. Now, he wanted to know *what* could cause certain genes to switch on or off, and in turn, potentially influence the health of their offspring. To find out, he placed a mouse embryo in a culture dish. And while it was a seemingly minor act, he discovered it triggered a "switch" that turned off certain genes. "After we had seen how relatively easy it was to change the switches in mouse embryos, we thought perhaps the same could be true of human embryos," Reik said in an interview.[30] So he turned his attention to mothers like Stephanie Mullins, who had her first child by in vitro fertilization. Was it possible that the IVF procedure she underwent to become pregnant—which included transferring the embryo to a petri dish—had something to do with switching genes on or off, as it had with mice embryos? And if so, might it have anything to do with her son being born with Beckwith-Wiedemann syndrome? Reik thought there might be a link, and a close look at the data revealed he was right: babies conceived by IVF treatment were three to four times more likely to be born with Beckwith-Wiedemann.[23]

Reik's discovery has profound health implications, because his findings mean it's possible that the IVF procedure—which includes a simple change in the environment of the embryo—switches genes on and off. But Reik's findings go even further, for they demonstrate a link between environment and throwing gene switches on and off in such a way that it can lead to *abnormal* gene expression. In other words, the IVF procedure itself—not inherited genes—could cause a "faulty switch" in the embryo that increases the odds of it developing BWS.

After discovering that environment can turn a gene on or off, there was still another genetic frontier to cross: In addition to DNA, could genetic switches that had been altered by environment also be inherited? If so, geneticist Marcus Pembrey might have the answer to the phenomenon he and Bygren had observed in Överkalix; the mechanism that has so far kept them from finding the answer to the question they were asking: How is it possible for the life experiences (such as diet, stress, air quality, and other environmental factors) of one generation to be "transferred" to future generations?

In the first few years of the 21st, when both Pembrey and Reik were making their discoveries, conventional genetics and its DNA-is-destiny dogma still reigned supreme. Although the concept of phenotype and the expression of traits had been known for decades, the scientific community thought it impossible that the mechanism that switched genes on and off could be inherited. Still—although it was verging on blasphemy—Reik wanted to know if this were possible. To find out, he would conduct another experiment. This time, he would take some mice whose gene switches had already been altered, and then breed them. "Our expectation was that as the altered genome was passed to the children, any [genes that had been turned on or off] would be wiped clean," clarified Reik.[31] But when the researcher looked at the gene profile of the offspring, he had to re-think his initial prediction, for the genetic switch in one generation was clearly present in the second generation. "You had dots that you were looking at, and every dot means a gene is on," Reik said. "Nobody had seen this kind of thing before." Because it was the first time such data had been presented, classic geneticists working on the Human Genome Project at the same time were having a hard time believing that the data were accurate. But they were wrong and Reik was right.

Previously perceived as impossible, non-DNA-based genetic changes—produced by environmental experiences—could be inherited, after all. It seemed as if epigenetic mechanisms had the ability to create "markers" on our genes that could "remember" an event experienced in one generation, and then pass the *effects* of that experience onto future generations. (Please see the sidebar, "Perspective: A Transgenerational View," for more about this.)

5

Some scientists have described the genetic marvel we've been discussing as "the ghost in your genes,"[32] while others have called it the "genie in your genes." [33] In the mid-1900s, British developmental biologist Conrad H. Waddington coined the word *epigenetics* to describe the still-unknown phenomenon of switching gene expression on or off.[6] Not only do epigenetic changes in our genes affect us, Reik's study with

mice revealed they are heritable and can be passed on through generations. Is it really possible that invisible changes that occur in gene function, but which do not alter the DNA sequence itself, can somehow
influence health for better or worse through generations?[34, 35] Might
the heritable ability of genes that have been switched on or off offer a
plausible explanation about how the health and lifespan of grandchildren in Överkalix were influenced by the nutritional environment their
grandparents had experienced?

Perhaps the best demonstration of how the new science of epigenetics is rewriting the rules of diet, heredity, and disease, is a landmark
study published in 2003 by Robert Waterland, a postdoctoral student
at the time, and Randy Jirtle, a professor of radiation oncology at Duke
University.[36] Waterland and Jirtle were especially interested in epigenetics and the way in which the epigenome might influence phenotype and gene expression. Given this, they focused their attention on a
particular strain of mice that carry the *Agouti* gene. The mutant gene
causes Agouti mice to inherit a yellow coat and makes them obese, rav-
enous, and prone to cardiovascular disease, cancer, and diabetes, and in
turn, shortened lifespans. Given the physical manifestations that Agouti
mice inherit, the question Waterland and Jirtle wanted to explore was
this: Would a mild modification in the diet of Agouti mothers affect the
genetic legacy of a yellow coat and susceptibility to disease they passed
on to their children? If so, it would mean that a subtle nutritional
change in the pregnant moms' diet could have an epigenetic influence
on her offspring that was so dramatic it might lead to normal weight, a
normal mousy brown coat, a disease-free life, and a normal lifespan.

To proceed, Waterland and Jirtle designed their deceptively simple
but groundbreaking study. Just prior to the mother mice becoming
pregnant, the scientists supplemented the mothers' already-adequate
diet with a group of four vitamins that are called *methyl donors*: folic acid,
B12, choline, and betaine. They chose these methyl-rich supplements,
because many prior studies had linked this particular methyl chemical
group with the power to launch epigenetic changes that switch genes
either on or off.[36] Here's how it works: The CH_3 methyl group—one
carbon atom linked with three hydrogen atoms and capable of forming
a fourth molecular bond—is part of the chemical composition of the
four vitamins. By giving their methyl group to an enzyme called *methyl
transferase*, the vitamins become methyl *donors*. Like an electrician connecting two wires, the enzyme then connects the methyl group to the
gene at the junction where two nucleic bases—cytosine and guanine—

meet. And when the methyl group, enzyme, and nucleic bases connect, genes are typically turned off. It's as if your genes are like the wiring in a house, with the methyl-donating vitamins turning some genes off and others on.

The methyl donors fed to the test group of Agouti mother mice in the study are quite common, so much so that they are found in foods like onions, garlic, and beets; and they are often recommended as supplements to pregnant women. Once a pregnant Agouti mother mouse consumes the methyl donors, they work their way into the chromosomes and then onto the Agouti gene in the developing embryo. Would the chemical switch made possible by the methyl group consumed by the mother mice silence the harmful effects of the Agouti gene in their offspring? Remarkably, the offspring in Jirtle and Waterland's study suggest this is exactly what happened. Unlike the yellow, obese, sickly parent mice that were given the methyl donors, most of their offspring had the normal brown coat of mice; they were slender; they weren't prone to heart disease, cancer, and diabetes; and had a normal lifespan. *Without changing the DNA of the mice, the methyl donors that had attached to the Agouti gene in pregnant Agouti mothers, suppressed its devastating health effects in the offspring.* And the profound transformation was due to a simple change in the mother's diet just before conception.

What's interesting about this study is that by every traditional genetic expectation, the mice should have been obese, have a yellow coat, multiple chronic conditions, and a shortened lifespan. But this isn't what happened; rather, the scientists' study revealed that seemingly small changes in nutrition can provoke an epigenetic change in the developing fetus that is so powerful it can alter its health and lifespan. In other words, the study created a clear connection between diet and its ability to silence the harmful effects coded in genes. The key point of Jirtle and Waterland's study is startling, for it raises the possibility that diet can "redirect" genetically inherited, DNA tendencies coded in our genes—so much so that health may manifest instead of illness.

6

While the Agouti mice study looked at the methyl-rich vitamins of folic acid, B12, choline, and betaine, and their power to launch epigenetic changes, methylation is but one mechanism that can switch genes either on or off. During the past two decades, at least four other key "switches" have been identified: histone modifications, chromatic factors, chromatic structure, and microRNAs (also called *miRNA*).[37] Of all the dynamics that determine epigenetic switches, perhaps the most compelling is the relatively recent discovery of the "gene regulator," microRNA. As scientists unravel more and more about the role of microRNAs in health and healing, their findings are undeniably gripping. Nobel Laureate David Baltimore described microRNAs as "a whole new biology."[38] Indeed, perceiving microRNAs as the primary force behind an "RNA revolution," medical and science writer Gary Taubes describes microRNAs this way: "Biology is reeling from the discovery that tiny snippets of RNA—DNA's overlooked partner—regulate everything from longevity to cancer."[38]

What is revolutionary about the simple, single-stranded "snippets" of RNA are their two unique roles. First, not only do they originate from what scientists thought was "junk DNA"—genetic material with no observed function—but unlike base methylation and the other epigenetic mechanisms, they operate *outside*, not inside, the cell nucleus. The second amazing role is that their main purpose is to control the amount of proteins that are created by a wide range of other RNAs. Victor Ambrose, a biologist at the University of Massachusetts, first discovered the existence of microRNA when he found it to be the cause of a mutation in the simple worm *Caenorhabditis elegans*. Ambrose's discovery was ignored for seven years until other scientists started to find microRNAs in other organisms, which suggested they play a still-to-be-determined role in biology. And when this realization surfaced, interest in microRNA took off like wildfire.

Today, more than 500 microRNAs have been identified in humans.[39] As research on them intensified, researcher David Bartel and colleagues at the Howard Hughes Medical Institute in Chevy Chase, Maryland, identified why these tiny snippets of RNA are, indeed, "a whole new biology": by regulating the creation of proteins, *microRNAs shape over a third of the human genome's expression*.[39, 40] And because they play a key role in regulating genes, and in turn, cell processes, such as proliferation, differentiation, and apoptosis (cell death),[39] *hundreds of microRNA remnants play a pivotal role in determining health and disease*. Because of this, their role in gene regulation isn't trivial. For as with other epigenetic mechanisms that have the ability to switch genes on or off, microRNAs influence whether certain genes over- or under-express themselves, and in turn, may cause cancer.[41]

The implications are enormous, for the presence of microRNAs in various cancerous cells not only helps to distinguish cancerous from normal tissue, but such information can be used to distinguish different types of cancer. In other words, the presence of microRNAs provides the mechanism to diagnose the type of cancer, suggest how it might progress, and offer hope for early and effective treatment. And once this is revealed, of all possible treatments, *diet* may be the most effective strategy for supplying specific nutrients that can both turn off cancer-causing cellular activity and turn on prophylactic effects.

We know about the possibility of such diet-gene-health interventions because of studies reviewed by Cindy D. Davis on mammals, which link diet with microRNA activity and cancer. For instance, Davis discovered that deficiencies in dietary folate, a B vitamin, can change microRNA expression so that it increases the growth of certain cancer cells. In contrast, when these nutrients are *added* to the diet, they *slow* the growth of cancer cells.[35] Davis also showed that another dietary ingredient, a derivative of vitamin A called *retinoic acid*, can modulate microRNA by influencing whether it switches genes on or off that affect the growth of leukemia cells.[39] And yet another study by Davis—this time on a naturally occurring flavanoid called *curcumin*, which is derived from a tropical plant in India and abundant in the spice turmeric—showed that it influences the expression of microRNA in human pancreatic cancer cells. Such research on specific nutrients adds to the wealth of evidence that diet is one of the most important and *modifiable* determinants of cancer risk. And as diet-microRNA studies progress, we'll learn more and more about the bioactive ingredients in foods that can *protect us at different stages of cancer formation.*

7

If you look closely at epigenetics, a key concept that makes it unique is that your genes do not necessarily determine your health destiny; rather, the environment with which you surround yourself—such as diet and lifestyle—may modify your genetic tendency, and in turn, your health. The impact of environment is especially interesting to consider, because it could explain, for instance, why identical twins, born with identical genetic profiles, don't get the same illnesses. Instead, one twin may get ill, while the other doesn't. Understanding why this occurs not only sheds light on the role genetics plays in our life, it also illuminates the powerful role environment plays in altering our genetic destiny. Waterland and Jirtle's study suggested it's possible to re-create the health destiny coded in our genes by changing the nutritional environment of pregnant Agouti mice mothers. But we still didn't know if altering the environment of human beings could bring similar epigenetic benefits. An identical twin study could give us some clues.

The largest study of this kind was a twin study led by Spanish geneticist Mario Fraga in 2005. Fraga wanted to see if changes in environment would create epigenetic changes in identical monozygous (MZ) twins throughout their lifetime. To find out, he recruited eighty sets of identical Caucasian twins from Spain between the ages of three and fifty years old; thirty subject pairs were male; fifty were female. After recruitment, Fraga administered an in-depth interview to each twin, asking about his or her health, nutritional habits, physical activities, medications, and tobacco, alcohol, and drug consumption; in other words, he wanted to know the details of the environment with which they surrounded themselves. At the same time, a blood sample taken from each twin provided lymphocyte cells that would be used to evaluate the twins' epigenetic profile over time.

Born with identical genes, you might expect that if one twin got a certain disease at a particular point in her or his life, the other twin would also be susceptible to the same disease around the same time. But this wasn't what Fraga found. Rather, his study provides an epigenetic explanation as to why identical twins not only do not get a disease at the same time, but why one may get sick and the other doesn't. What Fraga found was that while MZ twins are epigenetically indistinguishable during the early years of life, older twins revealed remarkable differences in their profile. In other words, as twins got older and experienced more and more life experiences that differed from one another, methylation and other epigenetic changes would switch various genes on and off. And these epigenetic differences in gene expression could only be explained by the long-term influence of various environmental factors, such as differences in smoking habits, physical activity, or diet. Says Fraga about the way in which environment swayed the expression of the twins' genes, "Epigenetic markers were more distinct in MZ twins who were older, had different lifestyles, and had spent less of their lives together, underlining the significant role of environmental factors in translating common genotype into a different phenotype."[42]

Fraga's study of twins tells us that not all organisms with the same genotype look or act the same way, because appearance and behavior are modified by environmental and developmental conditions. It also reveals life-altering implications for the question of how environmental events can create epigenetic triggers: Is the use of IVF justified if it causes epigenetic changes in infants? What role does food supply and food quality play in creating epigenetic alterations? Might pesticides and poor air quality create epigenetic shifts? How likely is it that diet and other lifestyle factors leave people susceptible to epigenetic modifications? And what about alcohol consumption? Drug taking? Smoking? Exercise? What role do they play in creating epigenetic variations? If environment affects the expression of our own genome and in turn, our health, what is our responsibility to ourselves?

And perhaps most important, if environmental influences we experience can trigger transgenerational effects, what is our ethical responsibility to future generations regarding the diet and lifestyle choices we make each day? Aware of the transgenerational influence diet can play based on his work in Överkalix, Marcus Pembrey offers this insight: "Our study has shown a new area of research that could . . . have a big impact on the way we view our responsibilities toward future generations."[43, 44] Clearly, the emergence of epigenetics raises many questions about how we live our lives. As compelling are the potential, promise, and hope of this emerging field.

8

Although still in its infancy, the new science of epigenetics is already rewriting the rules of heredity, disease, and health destiny. For it tells us that while a person might be born with a predisposition to a particular ailment, the tendency comes not only from genes inherited from parents, it may also be due to their diet, environment, and lifestyle. In other words, our health destiny and that of ensuing generations not only involves the faithful transmission of genes, it is strongly influenced by the quality of the food we eat each day and the environment that surrounds us.

The potential of epigenetics is so powerful that it not only is poised to change medicine as it is practiced today, it is creating a new nutrition paradigm for the twenty-first century. For it is revealing how a change in our food choices—a shift in what we eat each day—holds the timeless genetic secret to reprogram "health traits" we inherit through our genes, so that they express themselves through good health instead of illness. The implications of such science are life-changing, because it tells us that what we eat each day affects not only our health but that of our children and children's children—for better or worse. We have control over our health and whether we bring our children into the world with genetically coded health advantages—or not. In this way, surely epigenetics is the new science of self-empowerment.

Nutritional genomics. nutrigenomics. nutri-epigenomics. Human Epigenome Project.[45] During the past decade, as more and more scientists have been studying the effects of food on our genes, a lexicon of words that didn't exist a decade ago is entering medicine. Now that we know that environmental influences such as diet and lifestyle affect not only our health but also the full complement of genetic information our children and future generations inherit from us, more and more scientists are researching how individuals respond differently to nutrients in the food we eat (called *biological individuality*), as well as genome-wide DNA methylation patterns. Interest is building because of the potential that nutrigenomics has for preventing, managing, or treating chronic disease with small but effective dietary changes.

As a matter of fact, with the evolution of epigenetics, a paradigm shift in our understanding of medicine is taking place. Consider this insight from Dr. Andrew P. Feinberg, writing in the *Journal of the American Medical Association*: "Epigenetics, the study of non-DNA sequence-related heredity, is at the epicenter of modern medicine because it can help to explain the relationship between an individual's genetic background, the environment, aging, and disease." Realizing that this new medicine would integrate genetics with epigenetics,[46] Feinberg continues with this inspiring vision: "The most exciting medical idea in epigenetics is that it might be possible to intervene at the junction between the genome and the environment, to modify the effects of deleterious genes, and to influence the effects of the environment on phenotypic plasticity, perhaps influencing aging or mastering tissue reprogramming in regenerative medicine."[37]

What Feinberg is suggesting is that with our ability to turn to diet and lifestyle to reset our genetic expression for wellness, we are like pilots in charge not only of flying our own plane, but also of deciding the direction the plane will take. And because the decision often is in our own hands, epigenetic medicine has the potential to lead to health, healing, and wellness for the 90 percent-plus of us who *do not* have a single-gene disease that genomic medicine, discussed in chapter 1, is designed to treat. In this way, it puts us in charge of creating—and re-creating—our own health destiny. We first saw this phenomenon in the introduction chapter about the four generations of cats whose health turned around when Pottenger was able to "regenerate" and reverse their ailments through optimal diet. We saw evidence of this again in mice with the Agouti gene, who, with a simple modification in their diet, produced healthy offspring. The scientific advances made by Pembrey and Bygren's work in Överkalix added yet another dimension by demonstrating that the nutritional environment of one generation can reset genes and influence ailments over three generations.

Such studies are especially powerful and far-reaching, for they suggest that not only can diet compensate for a genetic tendency toward health problems, they highlight the health-changing, epigenetic core of epigenetic medicine: *that diet and other lifestyle choices have the potential to affect the genetic expression of some of the 25,000 genes in your entire human genome—even if you cannot, or have not—identified a particular gene that puts you at risk.* These studies tell us that we, too, can re-create our health destiny and that of our children by taking advantage of the principles of epigenetic medicine: choosing a way of eating and living that provides a "lighthouse," a direction you and your children can work toward to prevent, treat, or reverse health conditions you have, or for which you are at risk. Epigenetic medicine sets in motion the potential for you to re-set the expression of your genes so that they manifest wellness instead of illness.

How else might the future of medicine look as insights from epigenetic discoveries merge with advances in nutritional science? Feinberg has this vision: "One of the greatest promises of epigenetics for medicine is the possibility of new therapies [such as nutrition interventions] because epigenetic changes are by definition reversible."[37] The healing process depends less on wishful thinking, worry, or a magic pill, than on your *immediate creation of a healing environment that includes optimal food choices,* because in choosing nutrient-dense foods, you may be activating your "healing genes" and turning off your "illness genes." In other words, by turning to food to re-create your own health destiny and the health destiny of your children, you're putting epigenetic medicine into action.

Our understanding about how to apply such scientific discoveries to medicine and medical care is in its initial stages. Clearly, there are many pieces to the epigenetic medicine puzzle—some known, still more waiting to be discovered. But, sparked by the Human Genome Project, Pembrey's and Bygren's discovery about the transgenerational effects of one's nutritional environment, and Reik's realization that inheritance is not just about which genes you inherit but also whether they are switched on or off, a whole new frontier in biology has been launched. Pandora's Box has been opened, and there is no turning back to medicine as it was practiced throughout the 20th century.

In the next few chapters, we'll introduce you to researchers who are moving epigenetic medicine forward, for their studies further our understanding of nutrition and the epigenetic mechanisms that make it possible for food and nutrients to turn off "illness-oriented" genes, while turning on genes that enhance health and healing. As you'll see, the diseases on which these pioneers have focused their state-of-the-art scientific skills are the chronic nutrition- and lifestyle-based conditions that today, more and more, are threatening our health and that of our children: overweight and obesity, heart disease, diabetes, metabolic syndrome, and certain cancers. At the same time, each study provides a plethora of insights, replete with breakthroughs and practical, pragmatic insights.

We'll give you insights into additional lifestyle "ingredients" you need to reset your genes for wellness: stress management, physical activity, and social support. In this way, we'll empower you and your offspring with the evidence-based insights you need to reap the rewards of epigenetic medicine—now and through generations.

Perspective: A Transgenerational View

Doctors have known for decades that a mother's nutrition, especially when she's pregnant, is a powerful determinant of her baby's health. Given this, the landmark study in Överkalix, by Drs. Lars Olov Bygren and Marcus Pembrey, is especially remarkable, because it reveals a previously unknown epigenetic phenomenon called transgenerational response (TGR). According to Bygren and Pembrey, this means that "a mother's nutrition during her childhood can influence her child's risk as an adult for cardiovascular disease, diabetes mellitus and hypertension."[1] But the transgenerational response is even more far-reaching, because both a grandmother's and grandfather's nutrition during their pre-puberty years can, through epigenetic changes in the germ line, influence their adult grandchildren's risk for heart disease, diabetes, and high blood pressure; even their lifespan.[2] When are grandparents most susceptible to nutrition that can affect the health of their grandchildren? Called a slow growth period (SGP), the vulnerable, pre-puberty time for girls is 8–11 years; 9–12 years for boys.[3]

Here's another way of looking at the nutrition-transgenerational response link: Because of Bygren's and Pembrey's findings, we now know that the nutrition of the grandmother, while pregnant, not only influences the nutrition of the female fetus, but also the grandchild's birthweight.[4] We know, too, that males also play a pivotal role through the epigenes they pass on to their progeny, because grandfathers who over-ate during their slow growth period produced a lineage of males—meaning, grandsons—with shortened lifespans, and a tendency toward heart disease and diabetes. In contrast, the grandparents who had less food available to them during their slow growth period had grandchildren who lived up to 15 years longer than the grandchildren of grandparents who had normal crop availability during their slow growth periods.

In other words, because of Bygren's and Pembrey's findings, we know that not only is the nutritional status of both grandmothers and grandfathers during their slow growth period passed on to their grandchildren, it has the power to influence the health and longevity of both their adult granddaughters and grandsons.

"What If . . . " Scenarios As amazing as these findings are, it would be especially telling to know exactly what the grandparents who were coming of age in Överkalix at the turn of the 20th century were—or weren't—eating. But the detailed centuries-old registry doesn't reveal this. Simply put, we don't know much about their regular daily diet. Still . . . it's tempting to speculate, and to consider possible parallels that might shed light on the diet and escalating health problems that plague many in today's generations.

Here are some possibilities we've considered about the diet of grandparents during their slow growth period in Överkalix, and what it may have meant to the health of their grandchildren.

Healthy grandchildren possibilities

- What if, during the time of failed crops and scarcity, little or no potatoes or grains were available? As a result, people under-ate and weren't overweight, and they possibly turned to animal foods such as fish and pork that are higher in protein and fat.

- If food was scarce, did inhabitants forage for wild plants that included an abundance of green, leafy, highly nutritious, wild edible greens?
- We've known for decades that under-eating is linked to longevity. Did failed crops mean inhabitants consumed fewer calories?

Unhealthy grandchildren possibilities
- It's possible that cold-hearty crops such as rye and potatoes—which thrive in cool weather—were staples in Överkalix. If so, did carbohydrate-dense foods contribute to overeating and overweight?
- Might an overabundance of grain crops have contributed to a tendency toward insulin resistance, often a precursor to diabetes?
- Even though crops were plentiful, is it possible the soil was depleted and deficient, so that though inhabitants of Överkalix consumed a lot of food, they weren't getting adequate nutrition and, therefore, were malnourished?

If inhabitants in Överkalix consumed a diet closer to our hunter-gatherer ancestors due to failed crops, they were healthier, and the epigenes they passed on to their grandchildren led to health and a full lifespan. Not so for those who likely over-ate an abundance of grains and other carbohydrates, which may have grown in depleted soil that produced depleted nutrients in crops.

Relevance to today's diet Is there a parallel we can draw between the Överkalix study and today's diet in America? Can such speculative scenarios offer insights into today's standard American diet and the plethora of health problems to which it's related: obesity and overweight, heart disease, diabetes, certain cancers, high blood pressure, metabolic syndrome, attention deficit hyperactivity disorder (ADHD), infertility, depression, and more? Beginning in the 1960s, highly processed, refined, denatured food products and beverages started to become the norm. During this decade, we also started to eat a lot more of these processed food products. Isn't the time of overabundance in Överkalix—which led to grandchildren with ill-health and shortened lifespans—typical of

our overabundance? Might it be possible that whatever epigenetic mechanism was passed on to create unhealthy grandchildren a hundred years ago in Överkalix, is comparable to today's
grandparents, many of whom started to consume processed food
products in the '60s and '70s? In turn, children growing up in the
'80s and '90s not only inherited their parents' nutritional "processed food epigenes," but this generation consumed more calories than previous generations—and mostly from processed and
fast-food outlets.

Today, the typical diet for many children is high in sugar and
processed oils (found in such food products as potato chips and
French fries); cheap processed meat; processed oils and cheese;
lots of soda, and other food products (meaning, it's not real and
whole fresh food) ranging from refined and sweetened cereals
to pizza, chicken nuggets, and ice cream. What does today's diet
have to do with Överkalix and the unhealthy genes that were
passed on to grandchildren that made them prone to diabetes,
heart disease, obesity, and shortened lifespans?

We think two nutrition-related dynamics have created a situation that is playing Russian roulette with our children's health:
the marriage of epigenes passed on to children from parents and
grandparents who have consumed many processed, denatured
foods throughout their lives, with a predominantly fast-food diet
that passes as nourishment for many children today. Our children
are paying a high cost for the cheap-quality food we feed them
with such diseases as diabetes, overweight and extreme obesity,
and heart disease at earlier and earlier ages. And we have something else in common with the grandchildren in the Överkalix
study: For the first time in modern history, today's generation of
children is expected to have shorter lifespans than their parents.[5]
Surely this is too big a price to pay for the convenience and cost-
effectiveness of being a fast-food nation.

Chapter 3

Diet, DNA, and Disease

Over the past couple of decades, there's been a dramatic increase in what is often described as "diseases of civilization," such as overweight and obesity, diabetes, and their family member metabolic syndrome. From four- or five-year-old preschoolers[1] and teens to middle-aged and older adults, the number of people with these food-related chronic conditions has skyrocketed.[2] If you think your DNA (*genome*) has made you "genetically prone" to one or more of these common ailments, consider this: It's likely you can both prevent and reverse them by befriending your *epigenome*—the busy "Grand Central Station" where the food choices you make each day (such as fresh vs. fast food, balanced vs. imbalanced proportions of dietary fat, too many or too few calories, etc.) create epigenetic changes that switch genes off that can lead to illness, or turn on others that enhance health. Epigenetics is such a new science, though, that we can't yet say for certain the many ways diet affects the epigenome and in turn, chronic conditions. Still, what we *can* say is there are clues that your daily diet not only affects your risk of disease, but that you can turn to it to alter whether your genes express either wellness or illness . . . throughout life.

I

The evolution of the field of epigenetics, which we talked about in the previous chapter, says that while our DNA is hardwired, our *epigenome*—and the messages it gives to our genes—is more flexible. Rather, the food choices we make each day not only switch genes on or off but these food-DNA-disease changes can be short-term, long-term, or even last a lifetime. This means that we have more power than previously imagined to influence our own epigenetics, and therefore, whether our genes express themselves through wellness or illness. And one of the key mechanisms that make this momentous change possible is a *methyl group*, a simple basic unit of organic chemistry: one carbon atom attached to three hydrogen atoms. Once this methyl group attaches to a specific spot on a gene (a process called *DNA methylation*), it can actually switch the gene on or off, heightening, but mostly diminishing (silencing) the gene's expression, and in this way, influencing your health and the epigenome you pass on to your offspring.

Recall that, also in the prior chapter, we told you about the work of Randy Jirtle—a professor of radiation oncology at Duke University—and his then postdoctoral student, Robert Waterland, and their study about the power of DNA methylation to alter the physical expression of genes. In 2003, this innovative team wanted to know if the Agouti gene in mice—which causes yellow coats, a tendency to overeat, obesity, diabetes, and a shortened lifespan—could be altered if the diet of pregnant mice with the Agouti gene was supplemented with certain B vitamins (vitamin B12, folic acid, choline, and betaine), in utero. Would these vitamins attach methyl groups to the Agouti gene and silence its expression? And if so, what would be the outcome? What they discovered was epigenetics in action; the supplements that were given to Agouti mice turned off the Agouti gene, enabling their babies to be born lean and healthy, with normal brown coats. Not so for the mice not given such supplementation; their Agouti gene remained "turned on," and their offspring (as expected) had yellow coats, and became obese.[3]

Not only did Jirtle and Waterland's study demonstrate the concept of diet and epigenetics and how DNA methylation works to alter both physical characteristics and health, it offered an epigenetic explanation about why—and how—what your grandmother or mother ate while pregnant might affect your or your children's health. Recall we saw an epigenetic, transgenerational, diet-DNA-disease dynamic in "Pottenger's Prophecy," when the food Pottenger fed to cats over a 10-year period made an imprint on genetic expression (without changing DNA, the genetic code, itself), changes that were passed on for at least four generations. We saw a similar dynamic in "Epigenetics: A Family Affair . . . and Fare," when caloric scarcity or abundance in a generation of grandparents created epigenetic changes that influenced the health of their *grandchildren*—for better or worse. Clearly, the new science of epigenetics is revisioning the rules of diet, disease, and heredity. Moreover, some emerging new studies are giving us glimmers of insights, some early clues into how the food you eat each day changes the expression of your genes, allowing you to be healthy or making you susceptible to chronic ailments.

2

Not long after Jirtle and Waterland did their pioneering study on the Agouti gene, their colleague, Dana Dolinoy, a geneticist and professor of environmental health sciences, took the lead on an equally elegant and simple study that would shed still more light on the impact of diet and epigenetics. By focusing on obesity, not only would Dolinoy's study take on special significance because obesity has become an *epidemic* (more than two-thirds of Americans are either overweight or obese), but also because being overweight or obese can be the metabolic "tipping point" that makes you prone to chronic conditions that more and more of us are being diagnosed with today: metabolic syndrome, and its consequences—heart disease and diabetes.

Given her special interest in genetics and first-hand knowledge about the Agouti gene in mice, Dolinoy and her colleagues used an experimental design similar to Jirtle and Waterland's study to further explore whether certain nutrients switch off genes that prompt Avy mice with the Agouti gene to eat more and in turn, become obese. But Dolinoy wouldn't choose B vitamins as the methyl donors in her study; rather, her nutrient of choice would be *genistein, a major phytoestrogen in soy and other legumes.* Dolinoy targeted genistein, because researchers have known for quite a while that not only does dietary genistein seem to lower the odds of certain cancers (in Asians who consume soy as an integral part of their diet), it has also been linked to decreased body fat. But could genistein alter the susceptibility of Agouti mice offspring to become obese?

To find out, Dolinoy gave pregnant Agouti mice a diet supplemented with 250 mg/kg of genistein (based on levels in human adult populations that consume high amounts of genistein in their diets). Would this nutrient—like the B vitamins used by Jirtle and Waterland—affect the Agouti gene and ward off weight gain? Absolutely. "We provide the first evidence that *in utero* dietary genistein affects gene expression and alters susceptibility to obesity in adulthood by permanently altering the epigenome," writes Dolinoy.[4] Indeed, her study shows not only that *in utero* dietary genistein can induce epigenetic modifications and ward off weight gain in Agouti mice offspring, but this simple supplement can also prompt epigenetic changes that produce markedly different changes in appearance both during prenatal and postnatal development.

Dolinoy is quick to caution against oversimplified conclusions. "In humans, we don't yet know the places in the genome that are being modified by specific nutrients," Dolinoy said in an interview.[5] Indeed, we discussed this conundrum in "The Gene-Health Promise" with the metaphor of a large and intricate spider web, with each intersection of all the major and minor strands representing a single gene. With this image, it's easy to understand that if you disturb one intersection (gene)

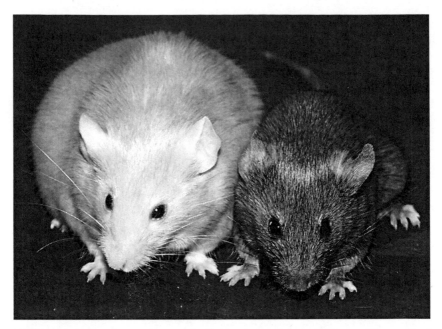

With no more than maternal dietary supplementation with methyl donors such as folic acid, choline, and betaine (Waterland and Jirtle 2003) or the phytoestrogen, genistein (Dolinoy, Wiedman et al. 2006), laboratory Agouti mice (left) gave birth to offspring (right) with normal brown coats, normal weight, and lower odds of diabetes, cancer, and shorter lifespans (Dolinoy, Huang et al. 2007). Reprinted with permission from the authors.

in the web, not only could one or more intersections (for our purposes, various genes) be weakened, torn, broken, or impaired, so, too, might one or more strands that are connecting the intersections.

Jirtle's Agouti mice experiments and Dolinoy's work on obesity are especially significant because they offer another clue about the reasons for the ever-growing girth in Western cultures. To date, researchers offer many theories for why we are so overweight, including why more and more children as young as four and five are obese.[1] Some say it's as simple as "calories-in, calories-out" (meaning that children should eat less and move more); others blame our "toxic food environment,"[6] fast-food society,[7] and pollutants and toxicants in our food and water supply, which work as *obesigens*. In our opinion, all these dynamics have worked together to create our obesity crisis. But Jirtle and Dolinoy's discoveries raise the possibility that grandparents' and parents' poor diet can create epigenetic changes that have made their grandchildren and children more susceptible to being overweight and obese. In other words, might diet-initiated epigenetic changes—due to poor diet—that have been passed on to our children be a major contributing factor to today's obesity pandemic? We think so.

But there are even more intriguing possibilities from Jirtle and Dolinoy's research, for their studies suggest that epigenes have the ability to re-establish a healthy state if we give them the right nutrients at the right time. Indeed, we saw just such a recovery for the first time in Pottenger's Prophecy, when the health of cats improved with each generation after they were fed an optimal diet. Does Jirtle and Dolinoy's research raise the possibility that human beings also have the potential to regain our health—even when faced with the genetic tendency to become obese? If so, then a fresh, whole, nutrient-dense diet—suggested by Dolinoy—may have the nutrients, *in the right ratio*, which can give our epigenome the chance it needs to recover from the effects of poor food choices, and in turn, allow us—and our genes—to heal and "reverse" overweight and obesity.

3

There is a disconcerting and somewhat tragic example of the diet/DNA/disease link in action regarding heart disease, albeit, not in ways we would expect, because the "additive" we're focusing on in the context of heart disease isn't a familiar vitamin or mineral; rather, it's an industrially produced, chemical compound called bisphenol-A (BPA), which we typically ingest through the food we eat and the beverages we consume. Indeed, most of us are exposed to the chemical because it is leached from hard, clear polycarbonate plastic, used in everyday beverage and food containers such as baby bottles, can liners, and the plastic containers used for microwaveable food. We're further exposed to BPA via other familiar items, such as dental composites, fire retardants in clothing, and paint and even the plastic in our telephones. Indeed, BPA is so integral to food and other household products that *up to 95 percent of us are continually exposed to the small, simple molecule*.[4]

Researcher Frederick vom Saal of the University of Missouri confirmed our high levels of exposure when he tested BPA in microwaveable plastics marketed as "microwave safe." What he found is cause for deep concern, for he detected high amounts of BPA—high enough to cause neurological and developmental damage in laboratory animals, including abnormal development of mammary glands, "identical to those observed in women at higher risk for breast cancer." Such findings prompted vom Saal to state "'There is no such thing as safe microwaveable plastic.'"[8]

Indeed, there may not be any level that's safe, regardless of its source. Consider this: while BPA does not accumulate in our bodies, as do many persistent organic pollutants (POPs) such as DDT, it easily enters into *all* of our cells. This is cause for concern, because it is a *xeno-estrogen*, meaning that although it is a foreign estrogen not produced by our bodies, it has estrogenic (hormonelike) properties, and has been found to disturb every developmental biological system in which it has been tested. In addition, because it acts like an estrogen, very small concentrations can disrupt the developing fetus. For instance, when researchers gave pregnant rats oral doses of BPA, the chemical entered the placenta and accumulated in the fetus.[9] In other studies with rodent mothers exposed to BPA, offspring had higher body weight, more breast and prostate cancer, and reduced reproductive function.

The impact of BPA is so all-invasive that John Peterson Myers, co-author of the landmark book, *Our Stolen Future* (about environmental pollutants and health) has said that

> 95 percent of Americans are exposed to Bisphenol-A levels which—when an adult mouse encounters (such levels), it causes insulin resistance . . . one of the central problems in metabolic disorder linked to Type 2 diabetes and obesity . . . And *Bisphenol-A alters the expression of at least two hundred genes* [emphasis added]. That's astounding. That's 1 percent of the human genome. It's a bad actor.[10]

Breast and prostate cancer. Reduced reproductive function. Insulin resistance. Type 2 diabetes. Obesity. And BPA alters the expression of at least 200 genes. The implications are clear: BPA disturbs every biological system in which it has been tested *in animals*—even at low doses.[10] But the question still remains: If BPA exposure raises the odds of risk factors for heart disease (and obesity, diabetes, insulin resistance, and so on) in *animals*, can ongoing exposure to BPA cause heart disease *in humans?*

4

To find out if BPA is linked to heart disease, epidemiologist David Melzer and colleagues at the University of Exeter in the United Kingdom conducted a population study which posed this question: Are high levels of BPA in our body related to coronary heart disease events, such as angina or heart attack? To answer this question, he used data from the U.S. National Health and Nutrition Survey (NHANES), from two time periods: 2003–2004 and 2005–2006, with more than 1400 men and women. Melzer then correlated measures of heart disease with BPA levels from urine samples taken from all the study participants. Was there any connection between levels of BPA in urine and the onset of heart disease? Absolutely. The more exposure to BPA, the more likely a person was to have heart disease.[11]

We now know there's a BPA-heart disease link, but is there an *epigenetic* dynamic at play? Given Myers's statement that "Bisphenol-A alters the expression of at least two hundred genes,"[10] it's likely that epigenetic changes cause genes to switch on or off that make a person more susceptible to heart disease. But this is speculation; we don't know for certain. This is because no experimental studies have been done on humans, BPA, and heart disease. After all, it would be unethical to expose people to potentially unsafe levels of BPA in order to test its effects on genes. Still, the question remains: Is it possible to turn to diet to prevent BPA-linked heart disease, as well as the plethora of other ailments to which it's been linked? While it's too early to say that diet can prevent the detrimental effects of BPA, there is an early clue that certain nutrients may be able to slow or prevent its epigenetic effects.

That preventing or reversing BPA's damaging effects may be possible is based on another innovative, experimental study by Dana Dolinoy, again with Agouti mice. We saw in the prior section on obesity that when Dolinoy fed genistein, a phytoestrogen from soybeans, to pregnant Agouti mice, it altered the susceptibility to obesity in their offspring. Might genistein also be able to ameliorate the negative effects of BPA on the offspring of Agouti mice? Armed with the knowledge that maternal BPA exposure reduced methylation of DNA at various sites on the epigenome, Dolinoy decided to evaluate the effects of maternal BPA exposure on the fetal epigenome. The question she was posing has special significance. After all, because of methylation, BPA can activate epigenetic changes in a mother, turn genes on or off, and in this way, affect what epigenes get passed down to offspring.

To proceed, Dolinoy assigned Agouti female mice to four groups, each of which was fed phytoestrogen-*free* lab chow. The control group, however, received *only* phytoestrogen-free lab chow, while the second group was fed the same lab chow plus *BPA* (50 mg BPA/kg); group number three was given BPA plus genistein with the lab chow diet; and the fourth group received the lab chow diet, plus BPA and the B vitamin methyl group (folic acid, B12, choline, and betaine). Each group would be fed its particular diet during three stages: prior to becoming pregnant, during gestation, and again during lactation.

When Dolinoy took a close look at the results, she discovered that the group given BPA *without methyl-donating supplements* was most likely to be born with the abnormal yellow coat color linked with obesity and other health problems, while those in the groups fed BPA plus genistein or BPA plus folic acid were more likely to be born with normal brown coats and reduced odds of related ailments, such as obesity, diabetes, and shortened lifespans. Concluded Dolinoy: "Maternal dietary supplementation, with either methyl donors like folic acid, or the phytoestrogen genistein, negated the DNA hypomethylating effect of BPA."[9] In other words, the potential epigenetic effects of BPA were diminished in the offspring of the mice whose mothers were given the maternal nutrient supplementation of the methyl group (folic acid, B12, choline, and betaine), as well as genistein.

While we've just begun to look at the potential effect diet has on protecting the epigenome and in turn, preventing heart disease and related ailments, this study raises the hope that good nutrition may ameliorate the epigenome-damaging effects of environmental toxins like BPA on our genes. At the same time, keep in mind that the Agouti mice were developed by inbreeding of a genetic mutation, and so what occurs in Agouti mice may have little relevance to humans. Because of this, it's too early to draw conclusions. However, what we *can* say is that for the first time Dolinoy's study does, indeed, raise the possibility that certain B vitamins and genistein may create epigenetic changes that may fend off some of the harmful effects of pollutants we ingest each day.

Until scientists unravel more of the diet-DNA-disease puzzle *in humans*, the nutrient-dense diet Dolinoy recommends may be a safe and smart step to take to switch on heart-healthy genes . . . and more. Another option: Consider taking appropriate dosages of balanced supplements that are optimal for you, based on recommendations by a qualified health care professional.

5

The statistics are daunting: Each year in the United States, 1.6 million *new* cases of diabetes are diagnosed in adults 20 years and older. These new cases join the 23.6 million children and adults in the U.S.—7.8

percent of the population—who also have diabetes. At the same time, an estimated 5.7 million Americans with diabetes are undiagnosed (meaning, they don't yet know they're diabetic), while 57 million (2.6 million of whom are teenagers) more have *pre*-diabetes.[12,13] Diabetes, a chronic condition, can manifest in three ways: when the pancreas no longer produces enough insulin (a hormone, or "chemical messenger"); when the body cannot effectively use the insulin it produces (*insulin resistance*); or when insulin production is impaired by a micro-nutrient deficiency, such as lack of chromium. Whatever the reason, the body isn't metabolizing glucose (sugar) effectively, and the end result is increased glucose concentrations in the blood. This matters a lot because excess glucose can damage blood vessels, and in turn, increase the odds of heart disease, kidney failure, and blindness.

For decades, researchers have known about risk factors that make diabetes more likely—such as a high-calorie diet, consisting of lots of processed grains stripped of their nutrients; lots of refined sugar; excess abdominal fat; obesity; vitamin D deficiency; lack of physical activity (less than three times a week); smoking tobacco; and race and ethnicity. And scientists have also long known that genes play a role, because people with a family history of the disease seem to be more at risk.

But today, more and more researchers believe that yet another key to type 2, or adult-onset diabetes, lies in *diet-related, epigenetic origins*, due to a poor diet based on an *imbalanced* intake of some macro-nutrients (fats, carbohydrates, etc.), and a deficiency of micro-nutrients (vitamins, minerals, etc.).

For example, since the late '90s, scientists have known that a high intake of dietary fat is associated with insulin resistance—often a precursor to diabetes. But an association between dietary fat and insulin resistance doesn't necessarily mean dietary fat is the cause of insulin resistance. Rather, it's possible that the fat-insulin resistance link is also due to the *conversion* of excess simple carbohydrates (from too much sugary soda, pastries, etc.) into saturated fat that is stored in adipose and muscle tissue. In other words, excess consumption of simple carbohydrates, which results in both circulating and stored body fat, could also be behind the increase in insulin resistance and diabetes.

Still, too much of the wrong kinds of dietary fat (highly processed and imbalanced) clearly play a key role. When researchers supplemented a regular chow diet for animals with high amounts of either fish oil (high in omega-3 fatty acids) or safflower oil (high in omega-6 fatty acids)—they found the high safflower oil (a highly processed polyunsaturated oil) diet raised insulin resistance; not so for the diet supplemented with omega-3-rich fish oil.[14-18] This tells us that the higher proportions of omega-3 fatty acids—found in fish oils, leafy greens, and walnuts, for instance—is healthful and protective. It also suggests that the *imbalance* and therefore lesser amounts of omega-3s and higher amounts of omega-6 fatty acids found in processed vegetable oils, such as safflower, may contribute to insulin resistance. Clearly, insulin resistance can be induced by high-fat feeding in animals, when the oil is *processed* safflower vegetable oil.

Are other types of fat also linked to insulin resistance and diabetes in humans? A study by Stephan Jacob, of the Department of Endocrinology and Metabolism and Radiology at the University of Tübingen in Germany, provides some insight. Jacob compared lipid levels within muscle tissue, as well as insulin sensitivity, of subjects with diabetic family members to those with no family history of diabetes. When he looked at the data, he discovered that those with a family history of diabetes had higher levels of lipids in their muscle tissue and more insulin resistance, compared to those with no family history of diabetes. These results are fascinating, because they suggest that *higher concentrations of lipids in muscle is a key mechanism behind insulin resistance.*[22] Apparently, too much fat stored in muscle is linked to diabetes. Is *epigenetics* involved in this link?

6

An innovative study by Romain Barrès and colleagues in the Department of Molecular Medicine and Surgery (MMK) at the Karolinska Institutet in Sweden has identified the epigenetic mechanism that links fat stored in muscle with increased odds of diabetes. His latest research suggests that muscle tissue exposed to high levels of circulating long-chain (palmitic) fatty acids may produce dynamic *epigenetic* changes that appear to make us more prone to diabetes.[24] Palmitic acid is the primary long-chain fatty acid that the body produces when excess fast-acting carbohydrates are not immediately used for energy.

To make the diet-epigenetic-diabetes discovery, Barrès and his team first wondered if the genes in the muscle cells of diabetics differed from those in healthy people. If so, did the epigenetic process of *methylation* have something to do with this modification? Barrès was specifically interested in muscle tissue because it has special significance for people with adult-onset, type 2 diabetes, in that their muscles have a reduced ability to consume energy in the form of glucose (sugar).

To find out if there was a methylation link, Barrès took muscle biopsies from three different groups of people: 17 healthy people; 17 people with type 2 diabetes; and 8 who were pre-diabetic, with early signs of insulin resistance. Then he conducted a genome-wide analysis to look for differences in DNA methylation in the three groups. When Barrès narrowed his focus to the *mitochondria*—the glucose-consuming, energy-producing units of the muscle cells—he discovered that those with diabetes had 44 genes with methylation differences, compared to healthy people. But what did this mean? The dynamic wasn't clear . . . yet.

To glean more information, Barrès focused his analysis on the PGC-1 alpha gene, a good choice, because it produces PCG-1 alpha, a protein known to control several energy production mechanisms in mitochondria, including glucose uptake. If the gene is unable to produce PGC-1 alpha protein, glucose metabolism is impaired. This in turn, leads to high concentrations of glucose in the blood, insulin resistance, diabetes, impaired energy, and so on. When Barrès assessed it in the tissue of diabetics in his study, he discovered a *hyper*methylation of the PGC-1 alpha promoter gene. Permanently switched off in diabetics, this ability of the gene to create the all-important PGC-1 alpha protein was shut down.

But how did the epigenetic marks "telling" the gene to shut down protein production get there in the first place? To find out, the researchers bathed the muscle cells from each of the three groups in three different media: glucose; long-chain fatty acids (saturated palmitate and monounsaturated oleic acids), and tumor necrosis factor, an inflammatory promoting *cytokine* (a protein, peptide, or glycoprotein molecule that communicates between cells), produced by various tissues in the body, including fat cells. What Barrès found revealed yet another important piece of the puzzle.

Given its key role in diabetes, you might expect glucose to play a major role in hypermethylation and switching off the protein gene. After all, high levels of circulating glucose have ravaging effects on our circulatory system and other tissues in the body. But this isn't what Barrès found. Rather, both the fatty acids and the tumor necrosis factor—but *not* the glucose—caused the PGC-1 alpha promoter gene to be rapidly methylated. And once it was hypermethylated and switched off, it no longer could create PGC-1 alpha, needed to regulate glucose uptake.

While it is risky to compare an *in vitro* study, which looks at cells outside the body, to what actually happens in muscles within the body, Barrès's findings suggest that an excess of both long-chain fatty acids (like the ones produced when we consume excess fast-acting carbohydrates) and inflammatory cytokines switches off the manufacture of a key energy regulatory protein (PGC-1 alpha), which in turn, impairs the regulation of glucose in muscle cells. These results are consistent with other *in vitro* studies showing that higher levels of membrane saturated fatty acids greatly impair the action of insulin, whereas the presence of *balanced* polyunsaturated fatty acids—especially of the omega-3 and omega-6 families—improve insulin sensitivity and glucose uptake.[25] Barrès's findings suggest yet another mechanism that may lead to diabetes. Given the role that long-chain saturated fatty acids play in diabetes, isn't it possible that the more adipose (fat) tissue we have, the greater the level of pro-inflammatory cytokines, and in turn, the greater the odds we'll develop energy-regulating genes that are switched on and methylating?

What is co-investigator Juleen Zierath's take on the research? Epigenetics, diet, and diabetes comprise "a much more dynamic process than we thought," she said. "The genetic causes of diabetes are important, but this shows us that epigenetic changes, which take place on top of our genes, can alter our physiology in critical ways."[26] As telling, their research shows that a poor diet works its way down to the epigenetic level, again suggesting that we have the power to improve or destroy our health destiny by choosing foods that reset our genes for wellness . . . or illness. Dr. Zierath explains the food-epigenetic-disease link this way: "We are not victims of our genes. If anything, our genes are victims of us."[27] In other words, we believe that the nutrient imbalances inherent in today's processed foods and in the typical standard American diet lead to impaired epigenes and in turn, not only to diabetes, but to many of today's chronic ailments. (Please see the sidebar, "Perspective: Another Fat-Diabetes View" for more about this.)

7

We have seen in this chapter how a number of seemingly minor changes in our dietary environment can have a dramatic effect on how—and whether—genes switch on or off, making us more or less susceptible to obesity, heart disease, and diabetes. Add large doses of specific supplements to pregnant mice with the Agouti gene that gives them a yellow coat and makes them obese with shortened lifespans, and their babies are born with normal brown coats, normal weight, and longer lifespans. Provide maternal dietary supplements of folic acid or genistein to mice exposed to bisphenol-A (BPA), and it raises the possibility that these nutrients prevent epigenetic changes caused by BPA, and in turn, it might reduce the risk of heart disease. Feed the right substance to the PGC-1 alpha gene linked with diabetes in humans, and it can switch on genes that regulate glucose, and in turn, diabetes. But these three chronic conditions have more in common than being diet-related diseases with roots in what we "feed" our genes. For decades, scientists have known they form a trilogy, key players in the *metabolic syndrome* (also referred to as MetS), yet another diet-DNA driven disease—though it's not yet clear if the syndrome is a disease or simply a constellation of risk factors.

The reason for the disease versus risk factor ambivalence is inherent in the definition of metabolic syndrome, which is based on five commonly measured criteria. If you have three or more of the following risk factors, you have metabolic syndrome:

1. Abdominal obesity, with a waist circumference of 35 inches or more in women, and 40 inches or more in men;
2. Elevated fasting triglyceride ($\geq$150mg/dl);
3. Low HDL cholesterol ($\leq$50 mg/dl in women, and $\leq$40 mg/dl in men);
4. High blood pressure ($\geq$135/85 mmHg)
5. High fasting glucose ($\geq$100mg/dl)

It's not hard to see the connection between the five risk factors for metabolic syndrome and their link to the three diet-DNA diseases we've discussed, obesity, heart disease, and diabetes. Have too much body fat around your waist (obesity), high triglycerides and blood pressure with low HDL cholesterol (three risk factors for heart disease), and high glucose levels (linked with diabetes), and you could have metabolic syndrome.

Perhaps the best way to explain the relationship between metabolic syndrome and the "trilogy" of obesity, heart disease, and diabetes is to liken them to a constellation. When you see a constellation of stars in the sky—say, the Big Dipper—your mind tends to connect the stars with invisible lines to create a picture. So, too, with metabolic syndrome: each disease—obesity, heart disease, and diabetes—appears to be linked, and each seems to be part of a pattern, but even so, they could be light years apart. This means we don't know . . . yet . . . if metabolic syndrome *is* a syndrome, with one disease leading to another, or if it's a constellation of independent imbalances.

But given what we're learning about metabolic syndrome, what we *do* know is this: the number of people being diagnosed with it is growing at lightning speed, and it has become a global epidemic.[28] When researchers at the Centers for Disease Control and Prevention compared the number of people in the U.S. with metabolic syndrome in 1990 to the number in 2000, they discovered that it increased from an estimated 50 million in 1990 to 64 million just a decade later. The conclusions of the researchers highlight the interrelatedness of obesity, heart disease, and diabetes and their link to metabolic syndrome: "Increases in high blood pressure, waist circumference, and [elevated triglycerides] accounted for much of the increase in the prevalence of the metabolic syndrome, particularly among women," the researchers write. In turn, metabolic syndrome "is likely to lead to future increases in diabetes and cardiovascular disease."[29]

But does metabolic syndrome have a diet-DNA link? We've seen that diseases that are part of the metabolic syndrome—obesity, heart disease, and diabetes (especially insulin resistance)—do, indeed, seem to have epigenetic underpinnings. French geneticist Claudine Junien recently proposed that individuals with metabolic syndrome have experienced improper "epigenetic programming" during their fetal and postnatal development due to inadequate maternal nutrition.[30] In this way, she believes, epigenetics may provide a link between genes and diet and how the two intertwine to predispose people to metabolic syndrome and its associated diseases.

Because metabolic syndrome is multi-causal with diverse clinical characteristics, understanding its diet-DNA mechanism isn't so easy. Still, there are clues that maternal nutritional imbalance during critical time windows of development may switch genes on and off, creating epigenetic alterations that predispose offspring to metabolic syndrome and that may even be transmitted to the next generation (transgenerational effects).[28]

How might nutritional factors in a mother create epigenetic changes that may increase the odds of her child developing metabolic syndrome? Peter Gluckman's theory of Predictive Adaptive Response (PAR) can give us some clues.[31] According to Gluckman, the nutritional milieu in a pregnant woman prepares her baby's epigenome to adapt to the same nutritional environment—from infancy throughout life—as it experienced in the womb. For instance, if the mother is poorly nourished, this prenatal deprivation sets the baby's epigenome for a lifetime of conserving nutrients from calories so that it can survive. However, if, throughout its lifetime, the baby/child/adult's calorie-conserving genes are faced with over-consumption, the genes will be super-efficient at conserving and storing the extra calories as fat. After all, based on the mother's malnourishment during pregnancy, the genes are expecting to be undernourished and are therefore set to hold onto extra energy. The end result: there's a good chance the person will develop obesity, heart disease, and diabetes; in other words, metabolic syndrome. Put another way, the baby's predictive adaptive response, based on its epigenome, is a mismatch with its calorie-rich environment.

What does Gluckman's predictive adaptive response model suggest about the reason for the present rapid rise in metabolic syndrome? Perhaps the growing numbers who have metabolic syndrome today have been epigenetically programmed—and therefore, are predisposed to the disease—because of their mother's nutritional deficiencies during their early development. Add their own poor, processed, Western diet during their lifetime, and you have a formula not only for metabolic syndrome, but also for its close relatives: obesity, heart disease, and diabetes.

While science is at the start-up stage in its understanding of the diet-DNA-disease connection, the studies we've just discussed give us some clues about what you can do right now to ward off ailments. First, as the emerging field of epigenetics continues to evolve, it's becoming clearer and clearer that the foods you eat each day are a more powerful determinant of a healthy epigenome—and in turn, health—than we ever imagined. This means that if you change your diet, you can influence your epigenome, and in turn, re-create your health destiny. Secondly, we're making this prediction: environmental pollutants in your food (such as BPA) may injure the epigenome—and your health—as much as, and sometimes even more than, a poor diet. Either way—whether your epigenome is damaged through diet or toxic ingredients humans were never meant to consume—the effects can be short-term; they can last a lifetime; or the damage can be passed on through *lifetimes* to unborn generations.

In a nutshell, metabolic syndrome is a multidimensional and multicausal disease that is a growing epidemic. More and more, it's being linked strongly to poor diet and inadequate maternal nutrition, which switch on health-harming genes that are passed on to offspring. We also know it tends to appear earlier and earlier in children born to mothers who already have metabolic syndrome; and that it tends to be more severe from generation to generation, likely because of the epigenetic marks passed on by parents to children during "critical time windows" during development and throughout life.

To ward off diet-DNA-related diseases, consider Dana Dolinoy's suggestion to consume nutrient-dense foods that are fresh and whole and pollution-free, because they are rich in the vitamins, minerals, phytochemicals, antioxidants, fiber, balanced essential fats, and more that your epigenome needs for health and healing. Our chapter 10 "Green-Gene Food Guidelines" gives you the in-depth tools you'll need to optimize what you eat, so that you can reset genes for health and healing, while "'Nourishment' Now" offers insights into how unwelcome and unexpected substances in food are creating changes in our epigenome in unexamined ways. In the meantime, in our next chapter, "Curtailing Cancer: Epigenetics in Action," we'll introduce you to a doctor whose comprehensive diet and lifestyle program has been shown to suppress the genetic expression of prostate cancer. And you'll meet a patient who has put the cutting-edge program into action and in this way, reset the "expression" of this dreaded disease. As you'll see, the key diet-DNA-disease *epigenetic* concept is this: To optimize how your epigenome functions each day, consider the *whole spectrum of naturally occurring nutrients in food* and their potential to heal. With such a strategy, you'll put the healing power of epigenetics into action.

Perspective: Another Fat-Diabetes View

It might be easy to interpret Barrès and Zeirath's study, which links the long-chain saturated fat—palmitic acid—to diabetes, to mean that dietary saturated fatty acids (SFAs) are a key player—perhaps even the key player—in the development of type 2 diabetes mellitus (T2DM). But this would be wrong, because there is much more to the story of how diet can increase insulin resistance, and in turn, the odds of diabetes. Undoubtedly, excess caloric intake, especially consuming too many processed and refined carbohydrates (chips, cookies and cake, white bread, sweetened beverages, and so on), are the typical dietary triggers that raise blood glucose and increase insulin resistance and ultimately lead to diabetes. Simply put, our body isn't designed to consume lots of carbohydrates—especially when they're refined. And when we do, our health pays a big price for it.

Consider this:

- The Paleolithic diet, on which human beings evolved and thrived, consisted of 22–44 percent of carbohydrates from total calories. Today, the average percentage of carbohydrates Americans consume is over 50 percent.[1]
- Most of the carbohydrates we consume are food products made from refined sugar and processed, denatured grains, meaning that the nutrient-rich germ has been processed out of the kernel, as has the fiber, which slows the metabolism of glucose.
- Today, Americans consume more food and calories than they did 50 years ago. Between 1970 and 2000, our average daily calorie intake increased by almost 25 percent, averaging just under 3000 calories/day.[2]
- The average American consumes 2–3 pounds of sugar each week, mostly in the forms of sucrose (table sugar) and high-fructose corn syrup. In the late 1800s, average consumption was 5 pounds a year per person; today, the figure has increased to an average of 135 pounds of sugar annually.[3]

The change in both the quantity (too many calories) and quality (from whole to refined and denatured) is the key link to increasing the odds of diabetes—for both yourself and your children—in sometimes unexpected ways. Here's why: When you consume too many calories in the form of processed, high glycemic-load carbohydrates, they are converted into long-chain saturated fatty acids, particularly palmitic acid. In turn, palmitic acid circulates in your blood and is then stored in your body in muscle tissue and around organs such as your heart. This happens even though the chips or cookies you consumed may have been "fat-free" or "low fat."

What this means to your health is this: Too much circulating palmitic acid—from too many dietary calories—is not only stored in muscle tissue and around organs, but also creates an inflammatory response that's been linked not only to diabetes but also to heart disease, some cancers, and metabolic syndrome. Diets high in these same long-chain fatty acids can exacerbate the problem.

Another way to look at the diet-diabetes-heart disease-fat link is this: The total amount of fat is not as important as the types of fat in the food you eat. This is because metabolic studies have revealed that different types of saturated fats have different effects on both health-harming LDL and total cholesterol levels. For instance, short-chain saturated fats (less than 8 carbon atoms) do not raise cholesterol levels; nor does stearic acid (18 carbon atoms). As a contrast, long-chain saturated fats (between 12 and 16 carbon atoms) increase LDL and total cholesterol.[4]

What does this mean to you and your health? The key dietary culprit may be consuming too much of a particular type of circulating long-chain saturated fatty acids, especially palmitic acid. This is likely if you: 1) eat a lot of high-calorie, refined and processed grains and sugar, which are converted into palmitic acid in your body, and; 2) if you consume an excess of palmitic acid-containing dairy and meat products.

Given that most Americans do, indeed, consume excess calories, mostly from refined, carbohydrate-dense foods, might this be a key reason 23.6 million people—7.8 percent of the population—have diabetes?[5] Or why Type 2 diabetes, which was extremely rare among youth younger than 10 years of age in the early '90s, is becoming more and more common? We think so.[6]

Chapter 4

Curtailing Cancer:
Epigenetics in Action

C an prostate cancer be reversed by diet and other lifestyle changes, such as stress management, exercise, and social support? And if so, might such comprehensive lifestyle changes have the power to turn off genes that are "expressing cancer," while at the same time, turn on genes that stop or reverse this disease with which one man in six will be diagnosed during his lifetime?[1] In a first-of-its-kind study, Dr. Dean Ornish and his research team posed these questions to men diagnosed with prostate cancer. In this chapter, we'll introduce you to the comprehensive and intensive lifestyle intervention that Dr. Ornish designed for men with prostate cancer, which appears to have *inhibited* (switched off) cancer-causing genes, while *activating* (switched on) genes that combat cancer. Such groundbreaking results suggest that comprehensive diet and other lifestyle changes can influence the way genes work—so much so that they may slow or reverse the progression of prostate cancer, sooner rather than later. But there's a caveat: Reaping the benefits calls for commitment to intensive and persistent adherence to each element of the program.

I

One sunny, spring day in 2007, Robert Caldwell, a 61-year-old academic, had a family meeting with his two teenage daughters and former wife in the kitchen of their home in Berkeley, California. As they sat around the kitchen table, Caldwell reflected that they hadn't been together like this for perhaps ten years. "I want to bring you up to date on a medical condition I have," he began. "It's potentially serious but it's not life-threatening." He paused before stating the reason for the meeting: "I have prostate cancer," he said. In response, Caldwell's oldest daughter shrieked; his other daughter "turned white—stone cold white," and the girls' mother instinctively brought her hands to her face. "This conversation with my daughters was by far the hardest part of the diagnosis," Caldwell said. At the time, one was in high school; the other was in college. "They were going to have to hear that their father has cancer—not as children, but as adults."[2]

It had been three months between the time Caldwell's doctor made the definite diagnosis ("Make no mistake about it; you have cancer") and his meeting with his family. Before telling them, he wanted to be clear about what it meant and what he would do about it. "I walked out of my doctor's office somewhat shell-shocked," he recalls. "Still, I knew I wanted emotional support and that I needed clarity about the next step I would take."

A diagnosis of cancer is life-changing. In the aftermath, anxiety and apprehension can be high-pitched; after all, it might literally mean life or death. From that point on, to assuage his concerns, Caldwell began what he describes as "rather intense research." His solution? To delve into the confusing field of treatment options for prostate cancer so that he could make the smartest choice for himself about how to proceed. Because the literature and medical opinions on treatment options vary, for Caldwell this meant ferreting out the top doctors in the field and then talking one-on-one with each.

"For starters, I checked out my health plan to get clear about the treatments it covered. Then I explored where the top doctors were located and whether I would have to go outside the Bay Area to find them," Caldwell says. He didn't have too far to go; some of the best cancer specialists were in San Francisco and in his own backyard—the East Bay. "I narrowed it down to four and made appointments with each." Over the course of three months, Caldwell was able to keep flowing a constant cycle of new information about treatment options for prostate cancer. After each discussion, he would seize on some new clue that would help him evaluate the treatment option that might be best for him personally. When he distilled his discoveries, three possibilities emerged: watchful waiting (observing whether the cancer stayed the same or progressed); removing the prostate through a radical prostectomy; or implanting radioactive seeds—also called seed implantation—which kills the prostate cancer cells.

To move closer toward a decision, Caldwell began by reflecting on what he had learned about his condition from the doctor who originally diagnosed it: The cancer in his prostate was slow-growing; only one small section out of twelve had cancerous tissue; it was in an early stage; and the position of the cancer cells rendered the cancer fairly safe. The location of the cancer cells is a key consideration when deciding on the best treatment. If cancerous cells are well within the organ's sac, as Caldwell's likely were, the odds of them spreading are low, but if they are positioned right next to the prostate wall, they could be poised to spread more easily by almost effortlessly passing through the wall. And there was another key consideration: Caldwell's Gleason score, a composite of how aggressive the tumor cells are, was on the low end.[3]

During the months of his investigation, even though Caldwell was discovering that his case was "conservative," each conversation raised different doubts about the best path to take. This is because "none were able to satisfy what I needed to know about outcomes," says Caldwell. In other words, would any of the procedures cure the cancer? Because of this, "I remained ambiguous" about what to do, he recalls, "until I received the most impressive advice—the opinion I needed to hear—from Dr. Peter Carroll, one of the oncologists I had seen. I asked him, 'If you were in my position and you knew I could tolerate the ambiguity of having cancer inside myself, would you have surgery or a procedure done?' Dr. Carroll's answer was unequivocal. He said 'No!'"

To Caldwell, Carroll's response made sense. And as a way of understanding why, Caldwell reflected on his particular situation by juggling such diagnostic concepts as "slow-growing," a "low PSA (prostate specific antigen] level," a "not-too-threatening position," "low Gleason score," and "early stage." He made his choice: he would opt for "watchful waiting." But this didn't mean he would just wait to see what would happen, that he would observe his condition passively. Rather, a fortuitous phone call to his friend, our book's co-author Larry Scherwitz, would catapult him onto a dynamic, proactive path that would change his life—and health—in ways he never imagined.

2

For more than 13 years, Scherwitz had been Director of Research and Co-Principal Investigator on Dr. Ornish's pioneering comprehensive program for reversing heart disease through lifestyle changes alone—without drugs or surgery.[4,5] This meant that not only was Scherwitz familiar with the program he had helped to design, he knew that Ornish and his team had applied the heart disease reversal program to prostate cancer. As with heart disease, the research they conducted was groundbreaking, not only because it revealed the beneficial influence lifestyle can have on prostate cancer,[6] but also because, for the first time, follow-up studies showed that diet and other lifestyle factors do, indeed, have the potential to determine how our genes express themselves, and in turn, whether prostate cancer progresses or not.[7,8] In other words, while it's not possible to change genes themselves, could the Ornish lifestyle-change program empower individuals to turn on genes that enhance health and turn off disease-promoting genes, and possibly change the outcome of prostate cancer? It was time to find out.

If you developed heart disease or prostate cancer prior to 1983, the idea that lifestyle could slow or reverse these diseases didn't exist. At the time, if you were diagnosed with heart disease, doctors around the world would first be likely to suggest a low-fat diet and exercise. If this didn't bring the hoped-for results, then they would likely treat the condition with cholesterol-lowering medication or, if they found plaque (blockage) in the arteries, with open heart surgery to increase blood flow to the heart. New evidence provided in 1983 provided an alternative when an additional, integrative medicine treatment option emerged for treating heart disease, as Ornish and colleagues published groundbreaking research in the *Journal of the American Medical Association*,[9] revealing that heart disease could be reversed through intensive and comprehensive lifestyle changes. Such a groundbreaking concept was validated further when ensuing studies conducted by Ornish supported the pioneering concept that lifestyle changes alone—without drugs or surgery— actually could reverse coronary heart disease.[10–12]

But Caldwell didn't have heart disease. He had been diagnosed with prostate cancer. So why did his exploratory conversation with Scherwitz about "watchful waiting" treatment options for his prostate cancer turn into a life-changing event? Because Scherwitz knew that Ornish and his team were in the process of applying their heart disease reversal program to prostate cancer. Would it bring results that could benefit Caldwell and other men diagnosed with the same condition?

To find out, the question the Ornish investigators posed was this: can intensive lifestyle changes slow the progression of prostate cancer? Ornish had answered this question with a definitive "yes" when he applied the same question to reversing heart disease. But would his comprehensive lifestyle-change program work its same benefits for men with diagnosed prostate cancer? Ornish and his colleagues thought this might be possible, because they knew that some doctors sometimes advise men diagnosed with the disease to make changes in diet, based on research studies that have suggested certain foods can slow the progression of prostate cancer.[13–15] But Ornish also knew that the impact of comprehensive lifestyle changes on prostate cancer—which included major dietary modifications—hadn't been evaluated yet. Rather, nutrition-related studies had been somewhat piecemeal in that they tended to explore the influence on prostate cancer of specific food macro- and micro-nutrients, such as omega-3 fatty acids and lycopene[16-18] or certain food groups, such as dairy and meat.[19-21] To find out more, Ornish would apply the same four key lifestyle factors for his study on men with prostate cancer that he had used for his heart disease reversal studies: diet, stress management, exercise, and social support.

3

In 2006, Ornish and his team set the revolutionary lifestyle-based research project into motion. Called GEMINAL, the name reflects the program: Gene Expression Modulation by Intervention with Nutrition and Lifestyle. The aim of the GEMINAL study was to evaluate the effects of combining intensive and comprehensive dietary and other lifestyle changes on gene expression in a group of highly motivated men with diagnosed prostate cancer. Each element of the program—combining a low-fat, plant-based diet,[20] lots of yoga-based stress management, daily exercise, and nonjudgmental emotional support among the participants—was set at an intensive level in order to maximize the treatment effect. Ornish and his team knew this was necessary because prior studies that had explored more minor lifestyle changes hadn't brought hoped-for benefits. Ornish and his research and clinical teams also knew that prostate cancer may be even more challenging to reverse than heart disease, because the risk factors linked with cancer aren't as clear as those for heart disease.

To appreciate the uniqueness of the program is to understand why it is revolutionary. Because of its potentially aggressive nature, almost all cancer is immediately treated with radiation, surgery, or medication—all, that is, except prostate cancer. This is because prostate cancer can be quite slow-growing, as was Caldwell's; when this is the case, "watchful waiting" is often the option-of-choice. In other words, because it can progress slowly, prostate cancer is the only major cancer in which watchful waiting is a treatment option. The innovative Ornish intervention was, in fact, a different "watchful waiting" program.

Until now, no one had ever tried to reverse prostate cancer by changing a combination of suspected risk factors. Ornish and his team would also do something else that had never been done: both before and after the three-month intervention, they would evaluate possible changes in gene expression, to find whether the intervention turned genes on or off.

Because lifestyle-based studies are quite costly and challenging for people to follow, Ornish started his study with a small, single group.[22-23] This first effort would be a pilot project, consisting of 30 men who, like Caldwell, had a diagnosis of low-risk prostate cancer that was slow-growing and located in a "safe" position that lowered the odds of it spreading; and the men would choose, on their own volition, to make lifestyle changes proposed by Ornish and his team, rather than proceed with other treatment options ranging from medication and radiation to surgery. When the study began, the volunteers, called research participants (RPs), had three things in common: They had a diagnosis of prostate cancer; they agreed to follow the study's comprehensive lifestyle changes; and, to assess the effects (if any) of the intervention on their prostate cancer, they would also undergo biopsies of non-cancerous prostate tissue before beginning the program and then three months after the intervention ended.

To launch the prescribed lifestyle program, the research participants participated in an intensive three-day residential retreat, so that they could learn, experience, and practice the program. Afterward, and throughout the three months, they kept in touch with a study nurse on a weekly basis; in addition, a registered dietitian, exercise physiologist, clinical psychologist, and stress management instructor were available for education and counseling. But the retreat served yet another purpose—perhaps one that was as powerful as learning the program itself: one of its major "side effects" was the social connection that the research participants experienced with each other. This meant that not only would they meet once a week for a pre-arranged social support session—along with eating, practicing stress management, and exercising together—but the program also gave them the opportunity to express their deepest fears in a safe and caring environment and to share the wisdom many had gleaned from their experience with prostate cancer. In this way, they were able to help each other in unexpected ways.[23]

Here's an overview of the four elements of the GEMINAL study, which the research participants practiced daily during the three-month duration of the program. Its core structure is based on what had proven promising in an earlier rigorous lifestyle study Ornish had conducted with men with prostate cancer.[6, 24]

Diet. The plant-based, whole-food meals—the core of the diet—were provided for the research participants throughout the three-month intervention. Breakfast, lunch, dinner, and snacks included lots of fresh fruits, vegetables, whole grains (such as brown rice, whole wheat, oatmeal, etc.), and legumes (beans and peas), plus a daily serving of tofu, a fortified and powered soy-protein beverage, and the following supplements: fish oil, vitamin E, vitamin C, and selenium. The food groups of nuts and seeds, dairy, fish, poultry, and meat were omitted, as were alcoholic beverages, junk food, sodas, and simple sugars.[25]

Quite a bit of research went into creating the rationale for such a diet. For instance, studies showed that men with prostate cancer often have low serum levels of the carotenoid lycopene; because it is abundant in tomatoes, tomato juice was recommended as part of the diet, because lycopene may inhibit the growth of prostate cancer.[17,18,26] Also included were omega-3 fish oil capsules, likely because of their anti-inflammatory benefits; the antioxidant vitamins E and C, and the mineral selenium, were used to neutralize free radicals, which have been widely implicated in a host of chronic diseases, ranging from cancer to heart disease.

If fruits, vegetables, whole grains, and legumes formed the core of the diet, what was the thinking behind omitting certain food groups? At first, milk was excluded during the intervention because studies were beginning to surface suggesting that conventionally processed dairy foods might contribute to the progression of prostate cancer. This suspicion received increasing, substantive support in 2007, after the program had been initiated, when a milestone meta-analysis of 13 independent case-controlled studies (a gold standard of high-quality research) showed a dose-response relationship between increasing milk consumption and a stronger likelihood of developing or having prostate cancer[26–32] although the findings are not always consistent.[34–36] Meat was omitted from the diet because many studies show a relationship between meat consumption and increased risk of prostate cancer,[19,37] while a diet that includes fish seems to have a protective effect by reducing the odds of prostate cancer.[38–40] (Please see the sidebar, "Perspective: A Re-Visioning of the High Fat-Low Fat View," for more about this.)

Stress management. As part of the program, research participants were required to practice gentle yoga-based stress management techniques, which included stretching, breathing skills, meditation, visualization, and progressive relaxation. They were asked to do this for a minimum of one hour each day. Yoga was used because it had been an effective stress-management component of Ornish's heart disease reversal studies (also called the San Francisco Lifestyle Heart Trial), wherein the minutes spent stretching and doing yoga poses (asanas), and practicing deep relaxation, breathing techniques, meditation, and guided imagery surfaced as the best predictor of reversal of coronary artery blockages.[41] However, the yoga component in the GEMINAL study differed in a minor way in that it emphasized some poses that would bring blood to the prostate area; and the focus during visualization shifted from heart health to a healthy prostate.

Exercise. Six days each week, research participants participated in moderate aerobic exercise that typically included walking an hour per day. The investigators included exercise in the intervention for many reasons: it can lower blood pressure, ward off weight gain, and boost immunity, making it easier for your body to combat cancer. However, intensive exercise may have another benefit of special interest to people diagnosed with prostate cancer: It has been shown to affect the gene expression profiles of circulating white blood cells (and various other blood cell types). White blood cells are a vital part of the immune system, which empowers your body to destroy cancer cells.

Social support. The fourth leg of the GEMINAL study required the research participants to meet for four hours each week to exercise, do yoga, share a meal and participate in a group support session. During this time, the research participants encouraged each other by discussing solutions to challenges. They also helped each other by sharing the feelings their condition provoked, such as fear and anxiety; at the same time, they expressed commonalities about how the diagnosis of prostate cancer had affected their lives. Perhaps most importantly in the group support sessions, they listened, carefully, to each other without judgment or the need to "fix" a situation, however challenging. Along with bringing the research participants closer together, their talk-time reinforced adherence to all four elements of the lifestyle program.[42] But it also served another purpose: the benefits of social support were well-documented by Stanford psychiatrist David Spiegel, whose research revealed that women with terminal breast cancer who participated in weekly social support sessions survived much longer than those without strong social support.[43]

The GEMINAL study seems challenging at the very least; perhaps it might seem like an extreme way to live. It's understandable. On the surface, GEMINAL may seem radical, severe, or intense, but it makes sense when we realize it is driven by an in-depth understanding and knowledge of what it takes to make a difference when a person has been diagnosed with a serious health threat. In other words, what the investigators learned from their prior relevant studies and their review of the literature on diet, lifestyle, and prostate cancer provided helpful clues and encouraging signs that prostate cancer occurrence, prevention, or progression is related directly to lifestyle changes that include what we eat, how we respond to challenges, how we move our bodies, and how much love and intimacy we have in our lives. As you'll see, it is these specific lifestyle components in combination that Ornish wanted to investigate to determine if they could reverse prostate cancer.

There was another reason, though, for such a thorough intervention. Ultimately, Ornish was exploring a lifestyle-based therapy for the treatment of prostate cancer. Given the more tenuous, still-unproven link between comprehensive lifestyle changes and prostate cancer, the investigative team knew they had to go for maximum lifestyle change—a total and comprehensive synergistic approach—in order to tease out whether lifestyle could reverse cancer. Conversely, if lifestyle-change had no affect on the progression of prostate cancer, then the comprehensive intervention would provide a more definitive test about its ineffectiveness than would a singular component, or a more moderate, multidimensional approach. Such careful thinking went into creating the GEMINAL study. And it was well worth it, for when the results were tallied, what they revealed was nothing less than revolutionary. Practicing the Ornish lifestyle intervention intensively can affect many genes that may, in turn, influence whether prostate cancer cells multiply and grow—or not.

4

Ornish interprets it this way: "Our genes are our predisposition, but they're not our fate," he said during a recent interview. After the research participants practiced the program for three months, Ornish discovered that some genes were turned on (expressed), while others were turned off. The genes that turned off were those that appear to play a critical role in the progression of prostate cancer.[44]

In other words, the GEMINAL study created an approach to treating prostate cancer by controlling genetic expression. The study raises the hope that by practicing its four lifestyle components intensively, it may be possible to activate the genes that fight the "runaway" growth of cancer cells and turn off the genes that promote their growth. "For me," Ornish said, "awareness is always the first step in healing. Just knowing these changes can make a difference so quickly can empower people and . . . motivate them to make these changes."[45-49]

But there's another powerful motivator you may not have considered. Recall that in the Introduction chapter, we discovered Pottenger's prophecy, which tells us that the food you eat influences more than your personal health—it empowers you to pass on either wellness or illness to your children and to future descendents. The GEMINAL study tells us that not only will a healthy lifestyle reduce your chance of a chronic disease—in this case, prostate cancer—if you are a male and you conceive male children, some of the changes in your genes may be transferred to them, meaning, they could potentially reap the rewards of your beneficial lifestyle with a reduced risk for prostate cancer, and perhaps other ailments. While, to date, studies haven't been done on transgenerational resistance to disease, theoretically, there's the possibility that parents who live a healthful lifestyle could, indeed, pass on epigenetic "codes" that help their children resist illness.

Reflecting on the results, Ornish said he is "impressed by how dynamic our bodies are. Instead of genetic nihilism—thinking there's nothing [you] can do—it's [inspiring] to know that if you can change your lifestyle, you can actually change your gene expression. And even if your mother, father, sister, aunt, and uncle all died of [prostate cancer] or heart disease, it doesn't mean that you have to; it just means that you need to make bigger changes than someone [without a hard-wired, genetic tendency] in order to prevent that."[50]

5

Back to Robert Caldwell. After consulting with top oncologists about treatment options, he had opted out of the conventional treatments of medication, or surgery and radiation, and instead, began to consider watchful waiting as an option. Was the GEMINAL program the "watchful waiting" approach that would work for him? Since the diagnosis, "I considered many options: yoga for cancer patients at a local medical center; a spiritual-meditation support group; and a writing program for cancer survivors, which I went to for quite a while," says Caldwell. After looking into an array of alternative options, he was convinced about the quality of Ornish's research, and confident enough about its results to commit to participating in an ongoing support group with others who were following the lifestyle-based program.

And so, after his friend, co-author Larry Scherwitz, consulted with Ornish's staff on Caldwell's behalf to ascertain whether Caldwell would be a good candidate for the GEMINAL program as a "watchful wait-ing" option (he was, because of the slow-growing nature and location of his particular cancer cells), Caldwell joined the weekly lifestyle-change support group, so he could practice and integrate the program into his everyday life. The group meets weekly in Sausalito, California, which isn't too far from the East Bay, where Caldwell lives; given his busy travel schedule, Caldwell knew he could commit to participating at least twice a month. During each get-together, one way in which he participates is by bringing a dish for the potluck meal. The meal is based on the program's dietary guidelines and is shared after the par-ticipants do group yoga but before the social support session.

Here's what Caldwell has to say about his experience with the pro-gram: "Getting diagnosed with prostate cancer has been quite a wake-up call. Knowing that it's reversible, that I have a measure of control over it, has made a strong impact. While I practice the whole program, for me, the key to success is the extent to which I can manage stress dif-ferently. With this in mind, I'm exploring how I want to re-design my life; I'm also looking at every part of my lifestyle so I can decide how I want to proceed. It's not just about reducing stressors," he continues, "nor is it only about having more control over my life. This program goes right to the heart of self. What is most important and what isn't?" Caldwell pauses before adding, "I suppose the program is guiding me to live my life as if it were a 'happiness practice.'"

There are a few striking things about the lifestyle program Ornish and his colleagues have created: it raises the possibility that a genetic susceptibility for prostate cancer can be prevented or reversed; that a diagnosis doesn't necessarily mean a lifetime sentence; and that genes, by themselves, may not determine health destiny. Rather, through the lifestyle choices we make each day, we may have the power to change our own health destiny. In other words, the lifestyle that comprises the GEMINAL study tells us we have a choice. By practicing its elements, we set into motion a synergistic dynamic—at least in noncancerous prostate tissue—that has the potential to prevent or turn around the progression of prostate cancer.[51] In other words, how we live our lives quite often is both the cause of, and solution to, illness or wellness. To address the issue, conventional health care has focused on prevention: don't smoke, lose weight, exercise, get vaccinated and screened, we're told. But Ornish has taken us one step further in seeking not only to prevent chronic disease, but also to reverse it. Because of his work and that of his colleagues, we now suspect that four major lifestyle components bring powerful, primal forces together: love and relationship; the drive for self-realization; making our lives meaningful; and enjoying—perhaps savoring—soul-satisfying food in the pleasing company of others.

Perhaps what we can learn from this study is that what distinguishes men diagnosed with prostate cancer who are on the GEMINAL program from patients diagnosed with prostate cancer who continue to live a more conventional high-stress, exercise-less, socially isolated, fast-food American lifestyle, is hope; the possibility they can cure their prostate cancer and, as powerful, help others do the same. And what's more, the men on the GEMINAL program don't just work harder at their lifestyle than others—they've also earned a sense of being in charge of a potentially life-threatening condition. In other words, they have replaced the option of watching the status of their ailment passively, waiting to discover if it's worsening or not, with lifestyle changes that empower them to feel in command of their disease—to believe they control it, that it doesn't control them.

What's more, the program has the potential to change lives to such a degree that Caldwell now describes his life and the lifestyle he's living as a "happiness practice." And there's more: while changes in his PSA levels raised questions, his latest biopsy showed no evidence of cancer. Being happy and discovering he is cancer-free. These are pretty powerful side effects for a "watchful waiting" treatment plan, aren't they?

Perspective: A Re-Visioning of the High-Fat, Low-Fat View

Most researchers and health professionals believe that dietary fat—especially saturated fat—was a key cause of heart disease. Indeed, the very low-fat mostly vegan diet that is part of Dean Ornish's intervention for reversing both heart disease and prostate cancer is based on decades of data linking diets high in fat with heart disease and other chronic conditions. Yet today, a new review suggests that the amount of dietary fat *per se* isn't the key culprit in heart disease. Rather, the quantity and quality of both fats and carbohydrates are the culprits.

There is an interesting example of this emerging new heart disease-dietary fat view in a review by Frank B. Hu and colleagues of the Department of Nutrition and Epidemiology at Harvard School of Public Health.[1] For instance, consider Hu's comment about a low-fat diet in his critical review about types of dietary fat and risk of heart disease: "Interestingly, in the control group [those not on the Ornish diet or program], coronary stenosis worsened (28% relative worsening) despite substantial reduction in fat intake (from 31% of energy to 25% of energy and LDL cholesterol (19% reduction)." Hu also questions the very low-fat Ornish diet because "even fatty fish and nuts, which have been documented to protect against CHD, are excluded." Still, it's important to remember those following the Ornish program achieved reversal of their disease even though they *didn't* consume "fatty fish and nuts, which have been documented to protect against CHD."

Might this mean that total fat intake by itself isn't the key point? For example, certain foods that are high in omega-3 fatty acids—such as fatty fish (salmon, etc.) and nuts (especially walnuts)—seem to provide protection. In other words, might both the *type* and *proportion* of dietary fat bring the best heart-health results? It's possible, and emerging research is providing clues that both an imbalance as well as the wrong types of dietary fats and carbohydrates in the foods we consume are major causes of not only heart disease, but other chronic conditions that plague us today.

Refined carbohydrates. In the chapter, "Diet, DNA, and Disease," we discussed the epigenetic link between metabolic syndrome and its members—central obesity, insulin resistance, elevated glucose and lipids, and high blood pressure—as a growing health problem. Is there a link between today's mostly refined carbohydrate diet compared to a diet that includes lots of whole grains, with the nutrient-dense germ and fiber of the kernel still intact? Iranian scientists were especially interested in exploring the refined-carbohydrate versus whole-food health link because heart disease is one of the major causes of mortality in Iran, and those with metabolic syndrome are at increased risk for heart disease.

To find out if there's a link, the researchers asked 827 Tehranian men and women, aged 18-74, to fill out a food frequency questionnaire. Their findings were unequivocal: The more refined grains consumed, the higher the odds of elevated cholesterol and triglycerides (risk factors for heart disease), high blood pressure, and metabolic syndrome. Conversely, those who consumed the most whole grains were least likely to have metabolic syndrome and related conditions.[2]

Refined fats. Is the quality—not necessarily the amount of fat consumed—a predictor of heart disease, metabolic syndrome, and related chronic conditions? To discover more, the same Iranian researchers who looked at the link between refined grains and increased odds of metabolic syndrome, took a close look at highly processed hydrogenated vegetable oils (HVOs) used extensively in Iranian homes; they then compared HVO consumption to people who consumed mostly unprocessed, non-HVO oils, such as olive and safflower oil.

Why was hydrogenated oil of interest? To turn liquid vegetable oil into a solid like margarine, it must be heated to high levels and hydrogen atoms need to be added to its fatty acids. This transforms naturally unsaturated fatty acids into trans fatty acids (TFAs), which correlate with higher levels of heart disease and other chronic conditions—from insulin resistance and diabetes to obesity and certain cancers. Here's another perspective: 4.2 percent of all calories consumed by Iranians are derived from TFAs, which is about twice the amount consumed in many developing countries.

At the same time, other processed vegetable oils that aren't hydrogenated, but that are heated to high temperatures to ensure a longer shelf life, create other health-robbing imbalances. During the heating process, health-enhancing omega-3 fatty acids are destroyed, leaving the oil with proportionally high levels of omega-6 fatty acids. As a matter of fact, human beings evolved consuming a 3:1 ratio of omega-6 to omega-3; with processing, though, the ratio in the typical American diet has changed to 14:1. And such high levels of omega-6, coupled with low- or deficient intake of omega-3, have consistently been linked with increased risk of certain cancers and other ailments.[3]

What conclusions can we draw from these studies? Given the profound nutrient changes in processed oils, it wasn't surprising when the Iranian researchers found high consumption of TFAs and HVOs was linked with increased risk of heart disease and type 2 diabetes.[4] This study also suggests that dietary fat, by itself, doesn't necessarily threaten health. Nor do whole carbohydrates. Rather, we need the right proportions of the three key fats—polyunsaturated fatty acids (PUFAs), monounsaturated fatty acids (MUFAs), and saturated fatty acids (SFAs)—as well as unprocessed whole grains and other carbohydrate-rich foods (fruits, vegetables, legumes, etc.) in their natural state and with the balance of naturally occurring nutrients intact. In other words, whole foods, balanced, essential fats, and oils lead to improved health; processed, refined, and imbalanced foods, fats, and oils lead to poorer health outcomes.

During the past decades, reduction in fat intake has been the main focus of national dietary recommendations. In the public's mind, the words "dietary fat" have become synonymous with obesity and heart disease, whereas foods that are "low fat" and "fat-free" are thought to be heart-healthy. In response to the low-fat campaign, the food industry has produced numerous commercial low-fat and fat-free products that are mostly refined carbohydrates and sugar. Ironically, while dietary fat intake as percentage of energy intake has slightly declined in the U.S. over the years, total calorie intake has increased. So, too, has the prevalence of obesity and type 2 diabetes. Has the tendency toward low-fat foods that, at the same time, are high in processed and refined carbohydrates, caused unintended health problems? We believe it may be part of the problem.

There's an expression, *caveat emptor:* let the buyer beware. When grocery shopping or eating out, we're suggesting this: let the diner beware.

Chapter 5

IT'S THE LIFESTYLE, STUPID!

Lifestyle. The statistics about it are daunting: 70 percent of all chronic illness—such as obesity, cancer, heart disease and diabetes—could be prevented through better lifestyles.[1] Yet only 3 percent of Americans take concerted action to stay healthy. This means most of us don't eat optimally, nor do we exercise regularly, de-stress, have many supportive relationships, and so on. This chapter is *more* than about lifestyle and the men and women who turn to it to prevent and reverse serious illness. It also introduces you to research scientists and to a growing body of evidence suggesting that the pattern of behaviors we call *lifestyle* may work together to influence whether your genes express themselves through wellness or illness. In this way, lifestyle is more, much more, than a mere word. For the lifestyle choices you make each day not only determine your health, they likely influence whether you pass on "healthy" or "unhealthy" epigenes to your children and grandchildren. In other words, it's the lifestyle, stupid.

I

In mid-1995, Cheryl Greene gave birth to her son, Austin. At the time, she was 40 years old, and delighting in both motherhood and her satisfying work as Executive Producer of DrGreene.com, the web site she had created with her husband, pediatrician Alan Greene. "It was a great team effort," Dr. Greene said in an interview.[2] It was so gratifying that "in early 1996, I said I can't imagine being any happier."[3] Shortly after expressing such joy, while nursing Austin, Cheryl found a lump in her breast. "On March 22, 1996, I was diagnosed with Stage III, high-inflammatory breast cancer," she said. "My doctor told me I would not live until the New Year." Austin was nine months old.

Because she was diagnosed at such a young age, Cheryl needed to make sense of what might have caused her breast cancer. It was especially unexpected, because she had no family history of breast cancer, nor did she have other risk factors, such as recent use of birth control pills, being overweight or obese, or use of alcohol. And then she remembered that as a kid growing up on a conventional grape farm that produced raisins, she had consistently been exposed to toxic pesticides. "My bedroom window was just feet away from the field," recalls Cheryl. "On Saturday mornings, I would lie in bed hearing the spray rig humming past my window . . . not realizing I was being exposed to all these toxins." But even back then, "high levels of toxic pesticides had already been linked to breast cancer," adds Alan. They had a clue.

Such insights helped Cheryl to make major lifestyle changes one year "after four surgeries, thirty-eight radiation treatments, and ten grueling months of chemotherapy." After this time, she was told there was no evidence of disease (NED), the term that has replaced "in remission." Thirteen years later, Cheryl still has no evidence of disease. As momentous, she and Alan attribute her success both to the excellent and extensive medical care she received, as well as to comprehensive changes she made in her lifestyle—especially in her diet. "I'm very lucky, I'm very blessed, I'm very fortunate," says Cheryl. "I know a lot of [her successful outcome] was the treatment I had. A lot of it was the *support group* I had. [And] we do not eat anything that is not *organic*," she adds. In other words, Cheryl attributes the 13 years she's had without evidence of breast cancer to the *comprehensive* lifestyle changes she made.

It seems that Cheryl successfully turned her life-threatening disease around in large part by availing herself of aggressive conventional chemotherapy and radiation treatments. But for all this, what really led to her beating the hopeless life-and-death odds she was given? The reasons why some people get sick and die, and others don't, is still mysterious. After all, like Cheryl, most of us are exposed to all kinds of carcinogens every day, but don't necessarily get breast cancer. And as we've seen, there was no history of breast cancer in Cheryl's family, meaning, the health of her parents—her genetic inheritance—didn't necessarily determine her health. And while conventional medicine provided powerful treatment options for her, it isn't designed to cure, prevent, or reverse most chronic illnesses.

While a key reason Cheryl eats organic food is to avoid cancer-causing pollutants and toxicants in food, there's yet another reason for "going organic": we now know that the food we eat each day can either prevent or contribute to the likelihood of breast cancer or other ailments. Confirms Alan: "Every bite of food you eat is an investment in your future, or it's a debt you're taking out. So make sure you're investing when you go to the grocery store."

Why, then, did Cheryl beat the odds—so much so that she did more than survive, she is thriving? The answer to why some of us get serious sicknesses and other don't is heavily dependent on how we live our lives each day. What (and how) do you eat? Are you physically active? How do you handle stress? Do you have social support? More than anything else, these kinds of environment-based *lifestyle choices* are what we have the most control over. Yet we often fail to give them the attention, consideration, and *action* they warrant—even though *they have the power to do even more than ward off or reverse an ailment*. Indeed, the lifestyle choices you make each day may be the most influential determinant of your "gene health," as well as whether you pass on healthy or unhealthy epigenes to your children and grandchildren.

2

March 27, 1513, is when Spanish explorer Juan Ponce de Leon is believed to have been in the vicinity of Florida, where he travelled to find the Fountain of Youth. At the time, the Fountain was believed to have waters that could "cure" old age, restore vitality, and bring eternal youth and life. Ponce de Leon never found the Fountain of Youth. Even so, the legend of the mythical spring lives on today, for many of us are still searching for eternal youth.[4] Here is how psychologist Dr. Mark Stibich describes the ways in which many of us search for rejuvenation today:

> In many ways, we are still looking for the Fountain of Youth. Researchers and drug companies are still searching for medications to make us live longer. Fad diets . . . and exercise routines all claim to extend life. In the end, a *healthy lifestyle* [emphasis added], positive thinking, and good relationships are our best bet for a long and happy life.[5]

What Stibich is saying is that the Fountain of Youth is a myth, a fictitious and made-up story about a place with magical, youthful powers. But the fact that the myth has existed for millennia in different cultures worldwide suggests that it speaks to an unconscious and deep desire that many of us have to stay young and healthy forever. He is also saying that science and technology have given us hope that the myth of the Fountain of Youth can be realized through quick-fix solutions: the magic pill will take off weight while we sleep, or the exercise machine will give us the "washboard abs" of a 20-year-old body builder. All the while, like Dorothy in the fable *The Wizard of Oz*, the healing balm we are seeking—the path to health and healing—has always resided in the timeless wisdom of our bodies. Give your body the lifestyle ingredients it needs and it can often heal itself. In other words, lifestyle is the path to restoring youth and vigor, but we've been looking in every direction for the Fountain of Youth, except the way we live on a day-to-day basis.

The famous sociologist Max Weber put the concept of lifestyle on the map in the late 1800s, when he defined it as a combination of social conditions and individual choices. In the Weberian view, this meant that a person's lifestyle is comprised of "life chances"—such as the opportunity to go to college—and "life conduct," the choices and actions each of us are free to make.[6] By the 1980s, the concept of lifestyle emerged in the scientific and medical arenas when Dean Ornish and his colleagues combined a seemingly disparate set of four health behaviors—diet, exercise, stress management, and social support—to show that when practiced together, they have the power to work synergistically to reverse heart disease and, as we saw in chapter 7, possibly even cancer through genetic changes.[7–10] Says Ornish: "We found that the more people change [their lifestyle], the better they get—no matter how old or how sick they were in terms of their heart disease, their prostate cancer, their diabetes, and so on."[11]

By illuminating the power of lifestyle to reset our genes for wellness or illness, in this chapter we introduce you to a new synthesis of lifestyle and health—with genes as a bridge between the two. What do you typically eat? Are you physically active? Is your life stress-full? How's your social life? Clearly, the marvel of lifestyle is the lifestyle choices you make each day can influence whether certain genes are turned on or off, and in turn, and quite possibly, your health. As incredible, the lifestyle "ingredients" you "feed" your genes create genetic expression that is dynamic: *changes take place in a minute, an hour, a day, a month . . . or throughout your lifetime.* And not only do they change quickly, they can go one way with a *poor lifestyle*, or they can be reversed with a *high-quality lifestyle*.

3

Are diet and other aspects of lifestyle the solution for the 95-plus percent of us who don't stand to benefit from genomic medicine because we don't have a single-gene disease? With this chapter, the future of epigenetic medicine, discussed in chapter 2, and its profound link to lifestyle is arriving. Through extraordinary studies, we are introducing the possibility that diet and other aspects of your lifestyle play key roles in re-creating your health destiny by resetting your genes—and our children's—for wellness. In other words, by presenting the possible mechanisms through state-of-the-art studies, we are offering a glimpse into how lifestyle can change your genes for better or worse.

In chapter 2, we discussed the emerging field of epigenetic medicine and the ways in which it integrates diet and lifestyle with genetic expression and in turn, wellness or illness. The pioneering studies we're telling you about in this chapter are signaling the direction we think the role of lifestyle will take as epigenetic medicine evolves. Right now, it's in its infancy. Still, we're giving you a preview of what's in store for you and your health in what an article in the *Journal of the American Medical Association* describes as "the medicine of the future."[12] And it is diet—as well as exercise, stress management, and social support—which comprises the core of a lifestyle Rx that brings gene-health benefits.

Consider, for example, the role of certain nutrients. In recent years, a member of the B vitamin family, called folic acid (also called *folate*), has emerged as an important player in cancers of the digestive tract. More and more, research is revealing an abundant supply can prevent these kinds of cancers, while deficiencies can contribute to their likelihood. In the search for a genetic link, geneticist Z. Attias and colleagues at Tel Aviv University wanted to find out if folic acid has the ability to turn off (down-regulate) the "over activity" of a particular gene called *IGF-IR*, which keeps cancer cells alive, productive, and multiplying. When they fed various doses of folic acid to colon cancer cells, they found that the more folic acid fed to the cells, the less active the *IGF-IR* gene.[13]

These findings have two significant implications about diet, genes, and health. The first is that adequate folic acid may actually be able to prevent colon cancer by turning off the *IGF-IR* cancer-causing gene. The bigger implication, though, is that a diet abundant in nutrients can contribute to health, while nutrient deficiencies may undermine health by allowing cancer-causing genes to run rampant. Prior to this study, scientists knew that folic acid deficiency could contribute to colon and other cancers, and that adequate supplies could prevent them. With this study, though, we now have a clear diet-*gene* link to health that we didn't have before.[13]

What's interesting about the diet-gene connection is that more and more, research is revealing the remarkable role particular nutrients play in compensating for genetic weaknesses and in turn, how food resets genetic expression by turning genes on or off. Indeed, diet seems to be a primary ingredient in the lifestyle-gene-health formula, as Drs. Marcus Pembrey and Lars Bygren (Chapter 2) discovered. At the same time, for decades, exercise has been a close "partner" with diet in the prescription for health. After all, doesn't the medical community often recommend them as a "pair" to treat chronic conditions, such over-weight and obesity, heart disease, and diabetes? We've already seen there is a clear diet-gene-health connection. Is it possible that there is also an exercise-gene-health link?

We get a clue with the exercise-gene expression study by pediatri-cian Peter Connolly done in 2004. Connolly and his colleagues at the University of California, Irvine, wanted to see if a single bout of intense exercise could influence or change gene expression. To find out, they asked a group of 15 healthy men, between 18 and 30 years old, to ride a stationary bicycle, vigorously, for 30 minutes. Prior to the intensive exercise session ("pre-exercise"), the researchers obtained blood sam-ples from each of the men. Then they took blood samples, again, after the 30 minutes of exercise ("end-exercise"); and again, one hour later ("recovery"). Not only did Connelly want to see what impact exercise itself had on the men's' gene expression, he also wanted to see if the impact lingered; if it continued to change an hour later; after what is called the "recovery" phase.

The results of the study were quite remarkable. When the research-ers looked closely at the blood cells from the three blood samples they had taken between pre-exercise and recovery, the effect of 30 minutes of heavy exercise showed strong effects on hundreds of gene responses. Perhaps predictably, most of the genes—311, to be exact—turned either on or off between starting and stopping the exercise. By the time the genes were measured again during the recovery stage an hour later, 553 genes had changed, although by this time, most had returned to pre-exercise levels.

What is incredible and notable about these findings is that the genes that were influenced by exercise were those in key systems that influ-ence health: those in our immune, inflammatory, and stress categories. But what especially surprised the researchers was that the exercise bout also affected a large number of genes in what is called the "cell-growth category," which is involved in the repair of tissue. This study revealed not only that heavy exercise turns a large *number* of genes on or off, it also *rapidly activates and deactivates genes* associated with stress, inflam-mation, and tissue repair, such as that which occurs during wound heal-ing. In other words, although the mechanism isn't clear yet, strenuous exercise changes the categories of genes that prevent the development of chronic *inflammation*, which more and more, is believed to be the underlying cause of many chronic conditions. The possibility that exercise can influence health and healing on a *genetic level* is of obvious importance to researchers, doctors, and health professionals—indeed, to all of us who are interested in the genomic response to physical activity, and in turn, the role it may play in preventing and reversing many health problems.

4

Over the course of this chapter, we'll be introducing you to key lifestyle-gene-health elements in addition to diet and exercise: a *stress* management technique that turns on health-enhancing genes, and studies showing the genetic benefits of *social support*. In examining such studies, we're finding that our epigenome is exquisitely sensitive to what we do on a daily basis; that it can react quickly, record what we do, and perhaps can even influence how the developing fetus adapts, based on its mother's diet. We're both awed and inspired by such dynamics, for as we get to know the "personality" of our human genome, it is telling us that our genes do not control us; rather, we control our genes—past, present, and future—by our experiences, our exposure to environmental influences, our diet, and our lifestyle.

Given the profound implications about the role genes and lifestyle play in heredity, health, and healing, we are realizing there is something profoundly limiting and incomplete in our ideas about the role of two of the most familiar elements: the *diet-exercise* duo. And perhaps nowhere is this more evident than in the tried, true, and *unsuccessful* advice we're given for weight loss. After all, aren't we typically told to cut calories and move more? And don't we assume that if we fail to diet and exercise and lose weight, it is our fault? But just as dieting, deprivation, and eating-by-number (counting calories, weight watching, counting carbs, figuring fat grams, and so on) don't work for long-term weight loss, more and more research is suggesting that exercise, by itself, isn't an effective weight loss strategy either. But isn't this in direct conflict with conventional weight-loss wisdom, which tells us that the more exercise you do, the more calories you'll burn, and the more weight you'll lose?

Preventive medicine physician Timothy Church, Chair in Health Wisdom at Louisiana State University, and his team, decided to find out why there's often a discrepancy between the amount of exercise dieters do and weight loss. The group they worked with included

464 overweight and obese post-menopausal women, each of whom the researchers randomly assigned to one of four groups. Group 1, who would be the control group, remained sedentary, non-exercisers throughout the study. Using stationary bicycles and treadmills, and working with a personal trainer, women in groups 2, 3, and 4 would do low-, medium-, and high-levels of exercise, and they would work out 72 minutes, 136 minutes, and 194 minutes each week, respectively. And the women would follow this routine three to four times each week over a period of six months.

To establish baseline information, at the start of the study, all women were weighed;, then weighed each week throughout the study. The women also were asked to keep a *food frequency questionnaire*: what and how much did they eat every day? The amount of time the women spent exercising wasn't the key measure; rather, the researchers predicted, beforehand, the number of calories each group would burn during each of the supervised exercise sessions. Another important aspect was the dietary guidelines of the study: there were none. Instead, the women were told not to change their dietary or physical activity habits (other than the supervised sessions).

The results of the study were completely unexpected. You would think that the women who exercised the most and who burned the most calories during exercise would be the ones who lost the most weight. But this isn't what happened; rather, the average number of pounds lost in each group was modest, at best: *high* exercisers lost 3.3 pounds; *medium* exercisers lost 4.6 pounds; *light* exercisers lost 3.1 pounds; and the *non-exercisers* lost 2 pounds. What's remarkable about this is that so little weight was lost for so much exercise. And even more surprising, those who did the most exercise didn't lose as much weight as those in the moderate exercise group. Even more unexpected was that a few women in each of the four groups gained weight; some 10 pounds or more. What happened here? Why didn't the group that exercised the most lose the most weight? Church speculates:

> Most exercise guidelines for weight loss recommend 200–300 minutes per week, and we provide evidence that this amount of exercise induces compensation (likely increased energy intake through food) that results in significantly less weight loss than predicted. If different doses of exercise result in different amounts of compensation, it is not surprising that when exercise studies of varying doses and duration are examined collectively, <u>*there is no relationship between exercise dose and weight loss*</u> [emphasis added].[14]

This study gives us two lifestyle-changing insights. The first insight is that it's easy to wipe out calories burned through exercise with "high-octane" foods. This finding has been so consistent and so strong for so long that psychologist Dr. Kelly Brownell, who has treated obese people for years, has renounced the exercise more-eat less food dogma, and instead, is focusing on food *quality* and *quantity* for weight loss.[15] The second lifestyle-based insight is that if you eat more because you exercise, or if you exercise so that you can eat more, you are not going to lose much weight—if at all. This became evident in Church's study, when he discovered that the exercisers tended to eat more, and virtually defeat their weight loss efforts. And the reasons they ate more after working out ranged from emotional eating to being hungry after exercise because it had stimulated their appetite. What's more, it's likely the "compensation" food they turned to isn't fresh whole food; rather, it's probably processed and calorie-dense carbohydrates.

Overexercising and overeating is exactly what happens to journalist John Cloud. For years, he has stuck to a comprehensive weekly exercise routine that includes a five-minute warm-up on the VersaClimber, 30 minutes on the stair mill, an hour with a personal trainer, a body wedge class, and a 5.5 mile run. Even though he's not overweight, and even though he exercises a lot, "I still have gut fat that hangs over my belt when I sit," he writes. And even though he gained weight for a two-year period when he "self-medicated with lots of Italian desserts," his usual post-exercise "reward" is a blueberry bar.[16] Church, the scientist who conducted the study on the seeming futility of exercising for weight loss, found a similar dynamic with some of his wife's friends who don't seem to lose weight even though they run an hour a day. The reason, he discovered, is their stop at Starbucks for muffins after their run.

5

That many of us reward ourselves with food for exercising—or other reasons—may not come as a surprise to you. After all, it's fairly common and routine for millions of us to turn to food for comfort. Feeling anxious? Try some potato chips or chocolate chip cookies. Have your feelings been hurt? Soothe yourself with ice cream. Want to celebrate a success; to reward yourself? Have a piece of choice chocolate or a "health bar." Clearly, turning to comfort food is so common, it's easy to consider it normal. But it isn't.

Meet EDNOS, the acronym for "Eating Disorder Not Otherwise

Specified." This term covers the gray area of disordered eating patterns that lies between optimal, healthful eating and serious psychological eating disorders, such as the "trinity" of anorexia nervosa, bulimia nervosa, and compulsive overeating. And a growing number of health professionals would say *most Americans* have some kind of undiagnosed eating disorder—which psychologist Dr. Susan Boulware describes as "'disturbed eating,' separating food from the physiological purpose of nourishing the physical body and using it to serve emotional and psychological needs."[17]

When health researchers and co-authors Larry Scherwitz and Deborah Kesten took a close look at "disturbed eating" and its link to weight, they discovered seven newly identified eating styles linked with overeating, overweight, and obesity: *Fast Foodism* (eating mostly processed, pre-prepared, and fast food); *Emotional Eating* (eating in response both to positive and negative feelings); *Food Fretting* (ongoing dieting and over-concern about the "best" way to eat); *Task Snacking* (eating while doing other things, such as working at your computer or watching TV); *Unappetizing Atmosphere* (eating while driving in hectic traffic or with unpleasant people); *Solo Dining* (eating alone more often than not); and *Sensory Disregard* (eating quickly or being too preoccupied to take time to taste flavors in food).[18, 19]

What's of special relevance about these overeating styles is *all of them are considered normal.* Think for a moment: most of us often eat fast or packaged food or comfort food to soothe emotions. Many of us diet, or eat while doing other things. It's typical to dine at a "table for one" in unpleasant surroundings. And eating quickly, not taking the time to taste flavors in food, is the norm.

We are especially excited to share these overeating styles with you, because—as with the four key lifestyle-gene-health "ingredients" of diet, exercise, stress management, and social support that are the focus of this chapter—we see the eating styles as a dynamic web of food-related choices, feelings, sensations, and social behaviors. *And five of the overeating styles*—Fast Foodism; Emotional Eating; Food Fretting; Unpleasant Atmosphere; and Solo Dining—*are linked with three of the lifestyle-gene-health factors of diet, stress, and social support.* Does their association with these lifestyle factors suggest that what we eat (diet), the emotions we bring to meals (stress), and our social environment (social support) also influence gene expression, and in turn, overweight and other chronic conditions? Surely, with the field of epigenetic medicine in its infancy, we can still only speculate.

What we *do* know, however, is that the traditional diet-exercise duo isn't bringing the weight-loss results we want. And we know that making subtle but significant changes not only in what you eat, but also how, why, when, where—even with whom—may lead to normal weight. In other words, overcoming the seven overeating styles isn't "just about calories or exercise, and our bodies know this," writes Dr. Christine Northrup. Rather, the opposite of the overeating styles— what we call *the Enlightened Diet*—"gives you exactly what you need to make eating what it was meant to be: a joyful, delicious celebration of life, nurturing, and friendship," writes Northrup.[19] In other words, to achieve a normal weight, change your relationship to food so your most-of-the-time way of eating becomes a social, health-enhancing, pleasurable experience. What a contrast to the unwelcome isolation and anxiety linked to traditional dieting and exercise . . . which doesn't work for most of us anyway.

6

We've just seen that diet and exercise are more, much more, than two often tedious, overly simplified elements of lifestyle. Rather, they are two critical lifestyle factors that have a powerful influence on the direction your genes take, and whether they express themselves through wellness or illness. In this way, the food you eat and the exercise you do raise the question: Are you eating and exercising in such as way that you're resetting your genes so that they enhance health? Or are you making lifestyle choices that invite illness?

Because we're most familiar with these two lifestyle "ingredients," many think that diet and exercise are the major elements of lifestyle associated with genes and health (and weight loss). But this isn't accurate, for *stress* is perhaps the most underestimated and neglected member of the lifestyle-gene-health family. Harvard cardiologist Dr. Herbert Benson discovered the potent role of stress through studies that began with meditation in the late 1960s. During this time, he observed Tibetan monks meditating in the wintry, freezing Himalayan Mountains with *wet* sheets covering their shoulders. What you would expect would be for the wet sheets to freeze and for the monks to be too cold to stay outside. But this isn't what happened. Benson was amazed as he watched steam rise from the wet sheets, and the speed at which the sheets dried. Somehow, the meditating monks not only warmed their bodies in sub-freezing temperatures, they actually dried the sheets![20] Clearly, meditation wasn't just some unfathomable, misunderstood practice done in the East; rather, it somehow enabled the mind to control the body—so much so that it could produce bodily heat in sub-freezing weather.

Intrigued, Benson returned to Harvard where he conducted studies to identify the mechanism at play. To do this, he attached electrodes to meditators to monitor what effect, if any, meditation had on the body. And what he found was remarkable: those who meditated by focusing on a singular thought or object experienced reductions in blood pressure, a slower heart rate, and slower brain waves. Such studies clearly demonstrated a *mind-body* connection—that the mind and body are one system. Benson called this *the relaxation response* (RR).[21] After conclusively proving the mind-body connection, he founded the Benson-Henry Institute for Mind-Body Medicine at Harvard Medical School. Its focus: bring stress and its evidence-based antidote, the relaxation response, into medicine.

Earlier in this chapter, we told you about the ability aerobic exercise has to turn on various genes within 30 minutes, and to turn them off in an hour or less after exercising. This is powerful knowledge, because it tells us that our genes are super-sensitive not only to our dietary environment—which is the major focus of this book—but also to movement and motion; that genes somehow "track" our activity level and in turn, influence the expression of genes throughout our entire body when we exercise. Does this also apply to stress, and the remedy of Herbert Benson's relaxation response?

We've known for decades that stress—an ongoing sense of threat, feeling overwhelmed, or anxiety—is linked with poor health outcomes.[22–23] From depressing your immune system and increasing blood pressure to heart disease—*stress can worsen existing ailments and cause others*. But, as with diet and exercise, recent studies suggest stress also turns genes on or off (up- or down-regulate) that make you more prone to illness.[24–26] But can the opposite occur? If stress is linked with worsening health, might *stress management* techniques such as Benson's relaxation response also turn genes on or off that threaten health, and in turn, prevent or reverse health problems? Mind-body researcher Dr. Jeffrey Dusek and colleagues decided to find out.[27] This would be an invaluable insight to discover, because it would mean the genetic effects of stress could be reversed with stress management.

The question the investigators posed is this: Can the relaxation response alter gene expression? To find out, they would test genes from blood samples taken from three groups of healthy people at the start of the study and eight weeks later. Group 1 consisted of people who had been practicing various relaxation response techniques—such as yoga, tai chi, repetitive prayer, deep relaxation, and breathing exercises—for a long time; they would continue to do so throughout the study. Members of Group 2 were new to the relaxation response; they would be trained in its techniques. And Group 3 was the control group: people in this group did *not* practice relaxation response techniques either before, during, or after the study.

The results were remarkable, for they provide compelling evidence—for the first time—that the relaxation response elicits changes in gene expression. And it gets better, because when the researchers conducted a refined analysis, they discovered that the genes that are turned on and off by the relaxation response influence many systems in our body, which in turn, influence disease and aging. And it gets even better: *the genes that were turned on and off during the relaxation response appeared to reverse the negative impact of stress* and related free-radical damage, a process that "rusts" cells and makes you more prone to ailments ranging from heart disease to cancer.

Such results suggest that if you do even a small amount of stress management each day, it can have a big effect on a cellular level—so much so that it may prevent or reverse various ailments. But a "weekend warrior" approach won't bring the benefits. Rather, sustaining these beneficial changes is directly linked to the amount of time you spend practicing stress management techniques. The longer you practice (both each day and throughout your lifetime), the more pervasive the benefits . . . for your genes, your cells, and your health.

7

In 1887, a physician named L. Emmett Holt identified a complex of symptoms linked to infants who "ceased to thrive." At the time, Holt equated infants who failed to flourish, and instead, experienced poor weight gain and failure to grow, with malnutrition—although it was clear to him there also were other causes. By the late 1960s, scientists had confirmed that malnourishment did, indeed, contribute to "failure to thrive," but they had also identified causes that had eluded Holt—and *parental deprivation* leads the list. Over time, a closer look revealed that both lack of food as well as "stimulus deprivation" could lead to all-encompassing "side effects" for a child—from interfering with her or his ability to absorb nutrients to depression and apathy. In other words, if a parent or caregiver is depressed or anxious, doesn't hold and nurture an infant, has poor parenting skills, feels hostility toward the child, or is perhaps highly stressed because of, say, financial or marital difficulties, some or all of these dynamics can contribute to poor growth during infancy and childhood.[28, 29]

The concept of failure to thrive begs the question: if substandard nurturing—both physically and emotionally—leads to poor health outcomes, would caring and loving comfort by friends and family—regard from people who value us—have the opposite influence? It appears so. And "social support" is the term used to describe the beneficial and positive influence that supportive surroundings can bring. Over the years, more and more research has demonstrated that social support can "neutralize" the negative effects of a wide range of ailments. For example, studies by psychiatrist David Spiegel of Stanford University showed that women with metastatic breast cancer who participated in weekly support sessions lived much longer than those who didn't participate in the social support groups.[30] And the often-called rabbit study by R.M. Nerem at the University of Texas revealed that rabbits fed artery-clogging food, who were talked to and touched while eating, exhibited less coronary artery disease than rabbits on the same diet who weren't nurtured while being fed.[31] Clearly, being surrounded by love and nurturance—or not—may not only influence wellness or illness; it may well have life or death consequences.[32]

Because of such studies, researchers have known for decades that social support is a critical component of a lifestyle that leads to well-being.[33, 34] But, unlike diet, exercise, and stress management—which we've seen are pivotal players on the lifestyle-*gene*-health field—it wasn't until 2008 that social support became the fourth key component of the lifestyle-gene-health package. This is due to the work of neurologist Patrick O. McGowan and his colleagues at McGill University in Montreal, who compared both the physical and psychological effects of *substandard* versus *quality* maternal care, first on animal pups and then on human beings.

The questions they posed are these: do pups and people who experience abusive and unloving maternal care (poor or nonexistent social support) respond by creating different genetic pathways than cared-for pups and children? And if so, would the difference have a life-long effect? To find out, the key response (*biomarker*) the team would study would be *stress-response* later in life. After all, if pups and infants are mistreated, surely it's a stressful experience. Could the stress response they learn in infancy carry into adulthood by turning on and off genes that may contribute to the production of stress-inducing hormones?

To find out, McGowan looked at two pathways in pups that determine whether particular stress-related genes are turned on or off when they have an affectionate mother. When the first pathway is launched, pups have an *affection-hormone-gene* response that increases *serotonin* (a hormone, or "chemical messenger," located in the brain) levels, which turn on a stress-related gene called *NGF1-A*. And it is this gene that helps to lower the levels of *cortisol*, a stress hormone that is released during challenging and threatening situations. The second pathway that is set into motion in "loved" pups is the turning on of another gene called *Nr3c1*. This gene, when it is turned on, supports NGF1-A in keeping stress hormones down *well into adulthood*.

What about pups born to unaffectionate mothers? McGowan found they don't experience such protection in response to stress, because they don't produce enough serotonin to turn on the *NGF1-A* gene that lowers cortisol. This tells us that lack of affection can reset the *Nr3c1* gene, making the unloved pups prone to higher levels of stress response throughout life. But there's a bright side: if pups of unaffectionate mothers are "adopted" by caring foster mothers within a week of birth, they grow up with the same "stress protection" experienced by pups loved by their biological mother from birth.[35–37]

The work of McGowan and his colleagues is brilliant. For the first time, he and his team used an animal model to define the molecular pathway linking lack of affection in pups to changes in genes, and in turn, heightened response to stress in adulthood. Would this also apply to adult *human beings* who were severely mistreated by their parents when they were children? Is there a parallel? When McGowan looked at adults who had been abused as children, he found that their *NGF1-A* gene, too, was more likely to be turned off, which suggests that abused children have "unaffectionate" hormone-gene mechanisms that are similar to the neglected pups.

With McGowan's landmark studies, we now have an explanation for how unaffectionate parenting can lead to genetic changes that lead to a lifetime of increased stress and depression in children.[37] Social support is now a piece of the lifestyle-gene-health picture. Add it to the three other elements of lifestyle—diet, exercise, and stress management—and we have an emerging integrative model of the role lifestyle plays in resetting our genes for wellness or illness.

8

If you ask Oscar-nominated actress Mariel Hemingway about her optimal lifestyle, she's likely to tell you she was motivated by genetics. Her family history includes suicide by her famous grandfather, author Ernest Hemingway; a mother who died from cancer; and two older sisters who suffered from mental illness. "Being in a family with serious addictions and mental illness led me to healthy, organic, and balanced living," Mariel said in an article about her healthy lifestyle. And while she describes food, exercise, silence, and home (different words for the same key elements of lifestyle—diet, physical activity, stress management, and family and friends—discussed throughout this chapter) as the four core elements that keep her happy and balanced, "healthy eating gets top priority."

And so it does. Not only does she have an organic garden, Hemingway writes cookbooks, encouraging people to eat locally grown, fresh and organic vegetables and fruits, whole grains, nuts and seeds, and eggs, as well as grass-fed beef that is hormone- and additive-free. And because she experienced inflamed, achy joints and fatigue when she ate processed foods, she specifically steers clear of what she refers to as "noisy," packaged food. Along with fresh food, exercise, too, is a natural for her. Having grown up surrounded by nature in a small town in Idaho, she continues to do regular physical activities, such as hiking and biking, which were part of her childhood.

Also integral to Mariel's lifestyle is quiet time, which she pursues with such stress management techniques as yoga and its "cousin," deep breathing. You can add cooking as part of her relaxation practice, because she finds it restful and relaxing—especially when her daughters, friends, and family are sitting and talking around the large farmhouse table in her kitchen, while enjoying one of her nourishing meals. "'Every person and every animal in my family passes through the kitchen at some point,'" reflects Mariel, "'because food is the centering point . . . the foundation from which everything else . . . can start.'"[38]

If we put Mariel's and Cheryl Greene's successful lifestyle stories together with the state-of-the-art research studies we've told you about that link diet, exercise, stress management, and social support with "healthy genes," we get a more complete picture of the path to lifestyle-gene-health success. Mariel and Cheryl were undoubtedly motivated to make lifestyle changes. Mariel knew it would be her path to overcoming her family's tendency toward the triple health threats of addiction, cancer, and mental illness; and Cheryl was a new mother and relatively young woman when she was diagnosed with advanced breast cancer. Their need and drive to overcome such adversity is clear.

But what truly distinguishes their health success is not only their determination; rather, it is the *comprehensive* lifestyle changes they made, which in turn, empowered them to re-create their health destiny by resetting their genes for wellness. Without going organic, integrating movement and motion into their lives, managing stress, and seeking social support, their health may have taken a different path. Seeking to understand her success, Cheryl knew she was "lucky" and "blessed." But she also said a lot of her good health fortune was "changing my lifestyle."[2] That doesn't mean she didn't take advantage of traditional and grueling medical treatment; it means she understands that the lifestyle changes she made took her genes on the path that leads to health and healing.

All the elements of lifestyle we've looked at so far are much more significant than what they tell us about health, by themselves. For what's pivotal to health success is this: like members of a family, the elements of lifestyle work in *synergy*, meaning, that when practiced *together*, we think the benefits are greater than if you did just one element in isolation. And the rewards—such as *preventing* problems (Mariel Hemingway's incentive) or *reversing* an existing ailment (Cheryl Greene's accomplishment)—are cumulative and can be quick, for it appears that when lifestyle turns on "healthy genes," the change can occur in a minute, hour, month . . . and over your lifetime. And this is what's amazing: *our genes are designed to adapt to the environment.* And our environment—especially diet and lifestyle—is what we create as well as what's around us. This matters a lot . . . not only for ourselves, but for the health and well-being we pass on to our children and grandchildren.

In Chapter 2, we saw the impact of diet over generations when we discussed the transgenerational effects of food availability on longevity in children born in the remote parish of Överkalix, Sweden. When their grandparents had less to eat, the grandchildren lived much longer than the grandchildren whose grandparents had an abundance of food. And again, in the same chapter, we saw the amazing effect of particular supplements on mice with a variation of the Agouti gene, which makes them prone to obesity, diabetes, and cancer. But the power of diet prevailed, for when pregnant Agouti mothers were given appropriate supplements, they were more likely to give birth to normal-weight pups that were healthy.

Aware that lifestyle is *the* path to the Fountain of Youth via its power to prevent, manage, or reverse chronic conditions often linked with aging, key thought leaders in medicine are recommending lifestyle as a key player in America's health landscape. Consider this suggestion in the Wellness Initiative for the Nation (WIN), proposed by the lifestyle- and integrative medicine-oriented Samueli Institute. The idea surfaced as part of a community discussion in response to a "call for ideas" for reforming the nation's health care: "Create an Executive office . . . specifically focused on developing policies and programs for lifestyle-based chronic disease prevention and management, integrative health care practices and health promotion."[39]

Or reflect on the "Take Back Your Health Act of 2009," a first-of-its-kind lifestyle-based bill by U.S. Senator Ron Wyden (D-Ore.), co-sponsored by Senators John Cornyn (R-Tex.) and Tom Harkin (D-Iowa). Says Wyden:

> This is a groundbreaking bill, based on the proven idea that lifestyle changes can improve the health of those with chronic disease if people stick with a program that has that goal in mind. The Take Back Your Health Act gets doctors and patients invested in the success of treatment, since doctors won't be paid unless their patients actually get better.[40]

Lifestyle is a powerful force. It is so influential that it determines our health. Its impact persists to such a degree that not only can it alter our genetic tendencies; we can pass on its effects from generation to generation. Our genes create the 100,000 proteins in our body. They help us digest food, repair cuts and wounds, make babies, communicate with one another. They make us susceptible to disease—or help prevent it. We help them toward their destination, or we derail them from reaching their goal based on our diet and other lifestyle choices. Such scientific insights about the gene-diet-lifestyle interconnection force us to consider our own responsibility about the diet and lifestyle we choose—not only because they are key "deciders" of our own health, but also because their "quality" persists in our children and grandchildren.

So far in *Pottenger's Prophecy*, we've seen that wellness or illness arises out of the steady accumulation of lifestyle choices, with a special focus on diet: the food you typically eat, what your parents ate before you were born, the gene-environment interaction you inherited, and the one you create for yourself everyday. The question we answer in the next chapters of *Pottenger's Prophecy* is what to eat so that each time you dine, you're resetting your genes for wellness. Is there an *evidence-based* way of eating that leads to "healthy genes," one based on insights gleaned both from our ancient ancestors and state-of-the-art Western nutritional science; one we can depend on to bring the health results we want? Yes, there is . . . if we take the time to understand the foods on which we—and our genes—evolved, and how what we ate—and thrived on for millennia—compares to what we're calling "'Nourishment' Now."

Chapter 6

FOOD, GENES, AND
HEALTH OVER TIME

For millennia, whole plant- and animal-based foods consumed by our ancient ancestors contained nourishing substances that not only sustained humankind but allowed us to flourish. During this time, the naturally occurring nutrients (protein, carbohydrates, fats, vitamins, minerals, and so on) in the food we ate entered into a dance with our genes. What are the foods and nutrients our genes have been dancing with for hundreds of thousands of years? And are the nutrients in these foods the same ones we still need today to be truly nourished? This question is pivotal, because if what now passes as food doesn't supply the nutrients our genes have been designed to metabolize, we are trusting—blindly—that our epigenome can keep up with the changes, and continue to keep us healthy. Can our genes change—or at the least, adapt to today's fast-changing Western diet? Perhaps what warrants even more speculation and consideration is this: What are the health consequences of stepping away from our ancestral sustenance; indeed, altering and ignoring what sustained, rejuvenated, and healed humans for millennia?

I

Seventy thousand years ago, heavy-boned, dark-skinned humans crossed the Indian Ocean from South-East Asia to Australia. Twenty thousand years later, the more delicately boned "Gracile" people joined their "Robust" family in Australia.[1] Originally called "Aborigines" (meaning, original inhabitants) by British settlers who discovered the Indigenous Australians in 1788,[2] these "first people"—with a population that ranged between 318,000 and 750,000 prior to colonization by Europeans—settled throughout Australia in the desert, inland, and on the coast.[3]

Depending on where they lived, the diet of the semi-nomadic Native Australians varied, especially as they moved across various areas and over the continent with the changing seasons. At any one time, inland inhabitants hunted small animals (possum, for instance), reptiles (lizards, snakes, etc.), birds, insects, and mammals (kangaroo, wallaby, koalas, etc.), and they foraged for fruits (berries, and so on), greens, and other vegetables. Those on the coast added shellfish and fish such as catfish, cod, and Gummy shark to the menu. Nutrition researcher Kerin O'Dea, who has studied the original Aboriginal diet, describes the animal and plant foods consumed by the physically fit and lean Australian natives as

> a varied diet in which animal foods were a major component. Despite this, the diet was not high in fat, as wild animal carcasses have very low fat contents through most of the year, and the meat is extremely lean. Everything on an animal carcass was eaten, including the small fat depots and organ meats (which were highly prized), bone marrow, some stomach contents . . . and blood. A wide variety of uncultivated plant foods were eaten in the traditional diet: roots, starchy tubers, seeds, fruits and nuts. The plant foods were generally high in fibre and contained carbohydrates, which was slowly digested and absorbed. Traditional methods of food preparation (usually baked whole or eaten raw) ensured maximum retention of nutrients. In general, traditional foods had a low energy (calorie) density but high density of some nutrients.[4]

O'Dea goes on to reveal that the naturally low-calorie diet, coupled with the intense physical effort the Natives put out to procure food, provided a natural barrier to weight gain. And not only was their low calorie/high physical activity lifestyle a barricade against obesity, O'Dea says the inherently high fiber diet from wild and gathered plant foods, "slowly digested carbohydrate, very low saturated fat, relatively high proportion of . . . polyunsaturated fatty acids, low sodium and high potassium, magnesium and calcium" protected the Aboriginal communities against non-insulin-dependent diabetes and heart disease.[4]

What O'Dea also reveals is that regardless of where they lived or what they ate, the Indigenous peoples were all unified as hunter-gatherers—the oldest human subsistence method—typified by nomadic hunting of wild game, fishing, and foraging for and gathering edible, wild plants from the land.[5] As with all indigenous cultures, for tens of thousands of years the Australian Aborigines were hunter-gatherers. Living in family groups and clans, men hunted for wild game and foul, relishing the rare find of a seasonal bird egg or honey, or an animal carcass with its not-typically-found or consumed small pockets of fat and organ meats from an animal's internal organs, such as liver, brain, heart, and kidney.

At the same time, women became so adept at searching for and gathering wild plants that, depending on what was available on a particular day or seasonally, up to 80 percent of food might be obtained by gathering rather than hunting.[6] More typically, though, hunter-gatherers consumed between 45 and 65 percent of their calories from animal prey or carcasses, says Loren Cordain, a research scientist and expert on the Paleolithic diet in the Department of Health and Exercise Science at Colorado State University, Fort Collins.[7] Regardless of the day's bounty, the food the women would fix for their family or clan would be baked or eaten raw. Says Cordain: "These diets provided balance in critical metabolic processes, favored health, and allowed our ancestors to thrive, reproduce, and pass their genes to subsequent generations. Modern humans are physiologically adapted to the diets of our ancestors, which shaped our genetic makeup."[8]

When Cordain took a closer look at the overall proportion of foods for hunter-gatherers, he came up with a plant-to-animal ratio of 45:65, suggesting most hunter-gather societies typically obtained more than 50 percent of their calories from animal foods such as fish, marine animals, fowl, meat, and internal organs. Of course, the animal food they consumed, and its balance of nutrients, varied due to environmental influences, such as latitude, season, and weather. As a contrast, only 14 percent of hunter-gatherer societies consumed more than 50 percent of calories from plant foods from stems, greens and leaves, fruit, wild grasses, and tubers (root vegetables, such as onions, potatoes, and so on). Scientists believe a key reason for the prevalence of animal foods is what is called the "optimal foraging theory": not only did hunter-gatherers seek animal food because the protein and fat in animals provides more calories (energy) than the calories derived from plant foods, it also took more physical effort for our Paleolithic ancestors to forage for fruits, vegetables, and wild grasses than to get their energy from animals they hunted or carcasses they found.[9] As a matter of fact, scientists coined the concept of "Ratio of Plant to Animal (P:A)" to compare proportions of plant-to-animal foods we consume.[7]

Reflecting on the diet of our ancient Paleolithic ancestors, Cordain tells us that

> the diets of historically studied hunter-gather populations provide important information regarding the limits and boundaries of the diets to which humans are genetically adapted. Our data clearly indicate that there was no single diet that represented all hunter-gatherer societies. However, there were dietary trends that transcend geographic and ecologic boundaries and represent nearly all the world's hunter-gatherers.[10]

What Cordain is saying is that he and his associates researched and created a representative breakdown of macro-nutrients (protein, carbohydrates, and fat), which they gleaned from data from 229 hunter-gatherer tribes—including Native Australians.

2

With the help of artifacts from hunting implements and bones to fossilized remains, Cordain estimated the percentage of calories from macronutrients (protein, carbohydrates, and fats) to which our ancient ancestors adapted.[7] Table 6.1, below, reveals a relatively high intake of protein, mostly from wild and lean animals. However, ancient ancestors who lived in northern latitudes (such as the Arctic), where plants were not available much of the year, consumed the highest percentage of protein (about 35 percent of total calories) from marine mammals, such as seal and whale.

Clearly, a high proportion of dietary protein from wild animals and fresh and saltwater fish played a key role in the hunter-gatherer diet.

Nutrient	Paleolithic Diet (% calories)
Protein[a]	19 – 35
Carbohydrates[a]	22 – 44
Total Fat[a]	28 – 58
Polyunsaturated (PUFA)[b]	25 – 40
Monounsaturated (MUFA)	16 – 25
Saturated (SFA)	10 – 15
Trans Fatty Acid (TFA)	0

[a] Cordain et al., 2000. [b] Eaton, 2006.

Table 6.1 **Macronutrient Content of the Paleolithic Diet (% total energy)**

At the same time, keep in mind that the plant-to-animal ratio varied depending on the average size of prey animals that were available on any given day or season to our Paleolithic ancestors. In the same way, the size of prey animals affected their percentage of body fat, and in turn, the protein and fat intakes in hunter-gatherers.

Regardless of protein and fat variations in available prey, it would be easy to interpret the hunter-gatherer diet to mean that consuming a diet of mostly lean, high-protein animal foods would be beneficial. But given what state-of-the-art nutritional science has learned about optimal protein intake, the idea that "if some protein is good, more is better," makes no sense. Indeed, consume too much protein, and it might actually make you sick. The anthropologists John Speth and Karen Spielmann discovered this when they documented what early American explorers described as "rabbit starvation," the nausea and possible death that can occur when humans consume too much fat-depleted lean meat of wild animals. "It is quite likely that the symptoms of rabbit starvation result primarily from the finite ability of the liver to up-regulate enzymes necessary for urea synthesis in the face of increasing dietary protein intake," Cordain says.[11] To ensure health, his guesstimate of a maximal "protein ceiling" humans can metabolize safely averages about 35 percent.

In contrast to a high intake of protein, carbohydrate levels are relatively low, because of the rarity of carbohydrate-dense wild grains (cereals) and honey; rather, carbohydrates came mostly from gathered fruits, greens, tubers, and nuts and seeds. With a range from 19 percent to 35 percent, total fat levels reveal the most variation. As with protein levels, dietary fat intake varied, depending on geography: those who lived in the far north consumed high-fat marine mammals for sustenance, while hunter-gatherers living in tropical and temperate climates turned to wild, lean game.

A closer look at the percentage of calories from macronutrients consumed by hunter-gatherers also has a lot to tell us about the types and proportions of dietary fat on which we evolved. As you can tell from the chart, clearly, polyunsaturated fats predominated, followed by consumption of foods high in monounsaturated fatty acids (MUFAs) and lesser amounts of saturated fatty acids (SFAs). Here is Cordain's reflection on the variation in SFA (up to 15 percent) intake of hunter-gatherers:

> The dominant (>50% fat energy) fatty acids in the fat storage depots (adipocytes) of wild mammals are SFAs, whereas the dominant fatty

acids in muscle and all other organ tissues are polyunsaturated fatty acids (PUFAs) and monounsaturated fatty acids (MUFAs). Since subcutaneous and abdominal body fat stores are depleted during most of the year in wild animals, PUFAs and MUFAs constitute the majority of the total carcass fat. Because of the seasonal cyclic depletion of SFAs and enrichment of PUFAs and MUFAs, a year-round dietary intake of high levels of SFA would not have been possible for pre-agricultural hominids preying on wild mammals.[12]

Of special interest are the types and proportions of fatty acids (the molecular building blocks of fat) eaten by early humans—regardless of their geographic location—because this information provides clues about the amounts and types of fats to which our human genes adapted. One of the conclusions to draw from the percentages in the chart is that early humans got most of their dietary fat from polyunsaturated fatty acids (PUFAs) and monounsaturated fatty acids (MUFAs), with relatively less saturated fatty acids (SFAs).

3

While protein, carbohydrates, and fat play key roles in the Paleolithic diet, "one of the most important medical findings of recent years is that eating a balanced ratio of essential fatty acids (EFAs)[13] brings your diet back in synch with your genes and helps you experience optimal health," writes Dr. Artemis P. Simopoulos, president of the Center for Genetics, Nutrition, and Health in Washington, D.C.[14] Obtained only through diet, the two families of the long-chain, polyunsaturated fatty acids to which Simopoulos is referring are omega-3 (n3) and omega-6 (n6). From supporting the cardiovascular, reproductive, immune, and nervous systems to producing prostaglandins that regulate heart rate, blood pressure, fertility, immune function, and more, these EFAs play a key role in health. They also play a powerful role in protecting us by sending messages to our genes. Simopoulos explains it this way:

> One of the reasons that our bodies are so finely attuned to the types of fat in our diet is that EFAs can "talk" to our genes, sending them clear messages to make more or less of certain vital proteins. For example . . . oils high in omega-6 fatty acids send a message to the genes to produce more of a cancer-promoting protein called ras p21. By contrast, omega-3 fatty acids render this protein inactive, possibly reducing the risk of cancer."[15]

What's pivotal to benefiting from these EFAs and enjoying good health is eating them in the right ratio. The ratio of omega-6 to omega-3 that sends our genes messages of good health is less than 4 to 1. "Not by coincidence," says Simopoulos, "this is similar to the ratio found in our evolutionary diet."[16]

Table 6.2, below, shows that our Paleolithic ancestors consumed a wide range of fatty acids, between 9 and 54 grams each day, and that the range of omega-6 to omega-3 ratios consumed by our Paleolithic ancestors was between 0.04 and 2.8—well within Simopoulos's suggestion to keep it to less than 4 to 1 (indeed, it's well on the low range). Whether our early ancestors obtained nourishment by eating fish, plants, or animals, they consumed abundant amounts of omega-3 fatty acids, and in a ratio that would promote good health.

Today, we are only 500 generations from the hunter-gatherer way of eating that sustained hominids for 2.5 million years. Put another way, 99.6 percent of the time we have been evolving into the humans we now are, we have consumed animal and plant food we hunted, fished, or gathered—foods that contained nutrients in the proportions Cordain identified.[8] We also know that the traditional diet of pre-agricultural humans—the hunter-gatherer, Paleolithic diet—is the diet we evolved on and for which our genetic profile was (and still is) programmed. Such a diet is characterized by lean meat and fish; a balanced intake of omega-6 and omega-3 essential fatty acids and monounsaturated and

Nutrient*	Paleolithic Diet (Range: Grams/Day)
Total Polyunsaturated Fat	9.0 – 54.3
Omega-6 (n6)	5.2 – 20.6
Omega-3 (n3)	3.5 – 25.2
n6:n3 Ratio	.04 – 2.8

* Eaton et al., 12–23.

Table 6.2 **Paleolithic Diet: Polyunsaturated Fat, Omega-6 and Omega-3 (Grams/Day)**

saturated fats; and a lot of leafy vegetables and fresh fruits and berries that provide high levels of vitamins E and C and other health-enhancing nutrients. In other words, Cordain's indirect reconstructions of Paleolithic human diets reveal consumption of foods that are nutrient-dense and jam-packed with vitamins and minerals in their proper ratio.[17]

With animal food providing up to 65 percent of the energy source, and wild plant foods comprising 35 percent of food,[7] the key nutritional lessons from this period tell us that protein is essential, as are nutrient-dense, carbohydrate-rich whole fresh fruits, berries, and vegetables; and that fats (mostly from wild animals and fish) we consume must be balanced in the naturally occurring ratio nature intended.

What worked nutritionally for millennia began to change gradually between 10,000 and 12,000 years when a food revolution changed hunter-gatherers to farmers and herders. Signaling the end of the Paleolithic era, this development forever changed the Paleonutrition way of eating—including the proportions of nutrients—that had defined us as healthy, thriving, human beings for most of our past.

4

For nearly two centuries, explorers, archeologists, and anthropological researchers have been trying to solve a mystery: How, and why, did our ancestors—who for 2.5 million years of evolution had survived and thrived as nomadic hunter-gathers—decide to domesticate plants and animals some 10,000 years ago, and in the process, launch civilization and the familiar food groups that comprise our diet today? During the past decades, scientists have gotten clues from fossil records uncovered in ancient settlements. What they think is likely is that the origins of agriculture—the decision made by humans to "partner" with the land by domesticating plants and animals—is believed to have become widespread sometime between 9000 BCE and 7000 BCE in the "Fertile Crescent" area in the Near East, a section writer Steve Gagné says, "stretches from the eastern shore of the Mediterranean Sea and curves around like a quarter moon to the Persian Gulf."[18]

The development of agriculture and animal husbandry was an especially unexpected evolutionary stretch for humankind because our Paleolithic ancestors expended a lot more energy gathering wild plants than they did hunting for wild game and animal carcasses. Cultivating (rather than gathering) plants meant planting seeds, then cultivating wild grains, vegetables, and fruits, and then harvesting them, activities that would require even more time-intensive labor. Given this, the agrarian transformation is not only astounding, the domestication of plants (agriculture) and animals (pastoralism) led to the evolution of towns, then cities. Over time, scientists coined the terms "Agricultural Revolution," "Neolithic Revolution" and "New Stone Age" to describe the period between about 8000 BCE and 5000 BCE that was characterized by the development of farming, managing animals for food, and the growing use of polished stone tools (to grind grains, for instance) and weapons for use in farming, animal husbandry, and food preparation.

At its core, the Agricultural Revolution is the story of the unprecedented development of agriculture and the domestication of plants (grains, fruits, greens and vegetables, beans and peas, and nuts and seeds) and animals (cattle, sheep, goats, and poultry). A gradual, evolutionary process, it originated in the Middle East; over time, as more and more hunter-gatherers gave up their ways of life, the revolution spread to Ancient India, Ancient Asia, Mesoamerica, Africa, and the Andes. But it produced more than domesticated plants and animals, for as our diet changed from wild plants and grasses and lean animal foods to fruits, vegetables, grains, beans and peas, nuts and seeds, dairy (mostly chicken eggs and cow, goat, and sheep milk), fish, pork, and cattle, the change in the composition of macro- and micro-nutrients—as well as the new types of food we consumed—created an evolutionary collision with our ancient genome. Our ancestral diet comprised animal and plant food we hunted, fished, or gathered—foods that contained nutrients in the proportions Paleolithic researcher Loren Cordain identified in the table shown above.

As a contrast, domesticated animal foods and cultivated plants—with a growing dependence on grains, and less diversity in both animals and plants—have only been part of human evolution for less than 1 percent of "human time," and our genes haven't had time to adjust. After all, consider milk from mothers, which, like all mammals, infants consumed for millions of years during the suckling period, then stopped after weaning. But with the domestication of cattle, for the first time, not only did humans consume milk from other mammals (such as cows, goats, etc.), we broke further with our evolutionary past by consuming milk and its products (such as cheese) well after weaning. Based on dairy fat residues found on pottery in Britain, scientists speculate dairying started sometime between 6100 to 5500 years ago. This means that the Agricultural Revolution is a mere few seconds in our evolutionary history, which means the genes of ancient humans didn't have time to adjust to their new diet. And their health paid a price for the new grain-based diet. Here's how Cordain describes the physical changes and "health fallout" of humankind's new dietary direction:

> One physical ramification of the new diet was immediately obvious: Early farmers were markedly shorter than their ancestors. In Turkey and Greece, for example, pre-agricultural men stood 5 feet 9 inches tall and women 5 feet 5 inches. By 3000 B.C., the average man had shrunk to 5 feet 3 inches and the average woman to 5 feet . . . They had more infectious diseases than their ancestors, more childhood mortality, and shorter life spans in general. They also had more osteoporosis, rickets, and other bone mineral disorders, thanks to the cereal-based diets. For the first time, humans were plagued with vitamin- and mineral-deficiency diseases. . . ."[19]

"What had gone wrong?" Cordain queries. "How could the benign practice of agriculture . . . have caused so many health problems?"

His explanation for the ill-health and disease is "the new staples, cereals and starches [that] provided calories but not the vital nutrients of the old diet—lean meats, fruits, and vegetables." Cordain goes on to clarify that

> the health picture got even worse . . . with the arrival of salt, fatty cheeses, and butter . . . Selective breeding—and the innovation of feeding grain to livestock—steadily produced fatter pigs, cows, and sheep . . . Most meat wasn't eaten fresh—fewer people hunted—but instead was pickled, salted, or smoked. Fruits and vegetables became luxuries—rare seasonal additions to the monotony of cereal and starch.[19]

Nutritional "deterioration" didn't stop with the Neolithic Revolution. A little more than 200 years ago, the human health picture went from bad to even worse with the arrival of yet another revolution that burst on to the evolutionary scene—for it would create an upheaval in our way of life that would transform food to "food products." On the slow clock of human evolution, this new revolution has been around for perhaps milliseconds. Still, it would enable human beings to create "food" that is incompatible not only with our early ancestors, but with our genetically determined biology.

5

What do machines and machine tools, manufacturing, steam power, and railways have to do with food? They are all part of the Industrial

Revolution that started in Great Britain in the late 1700s, which, in turn, led to the Second Industrial Revolution around 1850. By then, machines and the mechanization of a plethora of products—including the production of food—had spread throughout Western Europe and North America. Today, the world is still adjusting to the enormous, far-reaching effects of industrialization, which influenced virtually every aspect of daily life—including the food we eat each day. Today, not only are we well on our way to understanding how far today's industrialized foods have veered from our original hunter-gatherer cuisine—and how it affects our health—we are just beginning to surmise how utterly incompatible today's "food" is with our genes . . . and those we pass on to our children. In other words, the relatively recent foods that comprise the core of today's Western diet have given birth to genetic discordance; to resetting our genes so that they "express" themselves through chronic conditions (such as overweight, heart disease, diabetes, and cancer) that have become the norm for too many of us and our children.

The seeds of perceiving food as something that could be counted and measured—as well as today's Standard American Diet (SAD)—were planted when nutritional science was born in the eighteenth century, when chemist Antoine-Laurent Lavoisier defined the calorie, a measure of energy in food. The evolution of nutritional science continued in the 1840s, when German scientist Justus von Leibig isolated proteins, fats, carbohydrates, and minerals in food. But these discoveries didn't change our thinking about food much. It took the Industrial Revolution and the development of what was initially called "separated" food.[20]

Though roller mills—large cylinders that could crush wheat kernels and separate the flour, germ, bran, and other components of the grain—were patented in the 1750s, it wasn't until porcelain mills were introduced in 1870 that inexpensive white flour—in lieu of whole-wheat flour—became popular food for the masses. By the early 1900s, this separated food (what we now call "refined" or "processed") and ensuing nutrient loss resulted in diseases of malnutrition (such as beriberi and pellagra) throughout England and America and also countries such as Japan and China, where the population had turned from brown rice to milled white rice. We now knew what to do with the nutrients discovered in the mid-1940s: enrich white flour food products by adding back a handful of the twenty-five nutrients lost in processing. In this way, we could lower the odds of some deficiency diseases.[19]

Is it really possible to ensure health by restoring a limited number of nutrients to food that have been processed out? Recall that we mentioned earlier that white flour is made by first separating the three original elements of the whole wheat kernel: the white flour (endosperm), the germ, and the bran or outer shell. To create white flour, the life-giving nutrients found in the germ, as well as the fiber from the bran, are no longer part of the equation. Add denatured white flour to the missing fiber you need to slow down the absorption of food in your digestive system, and you've created a formula that increases the odds of weight gain, diabetes, and other chronic conditions. This happens because white flour food products are absorbed quickly by your body; in turn, the levels of glucose (sugar) and insulin (a hormone or "chemical messenger") in your body rise, along with the amount of circulating fat and glucose. Is this a threat to your health? Absolutely, because today in the United States, about 85 percent of the cereals Americans consume are highly processed refined grains.[19] And if you consider that such a high level of cereal consumption doesn't take into account white flour-based bread, pizza and pie crusts, cookies, cakes, pastries, pasta, and so on, that so many of us consume today, the health implications are compounded.

Clearly, the Industrial Revolution made white flour and its overconsumption integral to today's diet. But hands-down, the most toxic food "staple" that resulted from food-processing procedures, the human-made ingredient that has altered the crucial nutrient balance of the food we consume, is partially hydrogenated oil. Unlike naturally occurring PUFAs, MUFAs, and SFAs found in food, partially hydrogenated oil is an artificial creation that food manufacturers create by pumping hydrogen atoms into liquid oils (making them "partially hydrogenated") in order to thicken them, enhance flavor, and increase the shelf life of food that contain the oil. A side effect of its industrial roots, the process of hydrogenation changes the molecular structure of the oil to create health-harming trans fatty acids (TFAs). The molecular change is so alien to our genes that TFAs have been linked to diseases from heart disease and type 2 diabetes to obesity. Indeed, TFAs pose a higher risk to health than any other type of fat or processed food. For instance, not only does consumption of TFAs lead to harmful changes in serum lipids, systematic inflammation, and insulin resistance, but they have also been linked to increased risk of heart attack and death from heart disease. Says researcher Dariush Mozaffarian from the Harvard University School of Public Health: "The strength and consistency of the evidence for harmful effects of TFA . . . indicates little reason for continued use of partially hydrogenated oils containing TFA in food preparation and manufacturing . . . eliminating TFAs could avert tens of thousands of coronary events each year in the United States and around the world."[22]

The message is clear: trans fat harms health. Consider a study by Dr. Lawrence L. Rudel at Wake Forest University. Over a six-year period, he and his colleagues fed a 35 percent fat diet—and the same number of calories—to vervet monkeys, but with one difference: one group consumed a Western diet with 8 percent of calories coming from olive oil (made mostly of MUFAs), while a second group consumed a Western diet with 8 percent coming from industrially made TFAs. When the researchers compared the weights of the monkeys, those who ate trans fats gained four times more weight—especially in the belly—than the monkeys who consumed the olive oil-based diet.[21] Today, TFAs have been an addition to processed (cookies, cake, some bread, etc.) and fried foods (such as potato chips, fries, and so on) for decades. Still, given how hazardous they are to health, many restaurants and cities nationwide have banned their use in food, and legislation has been passed to prohibit them as a fast food additive.

What hasn't been banned is another health-robbing ingredient that was alien to our Paleolithic ancestors: sugar. Rather, "honey comprised 2–3% [of] energy intake" for our Paleolithic ancestors "as compared with the 15% added sugars contribute currently," states S. Boyd Eaton, research scientist at Emory University in Atlanta, Georgia, and author of the ground-breaking *The Paleolithic Prescription*.[24, 25] In 2000 in the United States, this translated into per capita consumption of more than 150 pounds of refined sugars, up from about 120 pounds in 1970, thirty years earlier.[19] The 1970s was a "sugar turning point" for yet another reason: food technology, huge crop subsidies for corn, and industrialization made it possible to manufacture inexpensive high-fructose corn syrup (HFCS). Today, super-processed HFCS is added to thousands of fast foods and beverages such as soft drinks. One reason why HFCS raises a health alarm is that your brain doesn't recognize that it's a food or that it has calories, although it is, indeed, calorie dense. Instead, your brain thinks you're under eating and starving; to compensate, it signals you to keep eating. In other words, HFCS ignites our hunger signals, and though you're consuming lots of calories, you're still hungry; in response to your activated appetite, you eat more . . . and gain weight.[26]

Clearly, since the inception of the Industrial Revolution, we have

1760 – 1840

changed from a diet of fresh, whole foods to the predominant ingredients in today's highly processed food products: denatured white flour, partially hydrogenated oil, high fructose corn syrup—and lots of calories. Cordain describes today's typical Western diet this way: "Food was processed in earnest by the mid-twentieth century with the invention of trans-fatty acids, margarine, shortening, and combinations of these fats mixed with sugar, salt, other starches, high-omega 6 vegetable oils, high-fructose corn syrup, and countless additives, preservatives, coloring agents, and emulsifiers."[18]

The message is clear: We have more than distanced ourselves from our nutritional roots. We have gone from millions of years of hunting and gathering wild animal and plant foods to domesticating animals and plants, and then adding lots of grains, milk, eggs, and fats as dietary staples. By the 20th century, machines made it possible to process these foods and create food products—from salami, bologna, cured ham, cheap meat and hamburgers, fried and frozen fish fillets, and macaroni and cheese, to French fries, corn chips, ice cream, cookies, cakes, donuts . . . and Twinkies. Wouldn't our Paleolithic ancestors be surprised—or perhaps more accurately, stunned—if they were to "time-travel" into today's supermarkets? Such a concept raises the question about whether our body and genes, too, are amazed at the work they have to do to ward off the health havoc linked to what passes as food today.

6

Was the switch to today's Western diet an evolutionary error of a magnitude we're just beginning to understand? Or not? The pioneering work of Canadian-born dentist Weston A. Price, during the early decades in the 20th century, can give us some clues about the Western diet-health link.[27]

Born in 1870 in a farming community near Ottawa, Price opened his dental practice in Cleveland, Ohio, in the early part of the 20th century. During those days, he observed a rapid increase in dental problems which captured his attention. Suspecting that the modern Western diet was the reason, he retired to travel the world in order to document the diets and health status of people who hadn't yet been exposed to modern foods. From the mountains of Switzerland and Peru to the Everglades of Florida and the bush of Australia, Price collected food samples, which a lab in Cleveland analyzed for macro- (protein, carbohydrates, and fat) and micronutrient (vitamins, etc.) content. He accomplished this by taking pictures of teeth and collecting samples of food, keeping careful records about what these cultures ate, as well as the nutritional quality of the food. Today, such data is especially invaluable—indeed, priceless—because the groups he studied have either vanished or adopted a Western diet.

What did Price find? People in isolated cultures who consumed a wide variety of traditional, fresh food-based diets (Price didn't identify a single ideal diet)—and who hadn't yet been exposed to white flour, processed vegetable oils, sugar, canned foods, and excess calories—showed virtually no evidence of tooth decay and malformed dental arches. What were these diets? Some thrived on mostly seafood diets, dairy-based diet, and diets wherein meat predominated, while others ate mostly fruits, vegetables, and grains. From the seafaring Hebrides to Inuit cultures with a diet of raw fish, wild game, fish roe, and blubber, Price noticed groups that ate mostly wild game were healthier than those who turned to grains and other plant foods as the basis of their diet. As a matter of fact, those he identified as being healthiest lived along the Nile near Ethiopia, living on diets comprised mostly of wild animals. He also found that groups held seafood in high esteem, and that organ meats (liver, brain, kidney, and so on) were especially prized. Taking a closer look, when Price analyzed the high levels of fat-soluble vitamins and minerals in organ meats, he coined the term "activator X" to describe the health-enhancing factor he identified (likely vitamin K2) in these foods. He also linked the higher levels of vitamins A and D in yellow butter produced by cows grazing on spring grass to good health. After years of research, Price made this simple, uncomplicated observation about optimal eating: the healthiest people ate traditional, fresh, animal and plant foods that were grown on nutrient-rich soils.

Earlier in the chapter, we discussed the semi-nomadic, lean, and physically fit Native Aboriginal Australians who ate just such a diet of animal and plant foods for thousands of years. But their idyllic diet and life changed suddenly when European settlers colonized the Indigenous Australians in the late eighteenth century. At the time, this included 500–600 distinct groups, speaking some 200 languages, with a total population somewhere between 300,000 and 800,000 people.[28] This ageless diet and lifestyle changed gradually for the Indigenous Australians with the colonization by the British; however, it changed drastically for 10–30 percent of Australian Aboriginal children who were removed from their families by government agencies and church missions, now called the "Stolen Generations." The key aim of this policy (which is now considered highly racist) was to assimilate Aboriginal children into European society and culture—which included an instant introduction to the Western industrialized diet.

It was during this time that Dr. Price visited the Native Australians and documented the healthy, straight teeth and jaws of the hunting-gathering Natives, compared to the crooked and deformed teeth and jaws of "Stolen Generation" children who had been forced to consume the Western diet. Loren Cordain has this to say about the findings: "Studies of their bones and teeth have revealed that these people were basically a mess . . . Instead of the well-formed, strong teeth their ancestors had, there were now cavities. Their jaws, which were formerly square and roomy, were suddenly too small for their teeth, which overlapped each other."[18]

Not only did their dental hygiene suffer. Without time to adapt to their environment, seemingly overnight, a culture that had been healthy for tens of thousands of years developed diabetes, obesity, heart disease, and other chronic conditions linked to the Western diet. Were the genes that once kept these indigenous people healthy unable to adapt to an almost-instant switch to a new diet and lifestyle? Were the genes that protected them from ailments and starvation when food was scarce and helped them to survive now being switched on to create obesity and their other diet-related ailments? New Zealand geneticist Peter Gluckman's "predictive adaptive responses" (PAR) theory, developed in 2005, may offer some clues.[29-31] Why, indeed, did the Native Aborigines develop "diseases of Western civilization" within two generations?

At its core, Gluckman's PAR model suggests that early environmental cues (in this case, a sudden dietary shift, change in physical activity, and stress due to being isolated from family; but also poor nutrition before or after birth) can switch genes on and off (the phenotype discussed in the chapter on epigenetics) in response to what the embryo, infant, or child expects in the future, based on the present experience. In other words, a predictive adaptive response provides protection based on what is predicted to happen—nutritionally—in the future. Given this, is it possible that when the Aboriginal children who were fed a malnourished Western diet grew up and the women became pregnant, the phenotype of the to-be-born embryo adjusted to the message of their parents' inadequate nutrition by anticipating continued malnourishment? If so, might this epigenetic change have slowed their metabolism so they could conserve calories and in turn, avoid starvation both while developing and after being born? According to Gluckman, such predictive adaptive responses, or PARs, are possible. Consider, for example, how especially advantageous such calorie-conservation would be for hunter-gatherer child-bearing women. If they can store fat when food is abundant, not having too much food later in their pregnancy might not present much of a problem for the developing fetus.

Does the PAR theory explain what happened to the Australian Aborigines when they became sickly after being forced to go from their hunter-gatherer diet to a processed Western diet? When you consider that Native Australians (and also indigenous groups in Fiji and Hawaii) experienced skyrocketing rates of chronic Western conditions after being introduced to the Western diet and lifestyle—when just a generation ago these diseases were virtually non-existent—it seems plausible that their genes simply didn't have time to make the modifications necessary to keep them healthy. Were their organisms predicting malnourishment and starvation—so much so that their epigenes created a way for their body to hold onto calories and the limited nourishment they did, indeed, receive? If so, the essential elements of PAR offer a likely explanation: survival.

7

Since Dr. Price studied the health of Native Australians in the 1930s after they had been consuming a Western diet for a while, scientists such as Loren Cordain have espoused the belief that the human genome hasn't had time to adapt, not only to the diet and lifestyle changes launched by the agriculture and animal husbandry revolution that began about 10,000, but even more to today's highly processed foods—those to which Native Aborigines were so abruptly exposed.

Still more advances in nutritional science during the last few decades have enabled Cordain and colleagues to identify seven specific changes that occurred because of our industrialized environment (defined by Cordain as "diet and other lifestyle conditions"[8]; for more about this, please see "It's the Lifestyle, Stupid!"). In other words, Cordain has targeted the key biological changes created by our denatured, altered, processed-food diet—changes that have likely occurred because today's Western diet collides with our ancient genome and in turn, our wellbeing. The seven features Cordain identified that are linked to today's altered diet are:

1. glycemic load (how much a food's carbohydrates quickly get into your fat cells);
2. fatty acid composition (omega 6 to omega 3 ratios and trans fats);
3. macronutrient composition (percentage of protein, carbohydrates, and fat);
4. micronutrient density (amounts of vitamins, minerals, phytochemicals, etc.);
5. acid-base balance (the proper pH balance between acids and bases);
6. sodium-potassium ratio (the proportion of sodium to potassium), and;
7. fiber content (the amount of indigestible carbohydrates such as cellulose).[8]

Writes Cordain's colleague, C.E. Ramsden, about the far-reaching food-gene-health implications of today's altered diet:

These drastic changes occurred over less than two hundred years, insufficient time for genetic adaptation. As a consequence, individuals consuming Western diets may no longer be consuming fatty acids within genetically determined ranges, disturbing metabolic processes ranging from inflammation and plaque rupture to thrombosis and arrhythmogenesis [irregular heartbeat]. These metabolic derangements play major roles in the modern epidemic of CHD [heart disease]."[33]

A closer look at Table 6.3, below, gives us an even clearer perspective about the changes wrought by today's highly processed Western diet. By taking out nutrients we need from processed foods, while at the same time adding nutrients we don't need, food manufacturers have created drastic changes in the proportions of key nutrients that more and more, are being linked to epigenetic changes and poor health. By comparing the percentage of total energy, based on macronutrients, in the Paleolithic diet (which we discussed earlier in the chapter) to the percentage of total energy from macronutrients in the modern Western diet, we can get a sense of just how radical these nutritional changes are. Not only have the proportions of PUFAs, MUFAs, and SFAs we consume changed drastically, but protein levels are much lower (15.4 percent); carbohydrate intake is much higher (51.8 percent); total fat (32.8 percent)—and the key types of fat—are in the low range; while consumption of toxic TFAs has gone from zero to up to 3 percent!

Perhaps nowhere is the collision between the artificially created proportion of substances in food more evident than in fatty acid composition (which Ramsden and Cordain identified as one of the seven altered nutritional characteristics in industrialized food). For instance, if you read labels carefully, as often as not the amounts of TFAs may seem small. But even small amounts of TFAs can harm both genes and health.

Consider, for example, the question posed about certain fats by molecular biologist Natarajan Saravanan and colleagues at the Indian Council of Medical Research in Hyderabad, India, about whether TFAs or long-chain SFAs switch on genes that increase insulin resistance,[34] the condition in which muscle, liver, and fat cells become resistant to absorbing circulating glucose. This is an important question to answer, because if our body becomes unresponsive to, or doesn't produce enough insulin, we're more prone to diabetes, obesity, and other chronic ailments. Do particular types of fat play a role?

Previous research had shown that an imbalance (meaning, high levels) of some long-chain SFAs and especially TFAs may decrease insulin sensitivity.[35,36] This matters, because insulin resistance increases

Nutrient	Paleolithic Diet (% total energy)	1995 – Present (% total energy)
Protein	19 – 35[a]	15.4[a]
Carbohydrates	22 – 44[a]	51.8[a]
Total Fat	28 – 58[a]	32.8[a]
Saturated Fat (SFA)	10 – 15	12
Monounsaturated (MUFA)	16 – 25	13
Polyunsaturated (PUFA)	25 – 40[b]	16.7[b]
Trans Fatty Acid (TFA)	0	2 – 3

[a] Cordain, et al., 2000.   [b] Eaton, 2006, 1–6.

Table 6.3 **Macronutrient Content of Paleolithic Diet Compared to Today's Western Diet (% total energy)**

the risk of diabetes, heart disease, and heart attack. However, here's the key point to consider: When high levels of long-chain SFAs were fed to rats, insulin resistance increased in muscle, liver, and fat tissue. In contrast, when the high-SFA diet was supplemented with omega-3 fatty acids from fish oil, insulin resistance decreased. This is a pivotal point to consider, because the typical standard, highly processed American diet has created a similar imbalance of SFAs to omega-3s. In other words, our processed-food fare has led to a change in the ratio of SFAs to omega-3s. SFA consumption hasn't changed for centuries, but now our diet makes most of us virtually deficient in protective omega-3s. Might this be the reason we have an epidemic of insulin resistance, and in turn, diabetes, in our population?

Saravanan and his team had already shown that feeding TFAs from partially hydrogenated vegetable oils to rats decreased their insulin sensitivity; so too did palmitic acid, the long-chain SFA the body produces when it consumes too many calories.[35] But now they wanted to know exactly how these fatty acids affected the expression of specific genes that determine insulin sensitivity.

To find out, Saravanan selected 12 newly weaned rats that were the same age and with the same genetic background; then he divided them into four groups. For three months, Saravanan fed the rats in each group a diet with the same number of calories and percent fat; the only difference in the diets were varying proportions of fat and types of oil. More specifically, rats in group 1 were fed a diet high in omega-6 fatty acids (38 percent); the second group was fed a diet high in palmitic acid, a long-chain saturated fat (46 percent); group 3 received a diet relatively high in TFAs (15 percent) and moderate amounts of omega-6 (10 percent); and the fourth group was fed a relatively high TFA diet (13 percent), with higher levels of omega-6 (19 percent).

After three months the researchers measured the gene-expression patterns of 12 different genes taken from fat tissues in each group of rats. Saravanan chose to assess these particular genes because they influence the metabolism that ultimately determines insulin resistance. His findings were revealing: When the time came to assess the effects of various fats on gene expression, Saravanan found that the diet high in long-chain palmitic acid modified two genes that increased insulin resistance. He also discovered the two diets in TFAs changed the expression of yet two other genes, which also contribute to insulin resistance.

What's intriguing and innovative about Saravanan's results is the discovery that TFAs and long-chain SFAs lower insulin sensitivity by two *different* profiles of gene expression. This is cause for concern, because it raises the possibility that when we consume foods that contain both TFAs and SFAs that include long-chain palmitic acid, insulin resistance may be increased even more than if we consume either fatty acid by itself. As disturbing, the diets that included increased amounts of omega-6 (linoleic acid) did not ameliorate the insulin-resistance effects of TFAs. On the other side, one type of fat in food—omega-3 fatty acids—acts to increase insulin sensitivity . . . that is, if your diet isn't too high in TFA- and SFA-rich foods.[33, 36] However, because none of Saravanan's diets contained omega-3s and all were high in starch (a carbohydrate), we do not know what effect SFAs would have on insulin resistance if the diet were more balanced. As it stands, we know that TFAs are never good and that diets high in palmitic acid may exacerbate the effects of high levels of refined carbohydrates.

Nevertheless, Saravanan's findings are consistent with epidemiological studies,[32] which have demonstrated that both the amount and types of fats we consume play a key role in changing how our genes affect our cholesterol metabolism as well as insulin sensitivity, and in turn, our health. And there's another powerful inference from Saravanan's research; one that has far-reaching health repercussions: our "old genes" haven't adapted to high levels of TFAs, a "new" man-made fat, and we are paying a high price for this with poor health.

8

Recall that earlier in the chapter, we discussed the notable essential fatty acids (EFAs), omega-3 (n3) and omega-6 (n6), which, when eaten in a balanced ratio, switch on genes that lead to optimal health. This isn't a surprise when you consider the ratio in Table 6.4, below, which shows that our Paleolithic ancestors consumed a balanced n6:n3 ratio that lies on the low end of the ideal range (0.04–2.8). Recall that such a low ratio falls well within the optimal less-than-4-to-1 ratio as defined by nutrition and genetics expert Artemis P. Simopoulos.

With the advent of the Industrial Revolution and the ensuing processing of omega-rich vegetable oils—such as corn and safflower oils that are so abundant in our diet today—the balanced ratio of EFAs on which our human genome thrived for hundreds of thousands of years changed drastically. In place of the ideal ratio of between 1:1 and 4:1 on which our ancestors thrived, today most Americans consume an n6:n3 ratio that is between 10:1 and 25:1. Not only does this mean we're

Nutrient	Paleolithic Diet (range: grams/day)	Western Diet range grams/day)
Total Polyunsaturated Fat	9.0 – 54.3	24.5
Omega-6 (n6)	5.2 – 20.6	22.5
Omega-3 (n3)	3.5 – 25.2	1.2
n6:n3 Ratio	0.04 – 2.8	16.7

Eaton et al., 1998, 12–23

Table 6.4 **Paleolithic Diet vs. Today's Western Diet: A Comparison of Polyunsaturated Fat, Omega-6 and Omega-3 (grams/day)**

consuming much too much n6, it also means that we are taking in too little n3. "It has been estimated that we are now eating one-tenth of the amount of omega-3 fatty acids required for normal functioning," says Simopoulos. "Alarmingly, 20 percent of the population has levels so low that they defy detection." Then Simopoulos provides this warning: "The admonishment to 'eat a balanced diet' makes no sense when our food has been stripped of one of its most essential nutrients."[13]

Indeed, the mix of deficient EFAs and an imbalanced intake of omega-6 and omega-3 suppresses the expression of health-enhancing genes so much that we're susceptible to serious food-related health conditions—from heart disease, cancer and insulin resistance to diabetes, obesity, arthritis, and other inflammation-linked ailments, among others.

As disconcerting as our imbalanced, deficient intake of EFAs is, EFAs are just part of profound changes in percentages of macronutrients and ratios to which anyone who eats a predominantly Western diet is exposed. The first column in Table 6.5, below, shows ranges of macronutrient values, based on an analysis of 229 different hunter-gatherer tribes. The wide ranges are due to geography and seasonal availability of various foods. Given this, it's likely the Paleolithic diet typically falls in the middle ranges in this column.

A closer look at the percentage of macronutrient levels of some

Nutrient	Paleolithic Diet	McDonald's Hamburger	Beef Franks	McDonald's French fries	American Cheese	Potato Chips	Margarine (with salt)
Protein	19 – 35[a]	19.6	11.35	4.8	25	4.8	0.16
Carbohydrates	22 – 44[a]	48.7	2.35	49	1.2	37.5	0.70
Total Fat	28 – 58[a]	33	30.26	46	74	60.4	81
Saturated (SFA)	10 – 15	10.4	12.4	5.9	47	6.7	15.2
Mono-unsaturated (MUFA)	16 – 25	11.3	14.7	22.2	21	26.6	38.9
Poly-unsaturated (PUFA)	25 – 40[b]	0.78	1.36	13.3	2.1	26	24.3
n6:n3 Ratio	1:04 – 2.8	n/a	1:4[c]	1:12	1:1.6[c]	1:34[c]	1:15
Trans Fatty Acid (TFA)	0	1.9	2.25[c]	0.37	0.0[c]	0.08	14.9

[a] Cordain et al., 2000. [b] Based upon S.B. Eaton's statement that the hunter-gatherer had twice the intake of PUFAs. Eaton et al., 1998, 12–23. [c] http://www.nutritiondata.com/facts. All other values calculated based upon the USDA's Nutrient Data Laboratory.

Table 6.4 Paleolithic Diet vs. Today's Western Diet: Comparing Polyunsaturated Fat, Omega-6 and Omega-3 (grams/day)

favorite, commonly consumed, highly processed foods in the Western diet shows just how far out of optimal "ratio-range" many processed foods have gone. More distressing are the exceptionally low polyunsaturated levels in modern processed foods—with only one food product, potato chips, even approaching the lower range of the Paleolithic diet. Still, this isn't a good sign, because not only are potato chips fried (increasing health-robbing TFA levels), the liquid vegetable oil(s) they're fried in have such high levels of omega-6 compared to omega-3 that they make potato chips a true health hazard. Finally, trans fats are nonexistent in the Paleolithic diet but are widely found in many industrially manufactured food products. What can we conclude from this brief window of comparisons?

You can see from the chart that if you frequently consume highly processed foods, you're eating a diet that deviates a lot from the proportion of nutrients on which we evolved and thrived. In other words, consume some commonly eaten foods and your diet is out of synch with the proportion of macronutrients our ancestors ate; eat fast- and processed foods most of the time, and you're threatening not only your own health, but probably that of your genes, as well as the genes you pass on to your future progeny.

9

What we've learned from the change in food choices over time is that human *epi*genes are highly adaptable to a wide variety of diets. We also know that we can adapt genetically more rapidly than the slow pace about which Cordain theorized. This is evident by what ethnobiologist Gary Nabhan calls "evolutionary gastronomy." Here's how Nabhan explains it: "The longer the chain of ancestors who lived in one place—exposed to the same set of food choices, diseases, and environmental stresses for centuries—the greater the probability that selection was both for a diet and for genes that worked well in that landscape."[39]

Humans have made major food-gene-health adaptations during three major epochs: the long-term Paleolithic era; the relatively recent agricultural transition era, and; the more immediate post-industrial era. During the millions of years on the hunter-gatherer diet, the structure of our DNA was formed, in large part to the types of foods available. Since the Neolithic Revolution and the introduction of new foods such as grains and milk from animals, our epigenome made further adjustments, depending on the length of exposure to these new foods. Today, during the more recent post-Industrial era, our genes—and health—are still reeling from the denatured changes in our diet that have occurred overnight on the evolutionary scale.

The message is clear: throughout our existence as humans, our genes have shown they are highly adaptable to the available food supply and a wide variety of diets. We've seen this with the great diversity of foods our Paleolithic ancestors ate. Whether eating a diet comprised mostly of animal foods or a diet of mostly plant foods, not only have our genes adapted over millions of years, their adaption to various foods and proportion of nutrients we consumed from various foods, have enabled us to thrive. One key reason is that as seasons changed, we ate a great diversity of nutrient-dense wild plants, depending on the climate (tropical, temperate, Arctic, and so on). For instance, in some areas, more than 100 species of edible plants might be available; or grass-fed, lean game; or fish from pristine waters. At the same time, people living in the far north depended mostly on marine mammals abundant in balanced fats, with fruits and vegetables being available only during the warmer months. Regardless of what became food staples, our genes adjusted.

A second message is also clear: with each major shift in the types and ratios of food nutrients, humans experienced adverse effects on their health. But still, our genes gradually adapted to our new way of eating and we continued to thrive. A good example of this is the way in which we have adapted to two nutrients in two of the "new" Neolithic foods: lactose in milk, and gluten in grains. Apparently, populations that were exposed to milk and grains for the longest periods of time have inherited the ability to metabolize these foods. Today, for instance, 85 percent of hunter-gatherer Australian Aborigines who did not evolve consuming milk consequently cannot metabolize or tolerate lactose (lactose intolerance) in milk. In comparison, 23 percent of the desert-roaming African Fulani tribe—nomadic herders who consumed milk from animals for thousands of years—are mostly lactose tolerant; while only 2 percent of Swedish people—who have been consuming diary as a staple for a long time—have problems metabolizing lactose in milk.[40]

But what about today's highly processed industrialized diet? This brings us to the question we posed in the introduction to this chapter. Are there health consequences to distancing ourselves from our ancestral sustenance; indeed ignoring, even destroying, what sustained, rejuvenated, and healed humans for millennia? Today, we and our genes are still reeling from the introduction of foods made possible by the Industrial Revolution. With this change, in an evolutionary "nano-second," we've moved from thousands of years of family farming to chemical-dependent factory farming, accompanied by depleted soil, diminished nutrients, and animal feedlots. Even more recently on the evolutionary scale, no longer are whole foods the norm; rather, they have been processed into industrial food products, filled with denatured food and imbalanced nutrient ratios. In response to this "diet," scientists have coined the phrase "diseases of modern civilization." Still, throughout this book, we have demonstrated that our genes are struggling to compensate epigenetically, but it's becoming harder and harder for our genes to continue to function and keep us healthy when they're exposed to a day-in, day-out, ongoing onslaught of imbalanced nutrient intake and manmade chemicals. We saw this with the stunning imbalance in essential fatty acids (EFAs) in today's typical Western diet; the off-the-charts percentages of macronutrients when today's processed foods are compared to Paleonutrition; and again with Saravanan's study, revealing that diets high in TFAs—large amounts of manmade toxic fats to which humans had not been exposed previously—create epigenetic changes that can lead to insulin insensitivity and in turn, increased risk of a plethora of chronic conditions—from obesity to diabetes and heart disease.

10

What this chapter reveals is that humans are highly adaptable and that we can thrive and be healthy on a wide variety of animal- and plant-based diets if the foods are fresh and whole and in their natural state, or if they are fermented (sauerkraut, for instance) or cultured (yogurt), and they contain a balanced and natural ratio of nutrients. Dr. Weston Price's work studying hunter-gatherer indigenous tribes "untouched" by Western diets, supports this nutrition-gene-health nugget. So, too, do his observations of the adverse effects of a sudden change in diet—such as when Aboriginal children were "stolen" from their centuries-old culture and forced, virtually overnight, to consume an inherently imbalanced and unhealthy Western diet for which our genes were unprepared. Reflecting on the health impact of such instant dietary and lifestyle changes, journalist and food expert Michael Pollan posits that

> Price eventually came to see the problem of diet and health as a problem of ecological dysfunction. By breaking the links among local soils, local foods, and local peoples, the industrial food system disrupted

the circular flow of nutrients through the food chain. Whatever the advantages of the new industrial system, it could no longer meet the bio-chemical requirements of the human body, which, not having had time to adapt, was failing in new ways.[41]

For the millions of us who typically consume what passes for food today, our bodies—and genes—do, indeed, seem to be "failing in new ways." This, Pollan clarifies, is the conclusion and consensus of Dr. Price and others who explored the pre-Western diet of not-yet-Westernized cultures in the early part of the 20th century: "The human animal is adapted to, and apparently can thrive on, an extraordinary range of different diets," says Pollan, "but the Western diet, however you define it, does not seem to be one of them."[41]

In pursuit of a better understanding of the genetic mismatch between the foods on which we evolved and today's Western diet, in the next chapter we are going to take you on a different food-gene-health journey. From timeless foods consumed by the Inuit in the Arctic to fish in Lake Michigan and corn grown in the rural mountain settlement of Capulalpan, Mexico, we're going to introduce you to the post-Industrial food fallout that is re-defining gene-health and "'Nourishment' Now" for human beings worldwide . . . in ways our Paleolithic ancestors could not have even begun to imagine.

Chapter 7

"Nourishment" Now

Since human beings have dwelled on the earth, wild roots, greens and plants, berries, fish, fowl, mammals, insects, reptiles, and pristine water have been available for nourishment. But both the kinds of food and quality that humankind depended on for millennia began to radically change in the mid-1800s with the advent of the Industrial Revolution and its "child," food processing. Since then—like a snowball increasing in size as it rolls down a steep hill—food has picked up a muddled brew of both intentional and unintended artificial chemical compounds that is turning us into incidental research subjects of a toxic food environment. Undoubtedly, much of the synthetic—and imbalanced—alchemical cocktail that has made its way into our food supply was initially created by industry with the intention of better feeding humankind, eliminating infectious disease, and prolonging shelf life. But more and more, both we—and our children—are paying too big of a price for relying so heavily on compounds we were never meant to ingest. For the food we eat today includes man-made chemicals that are playing havoc with our health; even threatening our lives and that of future generations. Trying to adapt, the genes that inform our miraculous bodies are responding in previously unimagined ways to what passes as "nourishment" now.

I

When most of us consider today's standard American diet, images of fast food, sugary sweets and beverages, and highly processed, refined food "products"—from chips, fries, pizza, and cookies to soda, Twinkies and candy bars—likely come to mind. So, too, does the link between the standard American diet and chronic health problems: obesity, heart disease, diabetes, and more. What is less known is that—in addition to ingredients that include both highly processed, *added* fats and oils, sugar and corn syrup, and so on to *deleted* nutrients (vitamins, minerals, etc.) from fast food—other invisible "ingredients" have become part of our food supply in the past decades that not only contribute to many chronic conditions but may influence our genes and in turn, determine whether we and our children are healthy. In other words, combine denatured, *processed foods* with *man-made chemicals*, such as *xeno*estrogens (estrogen-like hormones created outside our body) in water, animal feed, meat and poultry, and *pesticide- and herbicide-residues* on fruits, vegetables, and grains, and you have a food-formula that is threatening more than health: it is turning "healthy genes" into "unhealthy genes" that are unfavorably influencing the health and well-being of ourselves and future generations.

Consider, for instance, the processing of vegetable oils that emerged with the Industrial Revolution, and the impact that this seemingly simple change has had on our health. In the chapter "Food, Genes, and Health Over Time," we discussed the original, naturally occurring ratio of omega-6 fatty acids to omega-3 fatty acids, which averaged between 1:1 and 2:1 in the diet on which humans evolved and thrived.[1] Nourishment now, however, means that most of us consume foods from conventionally raised animals (beef, pork, etc.) that have been raised on grains high in omega-6, instead of their original diet of omega-3-rich grass. Add a high intake of still more omega-6 fatty acids from vegetable oils that have been processed from seeds (sunflower, safflower, etc.), and the omega-6:omega-3 ratio skyrockets from between 1:1 and 2:1 to between 10:1 and 15:1.[2]

Researchers have known for decades that consuming an *excess* of omega-6 fatty acids that are "out of balance" with omega-3 fatty acids increases the odds of a plethora of ailments from cancer to heart disease.[1, 3–5] What is relatively new, though, is the link between excessive omega-6 intake and DNA damage. One study that made this connection is by Jagadeesan Nair from the Division of Toxicology and Cancer Risk Factors in Heidelberg, Germany, in collaboration with colleagues from Finland and Sweden.[6] To find out if there is an omega-6-DNA link, at the start of the study Nair fed a similar diet to women and men in two different groups—except for one difference: one group received a diet rich in polyunsaturated fatty acids (PUFAs), with an *im*balanced omega-6: omega-3 ratio, while the diet of the second group was high in monounsaturated fatty acids (MUFAs), with a naturally *balanced* ratio of omega-6: omega-3. After the research participants followed their diets for 25 days, Nair looked at the white blood cells of the subjects to see if there was any DNA damage. Surprisingly, there was—but for women only. In other words, the males in the study showed no difference in DNA due to the type of fat intake, while the women consuming the diet high in omega-6 had DNA damage that was *40 times higher* than the women who consumed the balanced omega-6: omega-3 diet.

Based upon prior research, Nair hypothesized that only women were affected because their naturally higher estrogen levels somehow worked synergistically with the omega-6 to damage DNA.[6] Why might this happen? The DNA may have been damaged and in turn, destabilized, when omega-6 *combined* with an estrogen compound. The end result: a potentially cancer-generating miscoding of the DNA.[7,8] In other words, marry high levels of omega-6 with elevated estrogen levels, and a mutant gene is created that can't replicate accurately. This suggests that when an "estrogen storm" occurs in an imbalanced "fat milieu," it can cause DNA damage and increase the likelihood of cancer.

"DNA mistakes" due to an excessive intake of processed oils don't seem to be an anomalous event. DNA damage is also likely to happen with another key "fake fat" that's *added* abundantly to processed foods and beverages: partially hydrogenated vegetable oil, or *trans fatty acids* (TFAs). When the naturally occurring fatty acids—omega-6 and omega-3—in inherently healthy foods (olives, walnuts, wild salmon, and so on) are *cold pressed* under carefully controlled conditions, the *molecular structure* remains intact. But heat any unsaturated vegetable oil to above 140 degrees to increase its shelf life and its inherently unstable, unsaturated, carbon double bonds begin to twist and turn, ultimately transforming into molecular shapes that our bodies were never meant to metabolize. And one class of these changed fats, called *trans* fats, are more harmful to health than any other fat—so much so that there is a nationwide movement to remove them from processed food.

For years, scientists have known that this unnatural, processed, man-made fat may be the most health-damaging fat we can consume. Indeed, consuming TFAs has been linked with increased risk of Type 2 diabetes, certain cancers, heart disease, infertility, and more.[9-13] However, an understanding of whether TFAs have the power to switch genes on or off and whether that can lead to insulin resistance comes from Natarajan Saravanan and his team of molecular biologists in Hyderabad, India, at the National Institute of Nutrition.[14]

To find out if TFAs affect gene expression and in turn *insulin resistance* (a condition that occurs when cells find it difficult to metabolize glucose), Saravanan fed four different groups of recently weaned rats varying levels of different types of fatty acids (including trans fatty acids) for 25 days. What the team discovered is that the rats fed higher levels of TFAs had *three types of gene expressions* that raise insulin resistance: 1) up-regulating mRNA levels of resistin, a protein secreted by adipose tissue;[15] 2) down-regulating PPAR (peroxisome proliferator-activated receptor gamma), a nuclear receptor protein that regulates glucose metabolism[16]; and 3) down-regulating lipoprotein lipase, an enzyme that metabolizes lipids.[17, 18] In other words, because insulin resistance is linked with an increased risk of diabetes and heart disease, by identifying the genetic mechanisms that switch insulin resistance genes on and off, Saravanan's research helps to explain how consuming TFAs increases the risk of diabetes and heart disease.

A powerful genetic "imprint" is left by yet another ingredient added to processed food and beverages in abundance: sugar. This became apparent in a study by epidemiologist Lisa Giovannelli of the Department of Pharmacology in Florence, Italy, when she set out to establish which ingredients in food could cause DNA damage. To find out, Giovannelli collected dietary information via a food-frequency questionnaire from 71 healthy adults: 48 men and 23 women; then she measured their DNA damage. Giovannelli made the sugar-gene connection when her findings revealed that the more simple sugar (glucose) a person consumed from soft drinks, desserts, and other sweets, the more *oxidative* DNA damage occurred in blood cells (*lymphocytes*). In contrast, Giovannelli found that those who consumed more cruciferous vegetables (broccoli, cabbage, cauliflower, collard greens, etc.) had *less* DNA damage.[19]

How could sugar harm DNA and cruciferous vegetables protect it? A well-nourished body that has been fed with nutrient-dense, fresh whole foods has an abundance of circulating antioxidants such as beta carotene (a precursor to vitamin A), and vitamins C and E, which have the power to neutralize free radicals, the byproduct of breathing, eating, exercise; indeed, life processes. When too many free radicals are circulating and a person's diet doesn't include adequate antioxidants, the free radicals can oxidize, and in turn damage, cells and DNA. Add excess sugar consumption to the mix, which, when metabolized, creates a lot of free radicals, and your body is poised for still more DNA damage.

As interesting as this study is, it only raises the question about whether there is a link between sugar intake and DNA damage. This is because Giovannelli's study shows a *correlation* between sugar intake and oxidative DNA damage, and correlation does *not* mean sugar is the cause of the damage; rather, correlation simply suggests that there's some sort of association between sugar intake and DNA damage. On the other hand, a study by Kayoko Shimoi and colleagues from Japan showed a strong *cause and effect* connection between glucose and damaged DNA. Shimoi discovered this in an *in vitro* study when he administered high versus low amounts of glucose to cultured cells taken from the interior lining of the umbilical cord: the higher the levels of glucose, the more the oxidative DNA damage.[20]

Yet another highly processed sweetener—high fructose corn syrup (HFCS)—may also cause DNA damage. But it's not the HFCS itself that wreaks DNA havoc; rather, the damage is due to the chemical *hydroxymethylfurfural* (HMF), the syrup produced when HFCS is heated during processing or afterwards. This is of special concern because since 1968, HFCS has been used in disturbingly large amounts throughout the global food supply. Today it is found not just in sodas but in breakfast cereals, candy, breakfast bars, ketchup, pizza sauce, salad dressings, whole grain bread, and a thousand other products[21]— in other words, in the processed food products that are the staple of most Americans' diet.

That HMF may lead to DNA damage was recently discovered in a groundbreaking "bee-busting" study published in 2009. For years, thousands of honey bee colonies had been dying, but farmers didn't know why. The demise of so many honey bees had been creating a major problem because honey bees do more than make honey; they pollinate a wide variety of blooming fruit and vegetable crops, such as squash, apricots, and walnuts. Honey bees are so important to these crops that farmers often rent colonies from beekeepers or raise their own. Without the pollination process from honey bees, blooming fruits and vegetables crops can't and won't produce. Why were so many bee colonies collapsing? When researcher Blaise LeBlanc of the Carl Hayden Bee Research Center in Tucson, Arizona, studied the problem, she discovered that for years, commercial beekeepers had been feeding high fructose corn syrup to their bees when nectar from flower blooms was scarce. And the more HFCS consumed by the bees, the more likely they were to die. When LeBlanc took a closer look, she identified the culprit: HMF, the heat-induced toxicant from high fructose corn syrup.[22] Might such a strong chemical—so integral to processed foods—also have a detrimental affect on humans who consume HFCS? Possibly. When environmental toxicologist Louise Durling of Uppsala University in Sweden studied the affects of HMF on individual human cells, as with the honey bees, she found a strong dose-response relationship: the more exposure to HMF, the more DNA damage and cell death.[23]

What might be happening here? Why do high concentrations of processed omega-6 fatty acids, sugar, and HFCS cause DNA damage? Consider the complexity and the vulnerability of the DNA in our three trillion or so cells, which are constantly replicating themselves. Occasionally, they make mistakes; they are also subject to attacks on their composition and integrity from nutrient imbalances and oxidizing agents. To repair damage, correct unintentional mistakes, and replicate effectively, cells need to be nourished by a wide variety of nutrients in a proper balance. However, when DNA doesn't get adequate vitamins or minerals, or when it's exposed to imbalanced nutrients (such as an excess of trans fats) and toxicants, genetic damage accumulates; in turn, the likelihood of developing various ailments increases—from premature aging and cancer to depression and heart disease.

What we can draw from studies linking imbalanced intake of omega-6 fatty acids, man-made TFAs, HMF, and a diet high in sugar is relatively straightforward: humans are meant to consume fresh whole foods—with their natural ratio of nutrients intact—as often as possible. When we consume large amounts of ingredients that are processed and separated from their original form (such as sugar from sugar cane), heated at high levels (vegetable oils and HFCS), or created chemically (artificial TFAs), we are making ourselves vulnerable to dietary abuse that can stretch all the way down to the genetic level.

2

Nunavik—meaning "land of snow" and "place to live"—is an area of boreal forest, tundra, and arctic in the north of the province of Québec, Canada. If you were to visit this barely inhabited virgin territory of 193,000 square miles at any one time, you might experience the blanketing silence of the wild tundra, thundering hooves of a migrating caribou herd, polar bears that roam northern coastal areas, and wolves that scout conifer forests filled with pine, fir and spruce, or perhaps the slow, cracking drift of pack ice. You might also see the stunning 1300-foot deep meteorite-made Pingualuit crater, 2.14 miles (3.44 km) across, ; or, as a contrast, Mont d'Iberville, Québec's highest mountain peak. Or, during the cold, dark winter, the green, pink, white, and violet colors that comprise the northern lights might do a dance for you in the night sky.[24, 25]

Winter in this northern region is likely to bring an ice-covered ocean. Throughout the summer, though, temperatures that average 50 °F (10°C) allow the sea ice to thaw. During this time, Nunavik is gifted with extraordinary light, because the sun doesn't quite set; rather, it brushes the horizon. It is also during this time that the Inuit—the ancestral peoples who inhabit Nunavik—take advantage of their area's other natural resources for food.

Descendents of the 4000-year-old Thule culture who spread eastward from western Alaska around 1000 BCE, the Inuit of today inhabit the Arctic regions of Canada, Greenland, Russia, and the United States.[26] Considered nomads, most of the 10,000 or so Inuit inhabitants in Nunavik consume a mostly marine animal diet from rivers and lakes. To obtain nourishment in the hostile and isolated expanse of glaciers and frozen sea they call home, their daily fare is filled with Atlantic salmon, arctic cod, and other salt water fish; marine mammals, such as seal, beluga whale, polar bear, and walrus; birds; and land animals like caribou and musk oxen. They also enjoy lesser amounts of local plants, such as fireweed (a perennial of the evening primrose family),[27] grasses, tubers, roots, stems, and edible seaweed, [28–31] as well as berries they pick during the summer and store for the winter.

Believing that food from marine mammals, especially, keeps their body warm and that it makes them strong, energetic, and healthy,[32] Inuit take tremendous delight and pride in their traditional foods.[33] And they are right about what they knew instinctively about their traditional diet: with virtually no heart disease (until Western-style processed foods were introduced)[34–36] it does indeed seem to keep them healthy—even though their predominantly polyunsaturated-rich high-protein diet of sea mammals and cold-water fishes averages about 75 *percent* of daily calories from fat. To what can fat-phobic Americans attribute this "Inuit Paradox" (high fat intake, low incidence of heart disease)?[31]

When researchers took a closer look, they discovered the reason for the seemingly contradictory data, and it comes down to the kinds of meat and fat eaten. In other words, unlike most Westerners who consume *industrially farmed animal* fats and *processed* fats, the more healthful fat from which Inuits seem to benefit comes from the *types* of fat found in the *wild-animal fats* that constitute the core of their diet. For instance, many marine animals (fish and crustaceans) show a high proportion of PUFA (40 to 50 percent), moderate proportions of MUFA fats (30–40 percent), and a lower amount of saturated fat (22–30 percent).[37]

Not too long after the Inuit Paradox seemed to be solved, Dewailly made an unanticipated visit to the Inuit in Nunavik. Meeting with them wasn't part of his research plans. Rather, before deciding to go, his focus was on assessing contaminants in breast milk of mothers living in a heavily industrialized and polluted area near the Gulf of St. Lawrence, the world's largest estuary, the outlet of the St. Lawrence River, which drains the Great Lakes system and much of southern Canada and north-central United States and which suffers from heavy pollution. With this and other rivers and streams flowing into it, and a vast connection to the open sea, the Gulf is a semi-enclosed coastal body of water that covers 91,120 square miles (236,000 km^2). It is a repository of rich biological niches and diversity. Because of this, for millennia, the gulf was an important source of marine food for its indigenous peoples and the Europeans who settled its shores.

While conducting his survey on possible pollutants in breast milk, Dewailly was approached by a midwife from Nunavik. Would he be interested in obtaining samples of breast milk from mothers there? Thinking the isolated and industry-free North to be pristine and pure, he thought he could compare what he thought would be *undetectable* pollution levels in the samples of breast milk from mothers living in Nunavik to breast milk from mothers living near the polluted St. Lawrence River. He agreed to go north, albeit reluctantly.

After a few months, Dewailly and his team airmailed samples he collected from Nunavik to the lab for analysis. "Dewailly soon got a phone call from the lab director," writes Marla Cone in an article on Dewally's unexpected discovery. "Something was wrong with the Arctic milk. The chemical concentrations were off the charts," so much so that "the peaks overloaded the lab's equipment, running off the page." When they checked additional batches of breast milk, "the scientists soon realized that the peaks were accurate: *The Arctic mothers had seven times more PCBs* [a hazardous pollutant banned in 1974] *in their milk than mothers in Canada's biggest cities.*" [emphasis added][38]

It didn't take long for researchers to find explanations for the unexpected off-the-chart levels of PCBs found in the breast milk of Inuit mothers who lived in what was thought to be one of the—if not *the*—cleanest environment on earth. They discovered that not only PCBs but also a murky blend of many other pollutants were and are being transported to the Arctic by rivers and ocean currents, wind and air. Indeed, most of the contamination found in the Arctic food web was arriving from areas far outside the region, often from countries that produce large amounts of industrial and agricultural waste that are hundreds or thousands of miles away, such as the United States, China, and India. Such an abundance of synthetic, mostly unregulated, laboratory-made chemicals began to proliferate during World War II, when chemists and companies, eager to contribute to victory, invented compounds ranging from plastics and pesticides to solvents and insulators—any "materials that could be used to make more effective weapons, increase crop yields, and feed more soldiers," Gay Daly writes in a special report on the subject.[39]

But how did PCBs get into the breast milk of Inuit mothers in the North? Throughout the decades, as the pollutants travelled in and through various water systems, they became part of lake *sediment*, eaten by tiny microscopic organisms called *plankton*. In turn, the 450-plus species of small, shrimplike, fresh- and salt-water crustaceans (*mysid*) eat plankton. When smaller fish like smelt eat mysid, they are also consuming PCBs; as larger fish like trout eat smelt and mysid, they concentrate the fat-soluble contaminants in their own fat, and so forth and so on up the food chain, through larger fish to the sea mammals that eat them.[40]

It makes sense, then, that when blubber-rich Arctic marine mammals eat the many fish their immense bodies need to thrive, not only do they take in a lot of PCBs, the PCBs accumulate to high concentrations and remain stored in the mammals' body fat. By the time Inuit mothers consume the seals and whales and other mammals that constitute the core of their diet, they too store in their body fat PCBs and other pollutants that are present in their food. Now Dewailly understood what at first had confounded him and his colleagues: every time Inuits in Nunavik ate their favorite food—food that had been a healthful tradition for millennia—*they were storing an abundance of toxic chemicals in their bodies, which of course became part of mothers' breast milk.* (Presently, the only proven method for humans to eliminate stored PCBs is through mother's milk.)

Clearly, it is a sad irony: a remote region, with no signs of locally created pollution, can become one of the most toxic food environments on earth. Surely, this tells us that the interconnection among all living creatures—especially that between human beings and the animals and plants we eat and the water we drink—is a delicate, interwoven, related web. It also tells us that what passes as "nourishment" now is not an isolated Arctic problem. Rather, the quality of the food we eat—including the breast milk that is supposed to nourish, not harm, our children—is an "un-arctic," universal, human dilemma. For, as with the gene-food-health "web" relationship we discussed earlier, disturb one or more "food threads" from airborne synthetic chemicals in food we eat; water we drink; air we breathe; antibiotics and hormones in conventional meat, fowl, and feed; then add *imbalanced nutrients* and other *food additives* due to processing, and the entire banquet is altered in ways we—and our genes—are just beginning to understand.

3

Perhaps the best way to grasp both the food-health implications as well as the "genetic fallout" from today's chemical cuisine (which, for instance, the Inuit's centuries-old marine-based diet has become due to man-made pollution in water, wind, and fish) is to go back 50 years, when both scientists and physicians believed that the *placenta*—the protective organ that connects the fetus to the uterine wall—protected the baby from any contaminants to which the mother may be exposed; in other words, the medical community held that the placenta provided a barrier to any toxic foreign material in the mother, which had gotten there either through food intake or environmental exposure.

This belief was shattered in the early 1960s when thalidomide, one of the most globally successful pharmaceutical drugs used to treat morning sickness in pregnant women, was exposed as causing major birth defects. More and more, researchers were revealing its link to limb and organ malformations that occurred during the development of the fetus.[41,42] The results resonated worldwide: pharmaceutical drugs do indeed pass through the placenta to the unborn child. Almost 35 years after this devastating discovery, researchers would reveal that exposure to thalidomide in the womb caused limb deformity in *male* children, who in turn, passed their genetic malformations on to their children.[43] But at the time—the 1960s—the discovery that thalidomide passed through the placental barrier provided clues into the next "wonder drug" that also passed on health problems to unborn children.

Following on the heels of the thalidomide debacle, doctors began to prescribe DES (diethylstilbestrol) for pregnant women who were at risk for miscarriage or premature labor. Created in 1938 and approved for medical use in human beings in 1941, DES was the first synthetic estrogen—a hormone or "chemical messenger," secreted by the endocrine gland, which regulates how various tissues or organs function. But by 1970, clear cell adenocarcinoma (CCA), a previously rare vaginal cancer, started to appear in young women. It didn't take long for doctors to link this rare cancer to the DES the young women's mothers had taken while pregnant.[44–47]

Again, as with thalidomide, we had proof that DES passes through the placenta and affects the developing fetus. But the impact of DES differs from that of thalidomide in that the harmful health impact of this synthetic estrogen appears when "DES daughters" are adult women. DES is also the first drug to show that a synthetic hormone given to women while pregnant can have life-long health effects on their offspring—both daughters *and sons*. We know this because ongoing research has revealed that "DES sons" have a greater risk of conditions related to male sexual development and fertility, birth defects of the urethra, even breast cancer.[40] Still more recent research revealed that these adverse alterations may be passed on not only to "DES sons," but to their children.[48]

4

Since the end of World War II, some 100,000 synthetic chemicals, pollutants (waste products), and toxicants (such as pesticides and herbicides) have been released into our air, water, or soil. Of the 1000 or more different substances manufactured and released into the environment each year, most are not tested for safety.[49] Depending on where you live, either some or many of these compounds are in the food you eat, the water you drink, and the air you breathe. And, as we've seen with thalidomide and DES, many of them have the power to disrupt the body's exquisitely sensitive hormonal messenger system throughout life; especially during critical stages of fetal development. What's of equal concern is this: even when they're present in food or your body—even in microscope *parts per billion*—they can create disturbing biological changes; disorder in your body that is both immediate and long-term.[40]

Because many of these chemicals have the power to *disrupt* the hormonal messages that regulate the function of specific organs or tissues, they are called "endocrine disruption chemicals" (EDCs) or more typically, "endocrine disruptors." We saw how this "hormone havoc"[50] can lead to harmful health effects when estrogen-like DES was given to pregnant women to ward off miscarriage. Although the mechanism wasn't understood at the time, the scrambled messages sent by the synthetic estrogen put the children of these mothers at higher risk for reproductive disorders, cervical cancer, and other related ailments later in life.

How do endocrine disrupting chemicals work their damage? Hormones—most of which are created in various glands such as the thyroid—act in the body like messengers, to transfer information from glands to receptor sites in cells. In a way, they are like a circulating "key" seeking the correct lock. The way hormones work is not unlike old-fashioned telephone operators who managed elaborate, intricate switchboards well into the 20th century to connect callers with those receiving the call. Typically, one or more operators (hormones) would be responsible for connecting callers by inserting a cable with a plug at one end into a socket (cell receptor site) on the switchboard (a cell). Once the plug was "locked" into the correct socket, the correct connection was made, and the telephone of the person being called would ring. But if the operator scrambles the plugs and puts them in the wrong sockets, the connections can't be made and instead, havoc, misinformation, and incorrect instructions and cellular responses ensue.

In the same way, when hormones circulate in our blood, they are seeking their "socket," the right site on our cells to plug into so that their message can be both sent and received by our cells and body. When the connection is made, estrogens and other hormones are poised to start and stop a wide range of physiological functions, such as directing the development of tissues in the fetus or initiating childbirth. Or, in the developing fetus, they may assert their genetic influence by determining whether a baby will be physiologically female or male.

On the other hand, hormone receptors are not selective. Instead of "partnering" faithfully with their meant-to-be hormone, they accept a wide variety of synthetic hormone-like strangers into their receptor sites, thus blocking the message of the naturally occurring hormone. In addition, because these synthetic hormones are constantly present, they may attach at the wrong time and disrupt the precise timing of the developmental order. Such hormone "promiscuity" may have made DES daughters prone to cervical cancer by blocking their cells from getting the hormonal message for their genes to switch off cell division. As a result, unchecked cell proliferation may have initiated the first stages of cervical cancer.

Because of the devastating health problems author and health advocate Lindsey Berkson experienced as a "DES daughter," she became passionate about undetected toxins in everyday foods and hormone-based medications and the destruction they reap when they disrupt hormones. In *Hormone Deception*, her landmark book on the topic, she identified at least five different responses that can occur when "inappropriate orders" are given by synthetic hormones—including DES and PCBs and the thousands we're exposed to from fuels, pesticides, detergents, and plastics, and other substances that have entered our food supply. Berkson identified a range of problems that may occur when endocrine disruptors send the wrong cue at the wrong time. They can:

- mimic the natural hormones in our bodies, such as estrogens;
- antagonize (block) our natural hormones, such as androgens (male hormones), thyroid hormone, and progesterone;
- alter the way in which natural hormones are produced, eliminated, or metabolized;
- modify the number of hormone receptors we have and thus the amount of hormonal signaling in our bodies; and
- stimulate the release of hormones or other natural substances that affect the balance of our hormones in our bodies.[40]

As disturbing as these effects are, another issue is what biologist Theo Colborn calls "bio-magnification." Based on evidence gleaned from more than 4000 studies, her classic book *Our Stolen Future* reveals that "hormone-disrupting chemicals are not classical poisons or typical carcinogens." Rather, their biological impact is magnified. That is, even very small amounts of (say) DDT, DES, PCB, or dioxin can "rob human potential before birth" by damaging sperm count or by causing prostate and breast cancer, endometriosis, miscarriage, and learning and developmental disabilities.[51]

Consider, for example, a series of studies on endocrine disruptors and fetal health done in the 1980s and 1990s by psychologists Joseph and Sandra Jacobson, two researchers from Wayne State University in Detroit, Michigan.[52-54] At the time, scientists knew that endocrine disruptors cross the placenta and affect the growing fetus's sex characteristics and related organs, creating subsequent health problems. The Jacobsons wanted to see if synthetic chemicals that mimic hormones—substances found in products such as pesticides, flame retardants, and hormone-containing pharmaceuticals that found their way into water systems, and in turn into the fish that pregnant women eat—could affect the intelligence levels of their children.

To find out, the Jacobsons studied 242 new mothers who consumed two to three meals each month of PCB-contaminated fish (such as trout and salmon) from Lake Michigan for six years prior to becoming pregnant. Over a period of 11 years, the researchers compared the intellectual performance of children born to fish-consuming mothers to the children of 71 mothers who didn't eat PCB-laden fish from Lake

Michigan. To ensure reliability, at the start of the study, the Jacobsons measured PCB levels in the blood of the babies' umbilical cords. When the scientists compared the progress of the two groups of babies beginning at birth, then followed up at seven months, four years, and 11 years of age, the children of fish eaters averaged lower IQ scores and were twice as likely to be at least two years behind in reading comprehension when compared with children from mothers who did not eat PCB-laden fish. Perhaps even more telling is that children exposed to the highest levels of PCBs were three times as likely to average lower IQ scores, and they were twice as likely to be at least two years behind in reading comprehension when compared with children from mothers who did not eat fish caught in Lake Michigan.

Do endocrine disrupters affect intelligence levels of children exposed to them while in the womb? Joseph Jacobson is cautious about drawing definitive conclusions, because, he explains, early brain development is "such a complex process."[55] Still, because studies have shown that infants who consumed breast milk that had substantial levels of PCBs after being born did not show any adverse effects, exposure to PCBs during gestation may be more harmful than disruptors consumed after birth. This is of special concern because of a landmark endocrine disruption discovery made in 1997 by Frederick von Saal, a reproductive endocrinologist at the University of Missouri. He established it only takes extremely low levels of exposure—parts per billion and even per trillion—to have a biological effect at sensitive stages of development.[56]

Earlier in the chapter, we discussed the surprisingly high levels of PCBs found in breast milk of Inuit mothers in what was believed to be a pristine far North. This and other studies tell us that various levels of endocrine disruptors are not only present in Inuit through their marine diet, and in mothers who consume fish found in Lake Michigan, they are likely present in most humans as well. How much of these substances you have in your system depends on where you live, the source of the water you drink, and usual daily diet. Indeed, the number of contaminants, their growing presence in everyday foods and the health problems with which they're associated are pervasive both for ourselves and for our unborn or nursing children. But there's some light on the horizon: more and more, concerned scientists, activists, citizens, and organizations worldwide are taking action to turn the tide.[57, 58] Others offer specialized symposia for the economically depressed Inuit population on coping with the invisible contaminants that are threatening their way of life.[59]

5

What does the reality of endocrine disruptors tell us about "nourishment" now and the food-gene-health story? Endocrine disruptors may be a permanent part of our lives. So, too, are other persistent organic pollutants (POPs), the term for man-made compounds that remain in the environment, including in our food supply.[60] These POPs include agrochemicals, a generic term for a broad range of chemicals used in agriculture that typically protect fruit and vegetable crops from being ravaged by insects.

One of the first agrochemicals was hailed as a hero, believed to be capable of wiping out malaria worldwide. During World War II, it reduced typhus among troops. In 1948, Swiss chemist Paul Hermann Müller was awarded the Nobel Prize in Physiology or Medicine for discovering its ability to destroy arthropods, such as insects and centipedes.[61] And after the war, when agriculture started using it as an insecticide to destroy insects that were devastating fruit and vegetable crops, both its production and use increased dramatically. What's the POP? The chemical *dichlorodiphenyltrichloroethane*. More commonly called DDT, it is a synthetic pesticide–a human-made insect and bug killer—that has other "relatives": dieldrin, parathion, heptachlor, and malathion, each of which the United States Department of Agriculture (USDA) distributed for public use after the war.

How common are they in our culture now? Recall that during our discussion about lifestyle, we introduced you to Cheryl Greene, who at a young age was diagnosed with breast cancer. With no family history of the disease, and no other risk factors, she wondered what might have caused it. And then she remembered that as a kid growing up on a conventional grape farm that produced raisins, she had consistently been exposed to toxic pesticides on her family's raisin farm. Did a particular POP cause Cheryl's cancer? Her speculation that it did may have merit when you consider that, today, various POPs account for 38 percent of all pesticides in use throughout the world.[62] Indeed, when thousands of people were tested for exposure to 34 pesticides, 19 were found in the study participants.[63]

The pesticides that were of concern to Cheryl are synthetic (human-made) compounds created to control a variety of agricultural pests that can damage plant crops (fruits, vegetables, grains, legumes, nuts) and livestock (cattle, sheep, and pigs). Yet pesticides aren't all "bad" or harmful. Rather, they encompass several categories: *insecticides* for controlling insects; *herbicides* for controlling weeds; and *fungicides* for controlling mold and mildew. Along with synthetic pesticides not found in nature that are used for crop protection and malaria control, "some are made from natural materials, such as *pyrethrum* from the Chrysanthemum flower, and *neem oil* from the neem tree," explained David Granatstein, a sustainable agriculture specialist from Wenatchee, Washington, during an interview. "Still others, such as insect *pheromones* and *spinatoram*, are based on naturally occurring compounds, although they are manufactured synthetically."[64]

The use of pesticides and other agrochemicals started long ago as farmers searched for methods to control pests that caused serious economic loss or crop destruction. They were needed because "most crop plants aren't grown in their original environment—and therefore don't have the complement of organisms that can provide checks and balances against pests," Granatstein said. A good example, he says, is the relationship between the apple—which originated in Kazakhstan and is now grown all over the world in all regions—and the *codling moth*, an insect pest (the worm in the apple) that can damage 95 percent of the fruit on a tree if uncontrolled. When the Washington State apple industry began in the late 1800s, damage by this pest quickly became a problem and few control options were available. At the time, "synthetic pesticides were starting to be developed, and one material, *lead arsenate*, a combination of lead and arsenic, proved effective against codling moth," says Granatstein. Over time, the insect became increasingly resistant to this pesticide, and higher rates were needed to get control. But "lead arsenate posed a direct health risk to those spraying it, and since it does not biodegrade, it persists in the soil and can provide future exposure through dust or growing of crops that can take up lead or arsenate through their roots." The obvious problems with this type of pesticide led to the search for alternatives. And the development of DDT during WW II was considered a major step forward, because it controlled insects on a variety of crops, including codling moths on apples.

"At the time, DDT seemed to be a miracle," says Granatstein. "It is an organic molecule, so it has to decompose in the environment. This differs from lead and arsenic, which are *not* organic molecules; once they're in the soil, they're there for decades or more. DDT was inexpensive, and effective at controlling pests, so this seemed like great progress." Unfortunately, DDT and its breakdown products bioaccumulated up the food chain and were linked to negative impacts on bird species, including the American bald eagle.

In 1968, with the publication of her landmark book, *Silent Spring*, an unassuming, somewhat shy biologist named Rachel Louise Carson was the unlikely messenger who, in effect, created public awareness about DDT usage and its problems. How did Carson inspire modern America—indeed, the world—to change their view about the role of synthetic chemicals in the environment? Now considered a landmark—indeed, one of the most important books of the 20th century—*Silent Spring* called into question the sanctity of "better living through chemistry," E.I. DuPont's advertising slogan, which, for decades after World War II, reflected the public's unquestioned support for use of novel chemical compounds.[65, 66] With its exposé about environmental dangers and long-term health problems, including the *genetic* impact that use of synthetic pesticides can cause, Carson's work challenged the notion that "scientific progress" is always good and pointed out that science needs to look harder for the unintended consequences that its discoveries may bring.[67]

By 1972, DDT was banned for agricultural use in the United States[68] and subsequently in most countries worldwide.[69] Even so, DDT and its metabolite, DDE, are still in use in some countries and they remain very much a part of the global environment. More resistant to complete decomposition than originally thought, DDT has been categorized as a major POP.[70]

"The benefits from pesticides are significant, but they have to be weighed against the negative consequences for human health and the environment," says Granatstein. "If DDT wasn't a sustainable solution for protecting crops from destructive insect pests, what was?" Enter *organophosphate insecticides*. "Apple growers shifted to organophosphates for codling moth when they became available in the 1980s. These have low persistence in the environment, but can be acutely toxic and may kill non-target insects that help with natural biological control."

Today, the evolution of pest management continues with newer pesticides that regulate insect growth with little or no effect on mammalian species. For instance, some apple growers now control codling moth damage with the use of *pheromone mating disruption*, a mechanism that floods the apple orchard with a synthetic version of the female codling moth pheromone used to attract male moths for mating. This confuses the males; they cannot find the females, mating does not occur, and eggs do not hatch into worms that burrow into the fruit. "This is a non-toxic pest control method, but is not always sufficient to do the job," says Granatstein. "No doubt future developments will continue the journey toward more sustainable pest management in apples and other crops, while food production and quality are maintained, and the environment and human health are protected."

We don't really know what harm low, long-term exposure to endocrine disruptors and agrochemicals can cause to humans. Are there drawbacks to consuming fish, fruits, and vegetables, and other food that contain various amounts of POPs? In the 1960s, Carson stated

> . . . the central problem of our age has . . . become the contamination of man's total environment with such substances of incredible potential for harm—substances that accumulate in the tissues of plants and animals and even penetrate the germ cells to shatter or alter the very material of heredity upon which the shape of the future depends.[71]

Was Carson prophetic? Might food we consume that has been altered with synthetic chemicals influence our genetic heritage? Our link with both past and future? We've seen clues in the work we discussed by Francis Pottenger, who, in the 1930s, observed transgenerational changes in cats due to poor diet. And we saw a similar phenomenon with humans in Överkalix, Sweden, in 2003, when clinical geneticist Marcus Pembrey speculated that some kind of "imprinting" in a generation of grandchildren could be linked to diet and other environmental influences experienced by their parents or earlier ancestors. Do such studies suggest it's also possible that we pass on to our children . . . and to our grandchildren, even our great-grandchildren—non-DNA changes in our genes caused by endocrine disruptors and agrochemicals that have made their way into our food supply? If so, this would mean that synthetic chemicals we consume are doing nothing less than threatening human evolution.

Two related studies, done in 2003 and 2004, by reproductive biologist Matthew Anway and colleagues at Washington State University, Pullman, can give us insights into whether endocrine disruptors affects not only us, but generations to come. To find out, Anway posed this landmark question: Can the fungicide *vinclozolin*, which is commonly sprayed on grapes and other fruits and vegetables, cause non-DNA *epigenetic* changes that endure for at least four generations? At the time, Anway knew that vinclozolin, given to pregnant rats, caused reproductive abnormalities such as lowered sperm counts in the male offspring. Might it also affect future offspring?

Anway proceeded by injecting pregnant rat dams with moderately high doses of vinclozolin daily over a period of seven days. When the first litter was born, Anway observed the effects of vinclozolin on the sperm count of the male pups. Across the board, they all showed reduced sperm count and motility, as well as abnormally developed reproductive organs. When Anway bred the next three generations of males with females *not* exposed to vinclozolin, the males had similar sperm abnormalities.[72] In the second study, when he observed both male *and* female offspring of all four generations throughout their lifetime, he observed their health problems skyrocketed: offspring in all four generations had greater rates of prostate and kidney disease, breast tumors, and immune system abnormalities.[73] As you consider these findings, keep in mind that at least two other research groups were unable to replicate Anway's transgenerational results.[74,75] Nevertheless, Anway's findings are especially intriguing for two reasons: They tell us that, under certain conditions, exposure to synthetic chemicals during the fetal stage can cause long-term reproductive damage for generations, and that the damage that's passed on can manifest through a whole host of ailments.

What's concerning about Anway's findings is that while the dosage of vinclozolin he gave to pregnant dams is much higher than doses humans are typically exposed to, since the introduction of endocrine disruptors and pesticides in the environment, sperm count of males has decreased 50 percent worldwide.[76] Is this a coincidence? Not likely, given that some studies are finding a link between increased infertility and exposure to pesticides.[77, 78] Such statistics give all of us cause to pause, because even though the Environmental Protection Agency (EPA) and Food and Drug Administration (FDA) have established "safe" guideline levels for pesticides, many Americans have levels in their body that exceed the guidelines, [79] with children between the ages of six and eleven carrying four times the acceptable level. Do these data mean Rachel Carson was indeed prophetic when, in the early 1960s, she declared that toxins in our food and environment have the potential to alter the course of humankind? Absolutely.

6

By the 1990s, it became apparent that conventional corn and herbicide-based Roundup Ready soybeans, especially, are other key players in the story of "nourishment" now and the food-gene-health link. A key example of this new "gene-in-your-food technology" is native wild corn, which for centuries, has been a staple of every family's diet in Mexico. Grown in remote, rural mountains, Mexicans are proud that their country is the place of origin of all varieties of corn. So when local farmers from the rural mountain settlement of Capulalpan discovered strange-looking, less tasty, "alien" corn in their crops, they were alarmed.[80,81] Close scrutiny by Mexican and American scientists revealed the reason for the "mystery corn": it was contaminated by *genetically modified organisms* (GMOs). In other words, the scientists discovered a segment of the plant's genetic code had been modified mechanically by chemists in laboratories, so that the corn could resist insects and reduce the use of herbicides.[82] The "enabler" is a powerful new technology called *genetic engineering* (GE), the process of artificially modifying and manipulating DNA by inserting desirable gene components from one plant or animal into another. The promise of such science is that it produces higher yields with fewer pesticides.[83]

Finding genetically modified (GM) corn in the rural hills in Mexico was especially surprising because since 1998, Mexico had prohibited the cultivation of GM maize (although it is still imported from the United States for human consumption). It was even more unexpected because it was found 62 miles from the nearest GM crops. And not only Capulalpan was affected; strains of GM-tainted maize were identified in 15 of 22 towns in Oaxaca.[84]

At first the unintentional spread of GM corn that produced abundant crop yields seemed like a dream-come-true. But the dream turned to concern when it became evident that ripe GM maize was especially susceptible to local plagues and diseases. Not too long afterward, yet another clue that all was not right with GM foods emerged—this time with *intra*-species hybridization—offspring that occur *within* plants. This is exactly what occurred when the soil bacterium Bt toxin (*Bacillus thuringiensis*), found in every part of a GE corn plant with Bt genes, caused the unintended death to butterfly caterpillars that consumed milkweed plants infected by windblown pollen from Bt corn.[85] Indeed, Bt has been engineered into many other crops, such as apple, canola, potato, rice, and tomato.

Since the debacle in rural Mexico surfaced like an international dust storm, genetically modified crops have continued to spread to the four corners of the earth via the "unintentional presence" of GM organisms (GMOs) because of pollen and mixing.[86] But it has also spread through other natural means, such as wind-blown pollen and co-mingled seeds, and intentionally, through food exporters in North and South America and black-market plantings.

This controversial technology has its roots in "natural genetic engineering"—selecting the best seeds from the hardiest plants. For centuries, humans have altered the genetic characteristics of plants naturally by selecting seeds from plants with desirable physical characteristics, such as taste, size or color. Breeding plants for certain qualities leaped to another level in the 16th century when Joseph Gottlieb Koelreuter conducted the first systematic experiments in plant hybridization,[87] and later in the 19th century when botanist Luther Burbank inspired world-wide interest in plant breeding when he "married" two plants with different characteristics via cross-pollination to create a plethora of new fruits, plants and flowers. So exceptional was his work with plants that he was honored by an Act of Congress.[88]

Over time, both natural human selection and Burbank's hybridization and breeding techniques were so successful that they contributed greatly to creating today's abundant food supply. Although many proponents of GE claim it is a safe process that is comparable to breeding plants, this is not accurate. The genetic code of GM plants has been modified by humans, whereas hybrid plants create their own genetic structure. And GE modifies a small piece of the genetic code, often with little knowledge of how this will affect the full genetic expression of the organism. In contrast, plants that have been selectively bred work together as a whole organism in the way in which nature intended. In other words, genetic engineering is comparable to taking a perfectly written, beautiful poem, then adding a word in order to change a line in the poem—without understanding how it may alter the entire essence, purpose, and meaning of the poem.

As prevalent as GMO foods are, in Europe, they're also shunned by many as "Frankenfoods"[89] and some major food companies in America have stopped using them due to public protest.[90] What's all the brouhaha about? It's about the growing evidence of inadequate testing, junk science, and an expanding litany of health threats that GM foods could cause in both adults and children. For instance, when researchers Ian F. Pryme and Rolf Lembcke conducted *in vivo* studies about the possible health consequences of genetically modified food, they concluded that genetic engineering creates widespread *genetic mutations* in hundreds of thousands of locations throughout the genome.[91] Concerned about the effects such mutations can have on vulnerable infants and children, pediatric neurologist and researcher Dr. Martha Herbert—who is also a board member of the Council for Responsible Genetics—has said[92]

> There is a lot of evidence that food can affect health. Early diet can be related to later diseases. The doubling of childhood asthma since

1980 has been linked to early diet. Certain [GM] foods can trigger behavior changes in vulnerable children such as some with autism or attention deficit disorder. All parents . . . should be able to make choices about the ingredients in their children's food . . . [but] without labeling, parents have no way of knowing whether or not the soy formula they're feeding their babies contains untested proteins.[93]

Herbert is also aware of the potential GM foods have to create *epigenetic changes* by switching genes on and off: "The methods used to insert these genes can disrupt essential genetic function, changing which genes get turned on or how much they do. But genetically engineered foods aren't systematically tested for these kinds of changes."[93]

It is hard to look at such concerns and not eschew an untested technology that can cause what author and GMO expert Andrew Kimbrell describes as "toxic genes." For "the truth is . . . every time [corporate scientists] insert a novel gene into a plant cell," writes Kimbrell, "the gene ends up in a random location in the plant's genome. As a result, each new gene amounts to a game of *food safety roulette* [emphasis added], leaving companies hoping that the new gene . . . will not destabilize a safe food and make it toxic."[93] With such insights, it becomes easy to understand how an unnatural, untested food technology that was inconceivable three decades ago could "confuse" our genes and lead to food-related health problems for us and the genetic legacy we pass on to our children.[94]

7

Inspired by a small flock of chickens she had been keeping, Pearl Perdue and her husband Arthur founded Perdue Farms in Salisbury, Maryland, in 1920. At first, the company was a typically small, family-run farm that sold eggs only, but by the 1940s, ready-to-cook broiler chickens became its main focus. When the company was incorporated in the 1950s, Pearl and Arthur's son Frank took over the business.

What Frank may not have known—yet—was that around the time he took over leadership of his parents' company, two Harvard Business School professors, Ray Goldberg and John Davis, were launching a food production model that would transform Perdue Farms—indeed, American agriculture—in unrecognizable ways over the next decades. No longer would the poultry (and meat and pork) industry be dominated by small family farms or ranches that produced eggs, dairy products (such as milk), and poultry from free-running poultry that had been fed in the farm area. Instead, the professors' new venture, called *agribusiness*, created a concentrated, vertically integrated business model with increased food production and corporate profit as the key criteria.[95] In 1968, under Frank Perdue's leadership, Perdue Farms achieved full vertical integration. By 2005, it became the third largest producer of chicken broilers in America. (Tyson Foods dominates the production of chicken meat in the United States, followed by Pilgrim's Pride Corp.)[96]

Some call it "factory farming"; others coined the phrase "Concentrated Animal Feeding Operations (CAFOs)" and "crowded animal factories" to describe the way in which vertically integrated farming has evolved. However it's described, today's conventional agribusiness typically refers to a large number of animals—from chickens and cattle to dairy cows and pigs—that are raised in conditions designed to produce as much poultry, meat, pork, eggs, or milk as possible at the lowest possible cost.

Such feedlot operations have many "distinctive characteristics," one of which is animals being confined in cages, crates, or indoor sheds; in other words, crowded living conditions that increase the likelihood of both profit and fast-spreading infections. In response, farmers and ranchers infuse feedlot animals with *antibiotics* to prevent and treat diseases created by their living conditions.

An even more recent "characteristic" being practiced by Perdue AgriBusiness is the use of NutriDense Grain, described as "a nutritionally enhanced corn that contains a stacked set of output traits designed to enhance animal feed performance."[97] In other words, corn fed to animals raised in Purdue's feedlots is genetically engineered.

Yet another key characteristic is growth hormones, called *anabolic steroids*. While this term may be new to you, the concept of growth hormones is familiar, for we discussed synthetic hormones and endocrine disruptors, such as DES (the first synthetic hormone), earlier in the chapter. Of the six anabolic steroids fed to cattle *in combination*, three are synthetic hormones: synthetic estrogen (zeranol); synthetic androgen (trenbolone acetate); and the potent synthetic progestin (melengestrol acetate). The other three are naturally occurring hormones: estradiol, testosterone, and progesterone.

Administered to most conventional cattle in the USA to increase growth and development, measureable amounts of the six steroids are found in meat muscle, fat, liver, kidney, and other organs, *even though steroids are stopped two weeks prior to slaughter*, due to the FDA's Acceptable Daily Intake (ADI) that can be administered to cattle, and in turn, consumed by humans.[98, 99] Still, Dr. Shanna H. Swan of University of Rochester Medical Center, a professor of Obstetrics and Gynecology, wanted to know if there are long-term risks from steroids that remain in the meat that many Americans eat each day. The health problem she focused her attention on was male infertility. Was it possible, Swan wondered, for hormones in meat consumed by pregnant women to cross the placental barrier and in turn, affect sperm concentration and therefore fertility, in their *adult* male offspring? (Clearly, such speculation isn't too far-fetched, because we saw a comparable dynamic with DES given to pregnant women and its effect on adult DES sons and daughters.) If Swan could find a link, it could provide possible insights into the dramatic reduction in sperm count in men since farmers and ranchers have been administering these steroids to cattle and chickens many Americans eat each day.

To find out if pregnant mothers' consumption of beef that includes growth hormone residues and other chemicals is tied to their to-be-born sons' fertility, Swan studied sperm samples from 387 adult men, averaging 31 years of age, who lived in five cities across America: Los Angeles, Minneapolis, Columbia, New York City, and Iowa City. She also studied questionnaires the men filled out about their mothers' meat consumption while pregnant. When she scrutinized the results, Swan found that high beef consumption by pregnant women may indeed alter sperm production of the male fetus in utero. "The average sperm concentration of the men in our study went down as their mothers beef intake went up," Swan said of her findings. Of special concern is that "although sperm production occurs in stages—prenatal, during puberty, and into adulthood—the most important stage for developing semen quality occurs in the womb," Swan said.[100, 101] As disturbing, Swan found similar results in a subsequent study she did that linked lower sperm counts in men living in a farming community to exposure to pesticides.[101]

Whether the chemical is pesticides, antibiotics (antimicrobial agents), GMOs, or growth hormones found in feed, beef, chicken, pork, or dairy, what they have in common is this: when we consume conventionally raised animal foods—or even naturally occurring high-fat meat, such as marine mammals that have been the core of the Inuit diet for centuries—it is likely we are consuming varying degrees of toxins and pesticide residue that have accumulated in the animals' muscle, organs, and fat. In turn, these toxins circulate in our blood, and mount up in breast milk (as we saw with pregnant Inuit women in the Arctic), and are stored in our body fat. Isn't it disheartening that "nourishment" now has come to mean ongoing exposure to the chemical cocktail in food we consume each day? And that such chemical cuisine increases our susceptibility to infertility and other health problems that we can pass on to our children—especially at vulnerable stages of growth?

8

The idea of food as predominantly processed and as an alphabet soup of PCBs, GMOs, and other chemicals that are forcing us to play genetic roulette may seem incredible. After all, when most of us consider food, we most typically think of it in straightforward, simple terms, such as "food for health" or perhaps, as a delightful dinner. The idea that a complex cocktail of artificial chemicals has infiltrated our food supply is almost overwhelming. This situation evolved over decades from a complicated set of circumstances. The people and companies who have created what Yale psychologist Kelly Brownell calls today's "toxic food environment"[102] never intended to create a food supply that is actually altering our health and genes, yet this is exactly what has occurred.

The chapter on *Food Then* looked at the question of what humans ate for millennia, suggesting that in order to thrive as a species, food must be fresh and contain nutrients in the ratio nature intended us to eat it. We've looked at the Industrial Revolution in the late 1800s when food first started to be processed en masse, and then in this chapter, how it led, by the mid-1960s, to food processing and "chemical cuisine" that escalated at an unprecedented speed. But the core subject of this chapter is this: the more we distance ourselves from ancestral diets, the more we are likely to be eating a health-robbing diet that is far removed from the health- and gene-enhancing diets on which we evolved and thrived. Epigeneticist Juleen Zierath at the Karolinska Institute in Stockholm, Sweden, puts it this way: "We are not victims of our genes. If anything, our genes are victims of us."[103] In other words, we are giving our genes bad instructions each time we consume highly processed foods and the slew of chemicals that have come to comprise "nourishment" now.

Such insights shed light on the phenomenon we first revealed when we discussed Dr. Francis Pottenger's discovery, made in the 1930s, that an inadequate diet affects cats and their kittens over four generations; and then later in the book, when we showed that "Pottenger's prophecy" applied to people in Överkalix, Sweden—with the discovery that the diet of grandparents, especially during critical growth periods, likely created epigenetic, non-DNA changes, which, in turn, influenced the health status of their grandchildren born decades later. And this phenomenon is the core of this chapter; indeed, the entire book: food and other substances mothers- and fathers-to-be consume, can affect not only their own health, but can create either healthful or harmful changes in their reproductive genes they pass on to their children and grandchildren—and perhaps, beyond. Like looking into a crystal ball, these discoveries would offer clues to what the future holds—for us, our genes, and our health—when synthetic chemicals—especially those that mimic hormones—are into the foods we eat each day.

In the next three chapters, we will introduce you to people, guidelines, and a plan of action designed to replace the epigenetic expression of food-related chronic conditions with health, healing, and well-being. In "Food Pioneers," you'll meet visionary people who are living lives with "gene-friendly" food at the core, while our chapter on "10 Green-Gene Food Guidelines" offers new nutrition guidelines based on a distillation of three worldviews about nutrition: 1) ancient food wisdom that has contributed to health and healing for millennia; 2) nutritional anthropological wisdom; and, 3) state-of-the-art Western nutritional science. In other words, our "green-gene guidelines" are comprised of a distillation of Paleolithic, Neolithic, and ancestral diets, as well as diets based on research that have shown it's possible to empower genes to "express" wellness while "suppressing" illness. Then our chapter that poses the question, If not now, when? will give you ideas about how to put the pioneering concepts discussed throughout *Pottenger's Prophecy* into action.

Chapter 8

FOOD PIONEERS

In Chapter 7, we revealed that many of the diet-gene-health problems we encounter today stem from our present-day understanding—or more likely, our misunderstanding—about both the origins and quality of the food we eat. Since we cannot solve the health injuries linked to industrial agriculture with the same mindset that created them, we have to view food and eating in a new way. To shed light on this new view, we are presenting the true stories of five visionary "food pioneers": ranchers who raise grass-fed cattle in Wyoming; a New York City chef who creates soul-satisfying farm-to-table food; a physician who includes organic food as part of his treatment plan; a family that grows and raises their own farm-fresh food; and a unique Organic Farming major offered at a university. At the heart of each pioneer's view of food is not the old adage "you are what you eat" but rather "you eat what you are." The food pioneers you're about to meet express the depth of their concern for healing ourselves—and the Earth—by creating and eating high-quality fare. As you'll see, they are part of a swelling chorus of women and men who are passionate about a profounder and more meaningful relationship with true food and its part in re-creating our health destiny.

I

If you think that cowboys and Native American Indians were solely part of America's 19th-century past, consider this: most of the horseback-riding cowboys who drive and move a herd of 3500 Angus cattle and 2800 yearlings on the Arapaho Ranch in Wyoming are members of the Northern Arapaho tribe. In other words, they are both cowboys *and* Indians on the ranch they own.[1, 2] In the summer, up to 40 people work the ranch, while about half that number work during the winter months.[3] Says tribal member, cowboy, and assistant ranch manager Ransom Logan about his rugged outdoor life on the organic cattle ranch: "It's a pride thing. There is an unwritten code to what we do."[4]

The multitude of diverse tasks and long hours, passion for what they do, and commitment to quality care are clearly part of the ranch's invisible set of instructions, the "unwritten code" that Logan and the other cowboys follow each day. The seasons typically determine their tasks, which are based on the overriding goal of assuring quality. If you were to ride the range with the cowboys from sunrise to sunset at any one time, you might see them branding calves, checking cows for pregnancy, or herding cattle from pastures. And the cattle? What do they do each day? Their key responsibility is to graze on the grass that covers the almost 300,000 acres of hills, valleys, and mountains of the ranch. Given the extent and lushness of their surroundings, the "menu" of grazing grasses is abundant: prairie grass, June grass, Idaho fescue, Indian rice grass, and needle and thread grass.[4] When the calves are old enough to be weaned, the yearlings also graze on the grasses. In this way, the grasses become the sole source of nourishment for all the cattle.

The lives of the organic cattle that roam this range on the high plains differ quite a lot from 99 percent of their counterparts. What does an "opposite" life look like? Most conventional cattle live their lives in muddy, crowded feedlots; their diet consists of grains and growth-stimulating hormones designed to fatten them up; and they're given antibiotics to kill off unwelcomed bacteria, with the intention of warding off the diseases to which their cramped quarters and inadequate diet make them vulnerable. Not only were the grains and corn that constitute their diet subsidized by the government, but their feed was grown with the help of millions of tons of toxic chemical fertilizer. When it rains, the excess fertilizer washes into local waters; in turn, it may sicken and kill fish after it enters the water supply.[5] Because conventionally raised beef is high in fat that the animal has been "forced" to gain through added hormones in its food; because it is high in the kinds of fat that harm health (saturated fats); because it is "fortified" with antibiotics and harmful, toxic chemical fertilizers—not only is the 99 percent of conventional meat most of us eat increasingly bad for us, it can even be dangerous to our health.[6]

It's clear that the lives of cattle raised on the Northern Arapaho Indian Tribe's ranch live a different life. But they differ from conventional cattle and their "fallout" in yet another way. If grass is the staple for the ranch's cattle, flowering plants, called *forbs*, not only feed the cattle, but also the bighorn sheep, elk, antelopes, horses, and other range-dwelling animals that roam the land. The key purpose for their being on the land is to deflect predators such as wolves, bears, lions, and coyotes from turning to the cattle for "dinner"; this means that the various mammals give their lives so that the cattle can live and thrive.

In keeping with their deeply ingrained philosophy of living in harmony with nature, many of the Northern Arapahos who have worked as cowboys on the ranch take the predatory animals that kill their cattle and other animals on the ranch in stride. As a matter of fact, they welcome them. "The bears and the wolves, they were here long before our cattle," tribal leader Ronnie Oldman said in an interview. "They were brought to the border of extinction because of agriculture. I'm glad they are back."[4]

Ranch Manager David Stoner is a non-tribe member who works the ranch with nine mostly tribal cowboys. Described in an article as a 57-year-old "scrappy, ropy-muscled, hollow-cheeked cowboy," he reflects a regard for nature in line with the Arapaho:

> We're not fighting the environment; we're trying to fit inside the environment. Predators are "our brothers," and natural grasses are central to a "beautifully designed system" that takes energy from the sun and fixes nitrogen in the soil. Cattle help fertilize the land with their waste, and grazing helps spread seed. The cattle "are part of the system." They are "the reward that we can get for taking care of the land."

Holding nature in esteem. A symbiotic relationship with animals. Gratitude for Mother Earth and the nourishment she provides. For millennia, Native Americans have had a relationship with the land that encompasses respect and appreciation for all it provides. And it is these values that the Northern Arapaho bring to their ranch and to the cattle they raise on it.

The journey to their ranch and the value-filled livelihood they've created both on and from it wasn't an easy one. The original four groups of Arapaho evolved living on land located at the source of the Arkansas and Platte rivers. But the Treaty of 1851 changed their centuries-old "headquarters," and they began to share land with the Cheyenne, whose range encompassed large portions of Wyoming, Colorado, and western Kansas and Nebraska. The "living arrangements" of one of the groups— the Northern Arapaho Tribe—changed yet again in 1868, when members signed a treaty that placed them on Wind River, a lush and vast 2.2 million acre Indian Reservation in west central Wyoming.[7]

In 1940, with water for irrigation from the beautiful Wind River that flows through the reservation, the Northern Arapaho established the ranch on a large portion of the reservation. They would use it to raise Angus cattle that would thrive on the ranch's year-round native grasses and unspoiled water. Still, for almost seven decades after establishing the ranch, calves were sent to conventional feedlots for slaughtering. But a change was blowing through the land, for ranch manager Stoner, with his decades-long history of ranch management, a deep love for the land, and a strong philosophical appreciation for organic methods, had a different vision for the fate of the cattle he oversaw: they would be grass-fed throughout their lives, and they would be raised organically. No feedlots. No crowded living conditions. No grains. No antibiotics. No cruel, toxic slaughtering. Driven by compassion, concern, and sincerity, he delivered his dream to the tribe. They agreed. The ranch would go organic. It had found its niche.

During the next few years, Stoner, management, and the Northern Arapaho Business Council set their sights on turning their dream into reality. This meant spending years winding their way through layers of rigorous bureaucratic red tape in order to achieve Organic Certification from the United States Department of Agriculture. Then, in April 2009, the Arapaho Ranch—now the largest certified organic cattle operation in the U.S.—shipped its first organic, grass-fed cattle. One month later, the partnership they had established earlier in the year with California-based Panorama Meats made it possible to market locally raised beef produced at the ranch to Whole Foods stores in the Rocky Mountain region.[1] Panorama Meats, whose tag states, "organic grass-fed meats," is in perfect alignment both philosophically and quality-wise with the Arapaho Ranch. Not only is their beef organic, but it comes from family ranchers who raise free-range cattle in the American West. When the ranch achieved organic certification, Panorama showed its support with this statement:

> Sustainable range-management practices, preservation of native wildlife and a commitment to maintaining the land's biodiversity meant the tribe easily met the requirements of USDA Organic Certification in 2008. Today, Arapaho Ranch is the largest certified organic cattle operation in the U.S., with tribe members raising 3,500 Certified Organic grass-fed Angus cattle and 2,800 yearlings on one of America's last traditional cattle operations. Thanks to the Arapahos' careful monitoring of range conditions to prevent overgrazing and protect the land, their cattle have a reliable supply of fresh grass and forbs, which produce uncommonly high-quality, flavorful beef.[1]

Since "going organic," not only has the Northern Arapaho Tribe created meat that is less harmful to health, but raising organic animals allows the Arapaho to live in harmony with nature, which means remaining true to their Native American spiritual values. By merging their connection to nature with their strong belief in the sustainability of organic ranching, the cattle raised on the ranch benefit, the Arapaho themselves benefit, the land benefits, those who "eat organic" benefit, and so does Mother Earth—perhaps in invisible and immeasurable ways we may not yet understand.[8]

2

What do you create when you marry an "apricot epiphany" with a childhood spent on your grandmother's farm?[9] Answer: Blue Hill, a restaurant in New York City that offers a feast for palate, senses, and soul. From the start, Blue Hill's award-winning chef/owner[10] Dan Barber was passionate about all things *real* in food—flavor, freshness, fields, sustainability, local foods, greenmarkets, growing, soil quality, planting, harvesting, raising food animals, animal feed, compost, ingredients, preparation, cooking, aroma, dining atmosphere, and serving. His ardor extends to the presentation, textures, and tastes of meals—and to caring a lot about whether those who dine at his restaurant have at the very least a pleasurable experience. Indeed, what he really wants to know is whether they savored, relished, and took delight in the meal. "Clean plates don't lie," Barber writes. "That's what I say when waiters at my restaurant ask me why I insist on examining every plate that returns to the kitchen with the slightest bit of food on it . . . When the waiters reluctantly hold them up for inspection, it's as if I can see my reflection."[11]

The gold standard "reflection" of quality food and exceptional dining to which Barber holds himself began when he was a child growing up on his grandmother's Blue Hill Farm in the Berkshires in Great Barrington, Massachusetts. "'I loved Blue Hill Farm more than anything in the world,'" he would say years later.[12] He loved its green pastures and backdrop of blue hills, and even the nearby dirty and run-down dairy farm run by two brothers. But if Barber's passion for farm-fresh food was born on his family farm, his vision to create a restaurant that mirrored his reverence and love for exceptional food may have been ignited serendipitously just as he was ending a two-year stint as an apprentice chef in Provence, France. While browsing in a local farmers' market on his last day, his eyes lit on some apricots. "The fruit was like nothing I had ever seen: plump to nearly bursting, and blushed a deep red," he would write about the sensory-stopping experience.[13] But when he tried to select a ripe piece, the woman running the stand would have none of it. Instead, "she lovingly played her fingers like a keyboard over her small treasures, landing on one with her middle finger and tapping it several times very gently . . . Then holding it up to the morning light, she wrapped the apricot in soft tissue paper." Now she was ready to hand the fruit over to Barber. And then he took a bite. "I was at once entranced and utterly confused—not because I was tasting the best apricot of my life, but because I was tasting an apricot I had never imagined could exist."

In response, Barber's eyes welled up, in part because the flavor was so intense and exceptional, like nothing he had ever tasted, but also because he was "returning home to an unknown future." In hindsight, perhaps his strong emotional response was due to an unconscious understanding that not only had his future just unfolded in the perfection of the apricot, but he had found his destiny. When he returned to New York City, Barber merged his passion for perfect food with the love he had internalized for his grandmother's farm and land. The product of these two passions was Blue Hill, the first restaurant he created in April 2000 in collaboration with two family proprietors and co-owners: his brother, David, who is Blue Hill's businessman; and Dan's wife Laureen. Located on the basement level of a Greenwich Village brownstone, the understated but elegant atmosphere reflects Dan's natural, back-to-the-land food philosophy. Consider this description of the restaurant in *New York* magazine: "There is something easeful and secure about this uncluttered room with its warm umber banquettes. Part of that is due to a subtle but audacious dropping of an already low ceiling in order to create the intimate recessed lighting, causing the room to glow from an unspecified source."[12]

Not surprisingly, the restaurant's seasonal American *nouvelle cuisine* exquisitely complements the aesthetics. Just a few months after Blue Hill opened, restaurant critic Hal Rubenstein rhapsodized about Blue Hill's "sweetly soft asparagus soup," a salad with a "fresh-mowed taste," "lime-scented gazpacho," salmon with "a sweet, almost floral aroma," poached duck that is "delectable, delicate and sweet," "barely sweet turnips," and more. And this was just the beginning. Over the next few years, Barber went on to receive a plethora of awards: "Best New Chef" in 2002 in *Food and Wine*; part of "the next generation of great chefs" in *Bon Appetit's* 10th annual restaurant issue; *Time's* "100 Most Influential People"; "Best Chef: New York City" in 2006; and most recently, the 2009 Outstanding Chef Award from the James Beard Foundation.

With Barber's passion for quality and exceptional fare, the birth of

Blue Hill's second incarnation, Blue Hill at Stone Barns, was as natural as Barber's food philosophy. The seed for Stone Barns was planted when the patrician Rockefeller family decided to turn their sprawling farm in upstate New York, with its beautiful 1930s stone barn complex, into a dining destination. With such a vision, they turned to Dan Barber to develop what would become his second restaurant as well as a special center for food and agriculture. Located less than an hour's drive from New York City, the complex would reflect Peggy Rockefeller's and Barber's mutual commitment to, and passion for, food, farmers, and farming communities. Restaurant reviewer Adam Platt describes his first impression of the extraordinary establishment this way:

> When we first arrived, dusk was falling and the air smelled of freshly mown hay and traces of chocolate. The barns, which are modeled after structures in Normandy, were built in the twenties as a way of educating young Rockefellers about agriculture. They have impressive stone silos, and tall eves that are strafed . . . by flocks of swallows. The restaurant itself is located in the old dairy barn, which has been renovated into a polished, welcoming space, with lofty metal rafters, cream-colored walls, and high windows offering long views of the countryside.[14]

And then there's the food at the Blue Hill at Stone Barns. Described as "a self-sufficient agro-restaurant with its own state-of-the-art Rockefeller-built greenhouse, its own flock of hyperorganic chickens, its own collection of prize Berkshire hogs and even a few sheep,"[14] each dish on the menu reflects its natural source and surroundings. Add herbs from the herb garden on the property and you have a cornucopia of ingredients that pays homage to nature's remarkable bounty of flavor-filled food.

Indeed, the restaurant is the recipient of vegetables and livestock that evolved based on the surrounding farm's philosophy of "community-based food production and enjoyment, from farm to classroom to table." This translates into food that is "flavored" with livestock and crops that are raised in a symbiotic partnership with the environment; that is, the food is produced without the use of chemical fertilizers, pesticides or herbicides. At the same time, the Center's livestock are free-ranging animals (poultry, pastured veal calves, sheep and hogs), raised on a pastoral system of intensively managed rotational grazing. "In this way," says the Center, "we not only get healthy animals and high-quality meat and eggs, but also a beautiful . . . farm that can sustainably co-exist with the wild flora and fauna that surrounds us for generations to come."[15] Perhaps such depth of care infused into the food served at Blue Hill at Stone Barns led *New York Times* restaurant critic Frank Bruni to describe the meal he ate there as "food you'd almost rather hug than eat."[16]

Dedicated to ensuring that the original Blue Hill in Greenwich Village offers a comparable "Greenmarketeering" dining experience, Barber has developed an especially unusual hands-on approach for keeping his New York City staff on top of the Blue Hill craft and food philosophy: Every few weeks throughout the summer months, he and his cooks make a pilgrimage to the original Blue Hill, his grandmother's old farm in the Berkshire mountains, to plant and harvest vegetables for the restaurant. As Barber describes it, it's a tight routine: they depart for the farm right after the restaurant's final dinner service, "arrive by 2 a.m., enjoy a meal together, nap, break ground by dawn (to plant and pick plants planted on a prior trip), and head back to the restaurant by late afternoon."[17]

It sounds hurried, but . . . oh . . . what magic manifests as the cooks share food during their middle-of-the-night meal; magic appears in the space between bites of food and laughter; magic makes the transcendent meaning of Blue Hill crystal clear. Reflects Barber: "There are small satisfactions in this business of cooking—a perfectly roasted piece of sea bass, a soufflé that rises as if by prayer—but there are few pleasures. Among them is sharing food around a table of cooks. Every night we provide the conditions for other people's pleasure. But tonight it's our turn . . . We clink our glasses, laugh, and dig in." Truly, Barber is talking about both the *fare* and the *dining experience* inherent in the meals he creates from the heart; food that celebrates the senses; and, by merging love and artistry, satisfies the soul.

3

If a picture is worth a thousand words, pediatrician Alan Greene's depiction of a doctor's bag brimming with a cornucopia of fresh, organic fruits and vegetables says more than words. The medical bag—overflowing with carrots, green peppers, apples, herbs, and more—represents a core component of his life work: bringing "Dr. Greene's Organic Rx" not only to parents and their newborns but to the world at large. His motivation? As a father himself, he is devoted to making it easy for you and your children to get the most nutrition—and health—out of every meal, every day. The mission statement for the award-winning doctor's

Web site, DrGreene.com, puts it this way: "Our goal is to improve children's health by informing and inspiring those who care for them. By addressing the connection between the health of our children and the health of the environment, we strive to make a difference for both."[18] And the environmental influence on which he focuses the most—the one from which parents and children stand to benefit the most—is the quality of the food they and their children eat each day.

Dr. Greene's road to becoming an nutrition expert is especially laudable, because, though the general public has become more aware of advances in nutrition in recent decades, most doctors still do not offer practical and dependable nutrition insights to their patients, even though diet is a major cause of chronic conditions and many ailments such as asthma and ADHD that doctors are diagnosing more and more in children.[19-21] But not only is he an expert in all-things-food, he is uniquely knowledgeable about *organic* nutrition, because consuming fresh, nutrient-dense food that is additive-free is one of the most empowering steps parents can take to enhance their own health and at the same time, protect the health of their children.

The seeds for Dr. Greene's commitment to, and passion for, organic food were sown one afternoon while visiting a farm in New England. Here's how he describes his epiphany:

> It was a crisp fall afternoon on a dairy farm in the rolling hills of Vermont. I was walking through the pasture with George Siemon . . . who was talking about the dramatic improvement in health for a herd of cows when it transitions from being a conventional herd to an organic one. The veterinarian bills go down, the lifespan of the cows more than doubles . . . George than made an offhand remark about how no one really knows what would happen to a human today when switched to totally organic . . . As the day went by, I couldn't get this casual comment out of my head . . . Today, about 98 percent of foods in the U.S. are produced with the use of toxic pesticides, routine antibiotics, genetically engineered hormones, or genetically engineered seeds. What *would* it look like in 21st century America to choose only foods grown organically?...Back at the kitchen table, I posed the question to my family . . . They were excited to watch and learn with me. . . .[22]

Over the next year or so, Dr. Greene, his wife, Cheryl, and their four children embraced organic food enthusiastically. At the start of their journey, many questions loomed. Would "going organic" mean giving up favorite restaurants? Might it make it challenging to eat meals with extended family and friends? What about food expenses:

would they increase or decrease? Would he experience any changes in his body? Would other family members see changes?[22]

During Dr. Greene's experiment with "going organic," not only did he and his family get answers to their questions, but integrating organically grown food into his and his patients' lives became a key mission for him. Over time, his and his family's cautious but committed beginnings gave birth to covering "all things organic" on Dr.Greene. com, the impressive, comprehensive, interactive, and dynamic Web site he created in collaboration with his wife. Visit the site and you'll also find "Dr. Greene's Organic Rx" for parents and their children; an introduction to his active involvement with organic organizations; and his award-winning books, which he wrote to show new parents how to raise and feed "baby green." Explains Dr. Greene:

> With organic foods becoming more available, people are asking me all the time, which are the most important foods to buy organic? And it's a good question, because every bite of food we eat is an investment in our vitality and in the planet. Or it's a debt we're taking out. Or often times, both. I want to help you make your investment really count. That's why I created Dr. Greene's Organic Prescription."[23]

Dr. Greene's Rx is his thoroughly researched list of the top ten organic foods that can make a huge difference in your health, your family's health, and the health of the planet. He's quick to point out that his list differs from another list of foods-to-be-avoided with which you may be familiar: twelve fruits and vegetables many of us eat that, when tested by the United States Department of Agriculture (USDA), were contaminated with pesticides.[24] "It's a great list," says Dr. Greene, but "there's no discrimination made between which pesticides are the most toxic and which ones are less so." Dr. Greene's' list, on the other hand, takes the most toxic pesticides into account—and more. His "top 10" lists organic foods that are more nutrient-dense, reduce exposure not only to pesticides but to synthetic hormones and antibiotics in food, do not contain genetically modified seed or cloned animals, and avoid the use of petroleum-based chemical fertilizers that contribute to global warming.[25]

Here is Dr. Greene's "top 10" list of organic foods, which he describes as "a way to go organic at your own pace."[26] They are based on the degree to which you and your family could avoid health-threatening pesticides, hormones, antibiotics, genetically modified food, cloned animals, and chemical fertilizers by choosing *organic* forms of foods that are generally highly problematic. Listed in order of their toxic potential, they are: milk, potatoes, peanut butter, baby foods, catsup, cotton (cottonseed oil), apples, beef, soy, and corn. Because these so often contain substances that could harm your health, you should be careful to select organic versions of these products.

As more and more Americans become interested in "going organic" (often at the urging of their children) more and more acres in the U.S. have been devoted to growing organic food, "but now it's up to us," says Dr. Greene. For his part, his "top 10" list has been voted "best pediatric site," "one of the most influential forces in healthcare IT," and more.[27] His site also gives interactive chats with personal access to his dietary and health wisdom. He has also published two "baby green" books ("to help parents teach their kids to enjoy healthy foods, even before they're born"). But he's contributing even more to enhancing health through organics through The Organic Center and its Mission Organic 2010, an innovative campaign with the goal of healthier people and a healthier planet by increasing the consumption of organic food from 3 percent (its current level) to 10 percent by 2010.[28]

Former U.S. Surgeon-General Dr. Julius Richmond has said of Dr. Greene's book, *Feeding Baby Green*: "What's in this book could change the trajectory of children's health."[29] That is the exact point and purpose of Dr. Greene's work: go green and choose organic foods as often as possible, and you're taking a big step toward turning around the pandemic of ailments plaguing us and our children, ailments that are increasingly linked to a diet of conventionally grown and raised food. On the other hand, Dr. Greene's "top 10" organic prescription leads to the *antidote* for today's traditional diet: vibrant good health[30, 31]

4

The desire for their children, Jake and Eliza, to experience the realness that comes from living on a farm was enough to convince Malea and Edward Balmuth that they'd have to move. Malea, who grew up in Robinson, Texas, had spent her childhood and teen years on her dad's farm, delighting in its abundant vegetable garden. As a matter of fact, the garden was such a integral part of her life that Malea still embraces it—so much so that she and her family would drive from their home in Fort Worth, where they lived at the time, to her father's house twice each week to garden and enjoy the harvest. But the 200-or-so-mile-long round-trip drive was time-consuming. So when their children were about six years old, the family started to look for property that would enable them to create their own back-to-the-land living—which, of course, would be filled with farm-fresh food and a way of life that differed markedly from the urban lifestyle. But there was more behind their need to move from their home in Fort Worth to a family farm: "We wanted our children to experience nature. To know what it means to connect to the earth. To raise animals and grow vegetables," says Malea. Pausing, she adds, "And by growing our own produce and raising farm animals, we also wanted them to learn to be self-sufficient."[32]

In December 2005, their dream began to take shape when they found a property in the country that would become their future farm. Located in Hood County between Granbury and Fort Worth, the 21 acres they discovered—with its 6-acre spring-fed lake—embodied Malea and Edward's vision of growing and raising food on their own land. The chlorine-free clean water meant that the children could swim in the lake. Not surprisingly, given the size of the property, creating the farm and vegetable garden they envisioned would be a challenge for each member of the family. For instance, because of the poor quality of the soil, they had to amend the soil and add organic matter. To do this, "my father [Calvin Scherwitz] hauled in seven dump-trailer loads of llama manure," says Malea. Calvin's work was well worth the effort, because now when the family wants a salad, they go outside and pick the ingredients. And not only are the vegetables that they can enjoy year-round nutrient-dense, flavor-filled, herbicide-free, and organic, their herb garden too is filled with fresh rosemary, lavender, basil, thyme, oregano, lemon balm, and more.

The Balmuth family eats vegetables based on two growing seasons: spring and autumn. In late winter, they plant cool-weather vegetables that can withstand light frost, such as potatoes, onions, radishes, broccoli, and cabbage. Then in late April through May, they harvest these vegetables. When the weather warms in early spring, they plant heat-friendly vegetables, ranging from tomatoes, corn, squash, okra, and bell peppers to string beans, sweet potatoes, cucumber, and eggplants; fruit such as cantaloupe and watermelon also become part of the summertime harvest. "In September, we go back to the cooler season vegetables," says Malea, "planting lettuce and greens, which we harvest through March." This cornucopia of leafy vegetables includes mustard, kale, spinach, and Swiss chard. Reflects Malea, "For us, living with nature and with the cycles of the seasons feels right."

What also "feels right" is the demanding job of staying on top of a lot of details to keep the garden growing, and to care for the farm's food animals: 27 Nubian and Minimancha dairy goats and about 50 chickens. "When we first moved here, Jake was allergic to cow's milk. So one of our goals was to find a dairy source for him that he could enjoy," says Malea. Today, not only are Jake's allergies better, but everyone benefits from—and takes delight in—the goat milk. "The family uses it to make yogurt, cheese and kefir," says Malea. "And the ice cream we make with it—with additions of maple syrup, vanilla, and arrowroot—has become a family favorite."

As gratifying as the fresh food is, daily roles, chores, and responsibilities still lie at the heart of the farm's success. If you were to walk through the Balmuth farm early in the morning, you might see Eliza feeding the cats and dog, while Jake rounds up the goats for milking. Malea offers this scenario about a typical day on the farm:

> I'm the "overseer" in that I keep track of everything that has to be done. Right now we're milking three goats. Jake brings the goats to the milking stand in the morning. Eliza washes the bags to prepare them for milking, and when we're finished, Jake takes the "milkers" back to the field. After I strain the milk, I decide what we're going to do with it. Drink the milk? Make yogurt? If we have extra eggs from the chickens on a particular day, will Eliza make flan? Before the day begins, I also let out our free-range chickens for the day. If any of the eggs they lay are dirty, I boil them and give them back to the chickens for protein; nothing goes to waste. We mix our own chicken food, because this is the best alternative to using processed grains. To hold our grains, Edward built a huge wooden grain-hopper that's similar to the bulk food bins you'll find in many grocery stores. With eleven sections and little sliding doors, ours is eight feet long, four-and-a-half feet high, and one-and-a-half feet deep. We all take care of the animals. The children are responsible for changing the chicken water every day, and gathering the eggs—which is typically about one-and-a-half dozen each day. On the weekends, Edward cleans out the goat barns. Any manure we have is put into the compost pile, which we use to enrich the soil in our vegetable garden. All of us need to complete our tasks because lives—both of the animals and vegetables growing in our garden—are depending on it.

On the other side of the chores is the delicious fresh fare the hard work provides—sometimes in unexpected ways. For instance, Malea and the children set up a bartering arrangement with a nearby neighbor who has an organic strawberry farm. "We pick the strawberries, weigh them, and enjoy them. In turn, we give our neighbor farm-fresh, free-range eggs throughout the year," explains Malea. A great math lesson for the children!

But even with such "community exchanges," life on the farm isn't always so idyllic. Consider the unwelcomed surprise Malea experienced this October, about a month after she had planted seeds for salad greens in her vegetable garden. Because the family eats seasonally, they especially look forward to the first tomato; the first salad greens; the bountiful salad they can make from their vegetable garden in autumn and early spring. With such culinary anticipation, Malea takes careful precautions to protect the seeds and seedlings from unwelcomed "visitors." For instance, after preparing the beds and planting the fall greens seeds, she covers them with a fabric row cover; to further protect them, she blocks off the area with a portable fence. Reflecting on the special precautions she takes, Malea explains that "we have this one chicken that's always trying to find her way in."

About a month after her hard work getting the garden ready, the day arrived when the season's first salad greens could be harvested. In preparation, Malea made feta cheese and buttermilk from the goat milk, and she planned to make ranch dressing. But first, "I took my basket outside to harvest the greens, but instead of salad greens, I find this chicken and her rooster and hen friends; they had devoured most of the lettuce patch; at least all the lettuce that was ready. I fussed at the chicken." Then, putting her frustration aside, she returned to the patch and watered it. "I knew it would grow again."

Such setbacks are more than balanced by the unadulterated delight the family takes in food preparation, cooking . . . and of course, eating and enjoying the fruits of their efforts on the family farm. For instance, feeling somewhat lonely one day—largely because her unique lifestyle isn't shared by a community—Malea felt especially motivated to connect with her family by sharing a family meal they would create together. What would that special dish be? Lasagna—and they would invent it from the available food on their farm.

For starters, Jake made some mozzarella cheese from goat milk, while Malea took its byproduct, whey, and made ricotta cheese. At the same time, Eliza—who loves to bake—made fresh egg-based lasagna noodles with help from the family's pasta maker. To do this, she blended freshly ground spelt flour the family had purchased from a nearby grist mill with their own eggs. For the sauce, they turned to the tomato sauce Edward had canned in the summertime, made from yellow and red tomatoes grown in the vegetable garden. What else was added to the special dish? "We picked basil from the herb garden, as well as some Italian parsley," says Malea. Then they put the dish together and baked it. Everyone was more than ready for dinner. "When we ate the lasagna, it was truly amazing," Malea says.

> It tasted alive; special. Every ingredient was fresh and filled with flavor. Perhaps it also tasted exceptional because we had grown the ingredients on the farm, and each of us had contributed something from the farm to the lasagna dish. In retrospect, I suppose it comes down to a matter of both flavor *and* feeling—a feeling of being alive. After all, more than is typical, the dish connected us to what we do every day and to what is important in our lives: the connection to each other, the food, the land, and our home. This particular meal reminded us *why* we do what we do. It feels right.

Their farm-raised food also "felt right" to the judges who awarded Jake, Eliza, and Malea various awards, such as honoring them as "grand champions" for their cherry tomatoes in the 2007 Hood County Fruit and Vegetable Show.[33] Their first win wasn't a fluke, because the next year, they won the highest prize level for growing the widest range of entries. Speculates Malea about the win: "We do biodynamic agriculture, and that makes a difference." Indeed, it would. Developed in the early 20th century by Rudolf Steiner, biodynamic agriculture was the first ecological farming system. Over time, it has evolved into a specialized holistic method of organic farming, with an emphasis on the interrelationship among crops and livestock, recycling of nutrients, soil maintenance, and the health and well-being of crops and animals. With such an integrated farming philosophy, the farmer is also part of the whole.[34]

Today, at a time when the standard American diet is at the center of an enormous storm because of its link to poor health, it's easy to forget the significant role that true food-centered parents like Malea and Edward can play. Growing up with parents committed to giving them a set of food-related skills that enable them to plant, grow, harvest, raise, prepare, cook, and eat real food, Eliza and Jake aren't familiar with processed and junk food products that make up too much of America's diet. To highlight the contrast between the Balmuth's' philosophy of fresh whole food as compared to typical American fast-food fare, Malea shared this telling story:

> Not too long ago, Jake and Eliza were in a group with some other children. During this time, the adult in the group asked some food

questions: "Who likes pizza? Who likes chicken fingers? Who likes hamburgers?" All the children raised their hand—all except Eliza and Jake. Then she asked, "Who likes gazpacho?" a soup made of chopped tomatoes, cucumbers, onions, garlic, oil, and vinegar, that is served cold? In response, *only* Eliza and Jake raised their hands.

Reflects Malea: "We've become used to our own vegetables and eggs, and to making our own cheese. When we have animal foods, it comes from grass-fed beef or free-range chickens that are additive- and hormone-free. More and more, we prefer to eat the food that comes from our garden and farm animals. This is because everything that comes out of the garden tastes so much better than pre-prepared or packaged food." Clearly, Malea and Edward are raising children who are highly knowledgeable about real food—what it is, how it grows, and how to prepare, cook, and enjoy it. As parents, they care a lot about this, because they know it will make a difference in the family's quality of life, and in their children's well-being, now and in the future.

5

The concept of a "hands-on" education takes on a new dimension for students majoring in the nation's first organic agriculture program at Washington State University (WSU). Depending on where they are in their course work, at any one time, students may be found on WSU's four-acre certified organic teaching farm, planting, growing, tending, and harvesting vegetables, fruit, herbs, and flowers. Or perhaps they're distributing the organic food they've harvested to the on-campus food service, local food banks, and local farmers' markets. Or possibly they're focusing their efforts on the exchange-like arrangement they have with a hundred members of their community-supported agriculture (CSA) program. The organic farming major is unique in yet another way: Whether they're studying organic animal and dairy production, economics, marketing, crop production, food science, pest management, or soil management—whatever the topic, students have the option of tailoring their "hands-on" work to their particular area of interest.[35]

Training students in all things organic is an idea whose time has come. When the WSU program was approved in June 2006 by the Higher Education Coordinating Board in Washington, U.S. sales of organic food and beverages had already grown from under $4 billion annually in 1997 to $13.8 billion.[36] By 2008—just three years later—sales were projected to surpass $25 billion.[37] With such consumer interest in organics, what was seen as a niche market for decades, promises to turn from "trend" to "the norm" in the 21st century. And as we discussed in pediatrician Alan Greene's "organic Rx" section above, the growing interest in organic food is also reflected in The Organic Center's "Mission Organic 2010" campaign, which has the goal of healthier people and a healthier planet by increasing the consumption of organic food, from its current level of 3 percent to 10 percent by 2010.[38, 39]

"The organic agriculture major is a natural outcome of the growth of organic food," said John Reganold, director and founder of WSU's organic farming major.[40] As a Regents Professor of soil science and agroecology who specializes in sustainable agriculture, Reganold was acutely aware of the groundswell of interest in organic food. He also discerned that while interest in the organic food sector was growing, enrollment in traditional agriculture degree programs was diminishing, and he wanted more students studying agriculture and food production. Such statistics meant that organic food farmers and marketers did not and would not have enough people to work in the burgeoning field and needed more employees knowledgeable about the unique techniques used in organic agriculture. For Reganold and his colleagues, the solution was clear: offer an organic farming major. "'Part of the reason I wanted to have a major . . . wasn't just that students were interested, but it would also be a great job market,'" concurs Reganold.[41]

If organic agriculture appeals to students because of expanding economic possibilities, use of natural fertilizers, respect for farmland, concern for farm animals, and caring about quality vegetables and fruits—the consumer may have other considerations: the perception that organically grown food is healthier. But is it?

Although many of us know that conventionally grown food forms the core of commercial and familiar food products sold in grocery stores, fast food chains, and most restaurants, what is less known is that the vitamin and mineral content of these common foods have declined over time in both the U.S.[42] and the United Kingdom.[43] The declining nutrient levels in much of the U.S. food supply are due to what agronomists call the "dilution effect,"[44, 45] meaning, nutrient content in food has been weakened in direct proportion to higher yields based on a half-century of plant breeding and ever increasing use of fertilizers and pesticides.[46]

What about organic food? How does its nutrient content compare to commercially grown animal- and plant-based foods? Is it really healthier? Or is organic food only *perceived* as healthier? Since a review of the scientific studies comparing organically and conventionally grown plant-based foods hadn't been done since 2003,[47,48] it was time to find out. To put the plan into action, The Organic Center produced a 2008 study in collaboration with professors from the University of Florida's Department of Horticulture and three academics from Washington State University, including horticulturalist Preston Andrews.

The question the scientists posed was this: Are plant-based organic foods nutritionally superior to conventionally grown vegetables, fruits, etc.? To find out, the scientists looked at nutrient levels in 236 matched pairs of organically versus conventionally grown foods. At the same time, they controlled for such variables as soils, climate, plant genetics, irrigation systems, nitrogen levels, and harvest practices. When the scientists compared the two growing methods, they did, indeed, find that organic foods have more nutrients. And the difference was substantial: organic plant-based foods had higher levels of eight of eleven nutrients studied; and they also had significantly greater amounts of two naturally occurring, health-promoting substances called *polyphenols* and *antioxidants*.

As a matter of fact, on average, the study revealed that organic foods have a 25 percent higher concentration of eleven vitamins and minerals than their conventionally grown counterparts. "The hopeful impact of this study," Andrews said in an interview, is that it could lead to "a more nutrient-dense food supply throughout the world." And it can help *all* farmers, because they "can know what aspects of organic farming contribute to higher nutrient contents." Empowered with this knowledge, organic farmers can "build a better food supply."[49]

To date, the impact of organic farming methods and its link to superior nutritional quality has focused mostly on plant-based organic foods. But a comprehensive review on grass-fed cattle suggests that they produce meat that is leaner than conventional cattle that have been fattened up with grains and hormones. In addition, while there are small amounts of healthful omega-3 (the "good" fat) in both grass-fed and conventional beef, the grass-fed cattle produce a bit more.[50-52]

What both plant- and animal-based foods that have been grown and raised organically have in common is this: *Organic food is unequivocally higher in health-enhancing nutrients* than its conventionally grown counterparts, and most of it is almost or completely *free of pesticides, herbicides, fertilizers, antibiotics, genetic modifications, and other toxic additives* that contribute to chronic diseases.

Organic. Sustainable. Grass fed. Free-range. Local. Green. Each "food pioneer" you've met in this chapter has integrated foods into their lives that hold the timeless genetic secret to health and well-being. As with the "food pioneers" you just met, the next chapter is also pioneering in that it merges dietary wisdom that served humankind well for hundreds of thousands of years with state-of-the-art nutritional science and gene-health discoveries. We created the "10 Green-Gene Food Guidelines" to give you the scientifically sound nutritional insights, skills, and tools you need to ignite the mechanisms that lead to health and healing. In this way, the nutrition guidelines you're about to discover redefine the role of food and eating in your life, as well as the concept of what it means to eat healthfully and optimally.

There are yet more benefits: the "10 Green-Gene Guidelines" provide a genuine alternative to the eating-by-number, rigid and restricted diet and "food product" mentality that is contributing to—instead of turning around—the plague of obesity and other chronic food-related health conditions, such as heart disease, diabetes, and many cancers. In short, with the nutrition guidelines that follow, we are inviting you to become your own "food pioneer." All it takes is making simple changes in your food choices—a shift in what you eat each day. With these new and essential ingredients of dietary self-care, you will have the nutritional tools you need to enhance the health of your cells and genes, and in this way, re-create your health destiny.

Chapter 9

TEN GREEN-GENE
FOOD GUIDELINES

The original meaning of the word "diet" meant "way of life." In time, it came to mean a prescribed, regimented way of eating. Our Green-Gene Guidelines are based on the initial definition of dieting, for they are a way of life and eating that support the fundamental heart of this book: nutritional epigenetics. Our passion for this emerging new science might best be explained by science writer David Shenk, who describes it as a "new paradigm" that is "perhaps the most important discovery in the science of heredity since the gene."[1] Realizing how timely and newsworthy it is, *Time* magazine featured an article on epigenetics on its cover (January 18, 2010).[1] And an article in the prestigious *Journal of the American Medical Association* has called it "the medicine of the future."[2] At the same time, the National Institutes of Health (NIH) have poured $190 million into a nationwide initiative to discover how epigenetic dynamics control genes. The age of epigenetics has arrived. Yet the field is so new that there is no place to turn to find practical "how to" information about what—and how—to eat to live up to our epigenetic potential. That is—not until the "10 Green-Gene Food Guidelines" we've created for you in this chapter.

I

Because there's much dissonance between what we eat now and the foods we evolved eating, tapping into the power of food to reset genes for health and healing will make more sense if we begin by "reintroducing" you to your epigenome. Recall that in "Epigenetics: A Family Affair . . . and Fare," you met Swedish scientist Lars Bygren and British geneticist Marcus Pembrey, who recently made the paradigm-shifting discovery that our cells contain an epigenome that tells genes to switch on or off. A poor diet can inappropriately switch genes on or off—or worse still, permanently switch them on or off. On the other hand, a good diet can repair the switches, making them flexible to circumstances so that they switch on or off as needed to keep our health in balance.

Such a discovery is both revolutionary and heretical. Why? Because since Charles Darwin wrote *On the Origin of Species* 150 ago, it's been a scientific given that, through natural selection, genetic changes take place over many generations and through thousands of years. But the amassed evidence that is creating the new field of epigenetics changes this paradigm, for it is revealing that our environment—especially diet (but also stress and other elements of lifestyle)—not only influences our genetic code and the genes we pass on to our progeny, but the food and calories we consume each day can create immediate, epigenetic-driven patterns of response, which, like traits, can be long-lasting.

We saw the power of almost immediate epigenetic changes in the chapter "It's the Lifestyle, Stupid!" when we discussed state-of-the-art scientific studies showing that not only diet, but also exercise, stress management, and social support have the power to ignite lightening-quick epigenetic changes. We saw a similar (albeit, somewhat slower) dynamic in our chapter on epigenetics ("Epigenetics: A Family Affair . . . and Fare") when we revealed that the diet of one generation of grandparents created epigenetic changes that were passed on to their grandchildren, making them more susceptible to obesity, diabetes, heart disease, and a shortened lifespan. We saw this epigenetic phenomenon yet again in "'Nourishment' Now," when manmade chemicals in food consumed by parents switched genes on and off, ultimately leading to reproductive problems in both sons and daughters in a single generation. We also discussed the other side of the food-gene-health equation in "Curtailing Cancer: Epigenetics in Action," with the discovery that in only a few months, diet and other lifestyle changes can actually "silence" genes that may lead to prostate cancer.

In other words, the paradigm-shifting reality of epigenetics reveals that diet is more—much more—than (say) a way to lose weight, lower the odds of heart disease, or manage diabetes. Rather, it tells us that our DNA is not our health destiny; that the health tendencies we think we inherited from our parents are not written in stone. Instead, we now know that the foods we eat each day give us the power to create almost instant, systemic, long-lasting changes by giving genes the flexibility to enhance health. Put simply, we are not victims of our genes. If anything, our genes are victims of the food we eat and other lifestyle choices we make each day.

2

The sound diet plan and easy-to-follow guidelines you're about to discover will demystify the optimal way to eat to activate genes that promote health and healing, and in turn, a healthier life. Accomplishing this goal calls for nothing short of reclaiming the "green-gene" nutrition heritage that has served our genes and humankind for millennia. What is green-gene nutrition? It is an evidence-based approach to food, nutrition, diet, and eating, based on foods that contain the optimal and natural balance of nutrients that can restore our genes' youthful responsiveness and flexibility, and in turn, lead to health and healing. Also, our green-gene nutrition guidelines are based on three worldviews about food and diet: an integration of research findings from today's nutritional, biological, and genetic sciences; ancient Paleolithic (beginning 2.5 million years ago) and late Paleolithic (12,000 to 50,000 years ago) nutrition; and the foods we eat that emerged more recently (between 5000 and 12,000 years ago) during the Neolithic Revolution, which we told you about in "Food, Genes, and Health Over Time."

With green-gene nutrition as our base, we are reexamining and redefining optimal eating within the context of the types of foods and proportions of nutrients our genes evolved on and which—as we've seen in study after study throughout this book—today's Western nutritional, biological, and genetic sciences are validating. For example, recall that in "Food, Genes, and Health Over Time" we paid a lot of attention to the key nutrients in the Paleolithic diet. Then we compared the Paleolithic proportions of protein, carbohydrates, fat, and types of fat to the amounts in today's highly processed, denatured, imbalanced, fast- and pre-prepared foods that many Americans eat each day. We did this to highlight the dissonance between the foods and nutrients our genes need to keep us healthy compared to the proportion of these nutrients in the diet many of us eat today.

But we're not alone and lost at sea with this disparity. We have our genes. Trying to help us out of such clashing nutritional disharmony, our epigenome is continually attempting to compensate. But without the nutrients they need to do their job to protect us, our genes are either turned on or off inappropriately. In other words, a healthy epigenome is one that can stay flexible, turning on and off in response to each environmental input (such as diet), whereas an unhealthy epigenome gets "stuck" with switches that are permanently turned on or off. In turn, our epigenome is unable to do its job and respond both to our internal biological needs or external environmental influences.

What we've discovered throughout this book is that the health effects of a poor diet are worse, much worse, than we ever realized. We know this, because through epigenetic mechanisms from infancy to old age, our genes "remember" how they've been treated. This means that if you mistreat your genes through poor diet while you're young, this mistreatment will come back to haunt you when you're older by making you more prone to illness. And not only does this impact you and your health, when your genes aren't given what they need to be truly nourished and thrive, the gene "memory" may be passed on if you have children. We saw this exact epigenetic dynamic with Dr. Francis Pottenger's three generations of cats, some of whom were fed well, and others poorly; and again with grandparents and their grandchildren in the far northern region of Överkalix, Sweden at the turn of the 20th century. And we saw this yet again with the work of Dr. Weston Price, who documented the detrimental health effects that manifested in a single generation when Australian Aboriginal children who thrived for millennia on a hunter-gatherer diet were exposed to a denatured, industrialized diet. We think this dynamic is a key reason why more and more children as young as six, seven, or eight years old are being diagnosed with such "diseases of civilization" as obesity and diabetes and why, for the first time in generations, the current generation is expected to have a shorter lifespan than their parents.[3]

Surely the link between the highly processed, Western, fast-food diet and ongoing ailments in both adults and children has been well-documented. We believe there's more, though, to the manifestation of disease in such young children today based on what they eat each day. Given what we've been discovering in this book, isn't it likely that the epigenetic changes created by today's denatured diet—the diet on which many of today's parents were raised, the diet many adults and parents still eat today and continue to feed their children—has created the epigenetic tendency for obesity, diabetes and more, in both themselves and their children?

Given the unsavory link between poor diet and the expression of genes that make us susceptible to poor health, it's heartening to know that the epigenetic story also works the other way. In other words, while a poor diet can create inflexible genes that are unable to switch on or off when needed, we believe that consuming high-quality *real* food, which contains the naturally occurring ratio of nutrients our body needs, can help our genes regain and retain flexibility and in turn restore their ability to protect our health.

When you think about it, the remarkable ability of the body to recover over and over again is quite amazing. Clearly, we can turn around poor health in a short period of time when our genes and body are given the nourishment they need (more specifically, were intended to eat). Actually, this is exactly what nutrition researcher Kerin O'Dea discovered when she designed a brilliantly simple study with ten full-blood Australian Aborigines. Original hunter-gatherers who had been consuming a processed Western diet while living in an urban area, they were asked if they would agree to return to their traditional homeland in an isolated region of northwest Australia, and then live on the traditional hunter-gatherer fare that had been their main food for millennia. Middle-aged, overweight, and diabetic from the Western diet they'd been living on, they agreed to return to their original dietary roots and lifestyle in the coastal and inland bush for seven weeks. Such an agreement meant their diet would change—instantly—from mostly white flour and white rice, sugar, powdered milk, cheap fatty meat, potatoes, onions, and a limited amount of fresh fruits and vegetables, to freshwater fish and shellfish, lean birds, kangaroo, grubs (the fatty larvae of local insects), turtle, crocodile, kangaroo, yams and other vegetables, figs, and honey.[4] Here's how O'Dea describes other elements of the Native Aboriginal diet: "A detailed analysis of food intake . . . revealed a low-energy intake (1200 kcal/person/day). Despite the high contribution of animal food to the total energy intake (64%), the diet was low in total fat (13%) due to the very low fat content of wild animals."[4]

Over the course of the seven weeks, all lost weight steadily, and their biomarkers for diabetes (such as postprandial glucose clearance and fasting plasma insulin concentration) also improved. Perhaps the title of O'Dea's research article on the study best describes the results: "Marked improvement in carbohydrate and lipid metabolism in diabetic Australian aborigines after temporary reversion to traditional lifestyle."[4] As telling, since O'Dea's experiment, similar studies with Native Americans and native Hawaiians have produced comparable results.

3

So that you too can enhance your health by returning to your evolutionary dietary roots, we have created "how to" guidelines. As you look over the guidelines, keep in mind that they take on even more importance than (say) eating to lose weight or lowering cholesterol levels. Follow them and you will, indeed, lose weight, improve cholesterol profiles . . . and more. But you'll achieve even more benefits, for we're suggesting nutrient-dense foods, with minimal contamination, and in the balanced proportions that respect the initial integrity of our DNA as it evolved.

In this way, the Green-Gene Guidelines are not only about what to eat but also about how to eat to activate "gene health." As you'll see, the ten guidelines are a synthesis of the sound scientific studies discussed throughout this book.

1. Eat fresh whole food in its natural state as often as possible. Our ancient evolutionary diet brought a food lifestyle that ranged from lean wild meat to fat-filled marine mammals; fish; shellfish; tree nuts; vegetables; roots, leaves, and stems; fruit; berries; and occasional bird eggs. With the evolution of the relatively recent Neolithic Era, cultivated fruits, vegetables, whole grains, legumes (beans and peas), and nuts and seeds, were added to the human diet, while domesticated animals created an abundance of grass-fed beef, goats, and sheep; free-range fowl and outdoor pigs; milk, cheese from grass-fed cows, goats, and sheep; and eggs from free-range chickens, ducks, and geese. What all these foods have in common is that they are fresh and whole. Compared to today's industrialized diet, these fresh whole foods contain a balanced proportion of macro-nutrients (protein, carbohydrates, and fats) and micro-nutrients (vitamins, minerals, phytochemicals, and so on) on which our genes—and health—thrived.

2. Eat a wide variety of foods. Whether our ancient ancestors sat around the fire savoring their wild catch-of-the-day depended on whether hunters successfully procured meat from their day's hunt. Based on recent hunter-gatherer cultures, physician and anthropologist S. Boyd Eaton guesstimates that "daily success rates vary considerably, from over 75 percent for the Aché of Paraguay to around 25 percent for the !Kung San of Africa's Kalahari"; some hunters might return empty-handed. When meat was successfully hunted or a carcass was found, locale would have dictated whether choices ranged from wild and lean buffalo, boar, and deer, to venison, kangaroo, or zebra. In colder, coastal climates, fish and marine mammals, such as walrus, whales, seal, and so on, were dietary staples.

Except for the most extreme environments such as the Arctic, gatherers (usually women and children) could be counted on to acquire the day's bounty. Indeed, a day of foraging typically produced a staple of between 10 and 20 vegetables that were often supplemented with more than 60 harder-to-find vegetables. The time of year and season also played a key role in what was available for harvesting. Whether the gatherers found leaves, fruit, nuts, beans, tubers, bulbs, berries, and seeds, or stalks, roots, wild fruit, fungi, and edible flowers, the harvest was diverse.[5] Whatever comprised the day's fare—which might range from 25 to 30 pounds for a group—the fruits and vegetables were shared with immediate families and other members of the community.

Such a variety of fresh food is a far cry from the limited number of fruits and vegetables most Americans consume today (even when you add popular French fries as a vegetable). And the lean, wild, chemical-free animal foods on which we evolved are quite a contrast to the additive-laden processed lunch meat products (sliced and packaged ham, bologna, spam, etc.) that are a "side effect" (byproduct) of conventional animal foods.[6] To give your epigenome the nutrients it needs to encourage health and healing, commit to consuming an abundance of varied fresh, whole foods each day. Green-Gene guideline #1 can give you more ideas about how to get started.

3. Select organic, grass-fed, free-range, local and sustainable foods whenever possible. Organic. Grass-fed. Free-range. Locally raised. Sustainable. A lexicon of words have entered our food supply that didn't exist not too long ago. What's behind these relatively new food-related concepts? The "green" movement. With its focus on natural, environmental balance, it has been growing forcefully over the past decade. Why are we including these concepts in our Green-Gene Guidelines? Because a natural, balanced environment brings us closer to the type and quality of foods and the naturally occurring balance of nutrients humans consumed— naturally and as a way of life—for millennia. In other words, consuming organic, grass-fed, free-range, local, and sustainable foods leads us back to the food our ancestors— and genes—took for granted.

In contrast, most of the conventional animal foods we consume today come from feedlots that use antibiotics, hormones, and other chemicals in their feed and animals. And these chemicals have made their way into the conventional meat and dairy most of us eat. Add pollutants and toxicants sprayed on fruits and vegetables; byproducts of slaughterhouse waste that are in our water; genetically modified organisms (human-designed genetic changes in a plant or animal) that have infiltrated corn and soy especially; highly processed oils and grains; and a huge imbalance of nutrients both added to and taken out of food, and you have a "chemical cuisine" recipe for epigenetic disaster.

Here's a mini-primer for choosing foods that can help you optimize your diet; choices you can make each day that can serve as a guide for the Green-Gene Guidelines:

GO ORGANIC. To maintain the integrity of the food, organically produced foods are made without antibiotics, synthetic hormones, genetic modification, sewage sludge, irradiation, artificial ingredients, and preservatives; organic producers also exclude cloning animals. Look for the United States Department of Agriculture "USDA Organic" seal that says "100% Organic" or for the USDA seal on food with ingredients that are 95 percent organic. If 70 percent of ingredients are organic, they may be listed on the label.[7]

To find out if produce without the USDA organic seal is organic, former chef and cookbook author Jay Weinstein suggests checking the Product Look Up Code (PLU) on produce stickers: four digits means it's not organic; if the first number is nine, then it is organic; if the number is preceded by the number eight, it has been genetically modified. Weinstein offers these examples: conventionally grown gala apples will be 4956; organic gala apples will be 94956; and genetically modified gala apples would be 84956.[8]

Still, as you navigate your way through the supermarket, keep in mind that the "organic" and "conventional" farming picture isn't all about "good" versus "bad"; "right" versus "wrong." Consider these insights by soil and sustainable agriculture specialist David Granatstein, whom we first introduced you to in "'Nourishment' Now." With a background in organic agriculture and environmental science, when he started working in organics in the 70s, "the polarization was huge," he says. "Conventional agriculture was bad and evil; organic was good; it was black and white. Even the language is a problem. Conventional really means 'not organic', but represents a wide range of farming practices. And likewise not all organic farmers manage their operations the same."

After working in the field for years, Granatstein has found there is a large diversity of practices across farms, and that a continuum exists rather than an organic:conventional farming dichotomy. "Many 'conventional' farmers are making really significant strides in sustainability, but for them—for various reasons—organic isn't an appropriate choice; still, they are doing really good things." In the same way, "organic farmers vary in their degree of management and the environmental impacts from their farms." In other words, there's a wide spectrum; not all farmers are the same. In fact, to accommodate this spectrum,

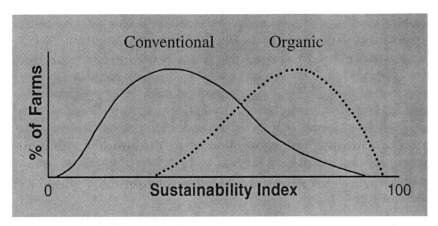

Figure 9.1 **Hypothetical Distribution of Farms on a Sustainability Index. Organic:Conventional Practices.**

Granatstein's graph shows that if you ranked farms across the country for sustainability (see the "Seek Sustainability" section, below, for more about this), with "zero" being the least sustainable and "100" representing "perfection," you would find both conventional and organic farms with both low sustainability and high sustainability. Clearly, there's a real crossover, and the degree of sustainability for both organic and conventional farms is constantly evolving. Reprinted with permission of David Granatstein.

the term "integrated farming" is sometimes used to describe farmers who are incorporating the best practices from both "organic" and "conventional" in their attempt to improve profitability and stewardship. For instance, both organic and conventional farms may—or may not—implement biological pest control, compost, cover crops, reduced tillage, and precision nitrogen management to naturally replenish their soils. Another key concept to keep in mind is that while farms that utilize an integration of best practices may not undergo organic certification, other labels identify their stewardship practices. A sampling: Food Alliance, Rainforest Alliance, Salmon Safe, Certified Humane, and LIVE (Low Input Viticulture and Enology, for wines).[9]

Granatstein created the graph above (Figure 9.1), to illustrate the diversity of farms relative to sustainability and the fact that some 'conventional' farms might rate higher than 'organic' farms, since organic certification is not a guarantee of sustainability.

A close look at Granatstein's graph reveals that organic farms are more likely to be "more sustainable" than conventional farms. The graph also reflects his opinion that sustainability is a long-term goal that encompasses economics, environment, and equity—making it so all-encompassing that our agricultural systems (much less our society) may never be able to achieve full sustainability. "Still, we can measure progress toward that goal by measuring strides made by organic and other defined farming systems that are attempting to move in that direction," suggests Granatstein. To reap the rewards of the organic:conventional farming "spectrum," ask your grocer where the food s/he sells comes from, and check with local farmers and ranchers about their farming practices. Then choose foods that come from sources with the best stewardship.

GET GRASS-FED ANIMAL FOODS. Cattle are grass-eating animals by nature. Grass-fed animals graze on grass-filled pastures and ideally are also "finished" on grass during the weeks prior to processing. A grass diet is beneficial because cattle and other ruminant animals have multiple stomachs that process food in different stages. When cattle eat grass, the digestion process starts in their first stomach, which has beneficial bacteria. But when they are raised in a feedlot and fed a grain-based diet—especially corn—the grain starts an infectious process in their first stomach that can ferment and create harmful bacteria. In turn, this makes the cattle sick and dependent on antibiotics.

Unlike cattle fed a mostly grain diet, grass-fed cattle produce milk and dairy products, such as butter and cheese, that can be a rich source of fat-soluble vitamins (E, A, K_2, and beta-carotene) and minerals (such as selenium).[10] And fermented dairy products (yogurt, kefir) from pasture-fed cows can be a rich source of K_2, which may lower the odds of clogged arteries and osteoporosis.[11, 12] But there's a caveat: levels of these vitamins decrease 50 percent or more during the winter months when grass isn't available for grazing, and animals are instead fed stored, dry feed, such as hay.

CHOOSE FREE-RANGE OR PASTURED POULTRY AND EGGS. Commercially produced chickens are raised entirely indoors with tens of thousands of other chickens in close quarters. Many consumers have the perception that free-range poultry means the bird was raised happily hunting and pecking in the grass in an open field. But the reality is that because the USDA definition of "free-range" is somewhat vague, the poultry can be labeled "free range" even if outdoor time has been quite limited, or if the open field or "range," is mostly dirt. This is quite an improvement over conventionally raised chickens that are raised in windowless buildings with tens of thousands of other birds raised on grains, antibiotics, and growth hormones, or birds living in stacked cages for egg production purposes. Pastured poultry, on the other hand, is yet another growing option that is defined as follows: "Birds are kept outside (as the season and daylight permit), utilizing a movable or stationary house for shelter, and they have constant access to fresh-growing palatable vegetation"[13] and insects. To ensure you're getting optimally raised and produced poultry and eggs, ask your grocer the source of your poultry and eggs, or contact the producer directly.

BUY LOCAL. Ever since Jessica Prentice coined the term "locavore" in 2005 to describe those who consume foods harvested within a 100-mile radius, the local food movement has been building momentum. Today, the meaning of "local" ranges from growing your own food at home, to buying food grown in your immediate community, state, region, or even country. More recently, the USDA suggested that 400 miles is the actual maximum distance for a food to be local. However it's defined, the key concept is simple: locavores consume food as close to home as possible. And there's a good reason for this: the nearer to you when food is grown, the fresher it can be, and the more likely it is to be nutritious. To get started, ask yourself if it's possible for you to buy locally raised, humane, and organic meat, eggs, and dairy. If you own your home, can you grow one or more vegetables in your yard? Or can you visit local farms for produce or buy locally grown fruit at your nearby grocer? Keep in mind that a key goal is to make food choices that reduce your carbon footprint. Whatever is easiest and feasible for you, personally, is the best way to begin.

SEEK SUSTAINABILITY. Simply put, sustainably produced food means the food was grown, raised, and produced based on farming and marketing practices that are able to be maintained over the long term—that is, farmers can make a living for their family; the land can be replenished with nutrients at the same rate—or better—than nutrients that were taken out; crops can provide nutritious food for the consumer; food is produced on soil without using huge amounts of petroleum energy for tilling and fertilization; and the environment is not degraded by the farming practices.

Buying local is linked to sustainability, but they're two different concepts. This is because it's possible to eat local foods that are grown or raised in ways that do, indeed, cause harm to plant or animal foods, the environment, and to us, the consumers who eat the food. Is the food you eat based on sustainability considerations? To find out, ask your grocer, or farmers at your local farmers market, how the poultry or animal foods you're buying were raised. And consider finding out the name and location of the farm that produced the fruits and vegetables you purchase.[14]

4. Consume quality food with the proportion of protein, carbohydrates, and fats our genes adapted to over the millennia. Today's industrialized diet drastically changes the original, naturally occurring proportions of the macronutrients of protein, carbohydrates, and fats in food. This matters, because the imbalanced proportions of macronutrients in a mostly processed, denatured diet create a formula for stressing our epigenome and producing ill-health. What has caused the problem is the marriage between conventionally raised animal and plant foods and further processing by food manufacturers of refined grains (into white flour, de-germed, GMO corn, and so on), vegetable oils that are heated and denatured (which creates a health-harming imbalance of omega-6 to omega-3 fatty acids), cheap meat (such as preserved and

Nutrient	Paleolithic Diet (% total energy)	1995 – Present (% total energy)
Protein	19 – 35[a]	15.4[a]
Carbohydrates	22 – 44[a]	51.8[a]
Total Fat	28 – 58[a]	32.8[a]
Saturated Fat (SFA)	10 – 15	12
Monounsaturated (MUFA)	16 – 25	13
Polyunsaturated (PUFA)	25 – 40[b]	16.7[b]
Trans Fatty Acid (TFA)	0	2 – 3

[a] Cordain, et al., 2000.   [b] Eaton, 2006, 1–6.

Table 9.1 **Macronutrient Content of Paleolithic Diet Compared to Today's Western Diet**

processed pepperoni, bacon, and so on), poultry (such as fried chicken McNuggets), and fish (farm-raised and often fried).

Table 9.1, previous page, illustrates how the proportion of macro-nutrients has changed over time. We first showed you this as Table 6.3 in "Food, Genes, and Health Over Time," and we're showing it to you here because it provides a clear snapshot of how today's industrialized diet has created drastic changes in the proportion of macronutrients on which our genes and body evolved. In other words, compared with our Paleolithic ancestors, today's diet has too little protein, way too many carbohydrates, and an imbalance of different types of fat.

Clearly, not only has this unholy union of conventionally raised and grown food with highly processed foods changed both the proportions and quality of fats and oils in the foods we eat, it has forced us to follow a "food detour" that has lead to a diet comprised mostly of lesser amounts of high-quality protein, refined carbohydrates, and an imbalance of fats. The end result: a formula for scrambled, crippled epigenes and increased risk for a plethora of chronic diseases.

PROTEIN. We discovered in "Food, Genes, and Health Over Time" that tribes all over the planet ate a higher ratio of high-protein animals compared to plant foods than we typically do today. A closer look at Table 9.1 shows the average Western diet has about 15 percent of total calories from protein, but our ancestors consumed between 19 to 35 percent.[5] The upper end of this range is not necessarily optimal, because too much dietary protein breaks down into urea, which can stress the kidneys and can cause weakness and nausea, even death. Given this, we suggest consuming not more than 30 percent of calories from protein.

Here's another key consideration: Because animal foods (meat, poultry, fish, dairy, and so on) have more complete protein than plant-based foods (fruits, vegetables, grains, legumes, nuts and seeds), the challenge is to find animal foods that are not contaminated with environmental pollutants and which are environmentally sustainable. Not only do most factory-farmed animals contain high levels of antibiotics and growth hormones, but our inland waters are polluted with contaminants, while fish stocks have been depleted in many of our oceans. Yet another consideration to keep in mind is that proteins in cultured dairy (yogurt, kefir, etc.) are more bio-available, which means that consuming cultured dairy lowers the odds of lactose intolerance and other digestive problems.

A cost-effective way to consume quality protein with minimal or no toxins is to turn to plant sources, such as beans and legumes, nuts and seeds. Consider wild fish twice a week, natural or free-range chicken, buffalo and other game meats, and lean cuts of beef, pork, etc., because toxicants and pollutants are stored in the fat of conventionally raised high-fat foods.

CARBOHYDRATES. With the major source of carbohydrates coming from a wide variety of fruits and vegetables, our Paleolithic ancestors ate more nutrient-dense, high-fiber carbohydrates than we do today. They also ate few wild grasses (grains), which were not available in quantity until the Agricultural Revolution. As a contrast, most Americans, today, eat fewer than five servings of fruits and vegetables and instead consume a high-carbohydrate diet comprised of food products such as potato and corn chips, cookies, cake, etc., that didn't exist until relatively recently in our evolution.

Because many of us still haven't had time to adjust biologically and epigenetically to today's processed grain-based diet, many of us have gluten sensitivity. Another piece of the puzzle is that most of us eat great quantities of simple and refined carbohydrates from grains and sugar, yet because we are not geared genetically either to the quantity or quality we're consuming, eating lots of processed grains has contributed to a host of chronic illnesses such as diabetes, obesity, and gluten sensitivity. If you are gluten sensitive, avoid grains high in gluten such as wheat, and consume low quantities of other forms of whole grains, such as brown rice or quinoa; better yet, turn to vegetables and fruits for high-quality, gluten-free carbohydrates. And choose high-fiber vegetables on the low end of the glycemic index, such as leafy greens (kale, collards, lettuce), cancer-protecting cruciferous vegetables (cabbage, broccoli, cauliflower, turnips), and alliums (garlic and onions).

Another lesser known reason to avoid a carbohydrate-dense diet high in processed grains and sugar is that when you eat more than your body needs for its daily energy requirements—as most of us often do—the excess carbohydrates are converted first into triglycerides and then into saturated fats that are stored in our body as adipose tissue (body fat). In turn, this increases the odds of overweight and obesity and related ailments. Excess body fat by itself might not be a problem if the type of saturated fat that is stored from excess carbohydrate consumption were not the long-chain palmitic fatty acids—a type of saturated fat that makes platelets sticky, also has been linked to heart disease and other ailments. Surely this is yet another reason to cut back on processed grains and sugar, found in many cereals, breads, chips, candy, pastry, cakes, pies, and more?

FAT. Here's a key concept you'll need to know for optimal gene-health: Of the three macronutrients, fat is by far the most contaminated with antibiotics, hormones, persistent organic pollutants (POPs, such as PCBs, dioxins, and DDT derivatives), and insecticides, which bio-accumulate in our bodies. This is because the most potent and hard-to-get-rid-of pollutants and toxicants in our food supply are fat soluble. This means they are stored in animal fat, and in turn, our body fat when we eat animal fat. Therefore, the source and quality of animal foods you consume—such as meat, dairy, and fish—are paramount considerations for achieving gene-health.

Another key concept is this: All food has fat—even, say, lettuce and kale. For instance, the total grams of fat in kale (based on 100 grams) is 0.70. Of this, 13 percent is saturated, 7.4 percent is monounsaturated, 48 percent is polyunsaturated, and the n6:n3 ratio is 0.138:0.180 (with higher amounts of omega-3s).

Just as the fat content in food varies, our Paleolithic ancestors' diets varied considerably in fat intake. What this means to us today is this: Depending upon our personal ancestral history, we can adapt both to high or low amounts of dietary fat. For example, those in the northern latitudes, such as the Arctic, had high intakes of fat from marine mammals—up to 58 percent of total energy—which was comprised of mostly monounsaturated and polyunsaturated fats, with just 8 percent of total energy coming from saturated fat[5]. Those living inland who ate land animals consumed lower intakes of fat in the range of 20 percent to 25 percent of total calories, with saturated fat intake depending upon the season the animals were killed (animals store more fat in the warmer months when grass and other foods are plentiful). If we consider wild meat sources only, such as buffalo, caribou, seal, grouse, and warthog, 30 percent of fat was polyunsaturated, 32 percent was monounsaturated, and 38 percent was saturated.[5] At the same time, oils from plant sources were—and are—primarily monounsaturated and polyunsaturated with few exceptions such coconut and palm oil.

A closer look at Table 9.1 reveals that the proportion of saturated fats hasn't changed much over time (we're just about in the middle range of our ancestors), but the percentage of poly- and monounsaturated fats has changed drastically. Clearly, this is due to the proportion of types of fats from wild animals, which are quite different from those most of us consume today from farm-animal fats and processed fats. In other words, our ancestors' diet was mostly mono- and polyunsaturated fat with lesser amounts of naturally occurring saturated fat. This differs from the proportions of fats most of us consume today.

Surprisingly, Table 9.1 shows we are consuming less fat than the amount consumed by many of our Paleolithic ancestors (32 percent vs. 28–58 percent, respectively). At the same time, while our consumption of saturated fat (SFAs) is in the same range as our Paleolithic ancestors (12 percent vs. 10–15 percent, respectively), we are eating somewhat lower amounts of monounsaturated fat (MUFAs), but substantially less polyunsaturated fat (PUFAs).

As you can see from Table 9.1, today's diet means slightly less monounsaturated fat, and substantially less polyunsaturated fats, more omega-6 and less omega-3, and more trans fats—mostly because of re-engineered vegetable oils and shortenings hidden in baked goods and snack food. To give you some perspective, margarine, shortenings and frying fats traditionally contain up to 19 percent industrially produced trans fatty acids (TFAs).[15]

It is the change in the quality of MUFAs and PUFAs that is wreaking havoc with our epigenome and health. This is because while we are consuming fewer PUFAs, the quality of the PUFAs we consume also has changed drastically in three key ways: 1) many of the nutrients (antioxidants, fat soluble vitamins, etc.) have been processed out; 2) the high heat at which processed oils are created produces TFAs and other health-harming molecules that are alien to our bodies; 3) the heat process also destroys omega-3, which in turn, changes the ratio of omega-6 to omega-3, tipping the balance to even higher health-robbing levels of omega-6. Add the relatively high intake of TFAs to today's diet, and you have a recipe for epigenetic malfunctioning. The guidelines in this chapter can get you started on turning the tide of such imbalanced proportions, while giving you practical insights into the foods you need to eat optimally.

5. Choose *only* minimally processed oils and fats that have retained their naturally occurring proportion of nutrients. Table 9.2, opposite, reveals that we evolved on a diet high in omega-3 fats, with lesser amounts of omega-6 fatty acids. Today's processed diet—with its high omega-6, low omega-3 ratio—is the inverse. This matters, because the ratio of omega-6 to omega-3 should be as close to a ratio of 1:1 and certainly no more than 4:1. This is because a balanced omega-6 to omega-3 ratio promotes a non-inflammatory state in the body, while tilting the intake toward a higher level of omega-6 promotes an inflammatory state that leaves us vulnerable to ailments from arthritis, asthma, and

Nutrient*	Paleolithic Diet (range: grams/day)	Western Diet (range: grams/day)
Total Polyunsaturated fat	9.0 – 54.3	24.5
Omega-6 (n6)	5.2 – 20.6	22.5
Omega-3 (n3)	3.5 – 25.2	1.2
n6:n3 Ratio	0.04 – 2.8	16.7

* Eaton et al., 1998, pp. 12–23.

Table 9.2 **Paleolithic Diet vs. Today's Western Diet: A Comparison of Polyunsaturated Fat, Omega-6 and Omega-3 (grams/day)**

fibromyalgia to heart disease, diabetes, obesity, and high blood pressure. Add a diet of highly processed foods, filled with carbohydrate-dense sugar, white flour, and other processed grains, and you have a recipe for ongoing inflammation and related ailments.

The key culprit causing this pro-inflammatory, gene-health imbalance and debacle is the denatured Western diet with its high intake of highly processed vegetable oils (safflower, corn, cottonseed, soy, and so on), particularly margarine and other hydrogenated oils. This is because the processing leaves high levels of omega-6 fatty acids, which are converted into high levels of arachidonic acid (AA) in the body. Food we eat from cows fattened on grains that are high in saturated fats and loaded with omega-6s compound the omega-6 and ensuing AA overload. And it is the excessive amounts of AA and the imbalanced, high levels of omega-6 in the Western diet that contribute to our chronic inflammatory degenerative diseases.[16]

The low levels of omega-3s in most Americans' diet—which is obvious in Table 9.2, above—take on even more significance when you realize the degree to which adequate intake of omega-3s contributes to the gene-health equation. For instance, in "Diet, DNA, and Disease," we told you about recent research which has linked higher blood levels of omega-3 fatty acids to protection against cellular aging. The key mechanism: like the ends of shoelaces that keep shoelaces from unraveling, adequate omega-3s influence telomeres—the tiny units of DNA at the end of each cell's chromosomes—which play a key role in cell division, and in turn, slowing or accelerating biological age.[17]

Some quick tips to "ramp up" omega-3 levels, and to restore the balance between omega-6s and omega-3s:

· Seek the highest quality, organic, cold-pressed oils.
· Shun processed vegetables oils that have been made to have a long shelf-life.
· Avoid all trans fats and partially hydrogenated fats.
· Avoid grain-fed beef and poultry, and eggs that come from grain-fed poultry, whenever possible. This is because grain-fed animals produce imbalanced, high levels of omega-6s.
· Another tip to consider: Be sure grass-fed beef is 100 percent grass-fed, and isn't "finished" with a grain diet.

6. Choose plant and animal foods that have been grown or raised on sustainable and nutrient-rich soil. Just as our bodies need a balance of the 50-plus essential macro- and micronutrients to be healthy, the soil our food is grown on also needs complete nutrition. Nutrient-rich soil contains organic matter (humus), it's alive with organisms (worms, bacteria, etc.) that are breaking down humus into useable nutrients for roots to absorb, it has a balance of trace minerals, and it is abundant in nitrogen, potassium, and phosphorous.

When it was founded, the United States had some of the richest soil in the world, and it contributed an inestimable amount to our prosperity. With such a gift, American farmers have been among the most productive in the world. Unfortunately, during the 20th century, our soil-rich heritage began to change because of poor soil management by farmers. Soil was overworked, laid bare, made susceptible to wind and soil erosion, no longer crop-rotated, and depleted of trace minerals and other nutrients. The bottom line: minerals in soil need to be replenished by nitrogen-fixing cover crops and/or other organic matter, crop rotation, and prevention of water and wind erosion. Without these rebuilding techniques, not only is soil depleted, but nutrients won't be available in the plants grown on it; nor will nutrients be there for the animals that eat the plants.

To replenish the major nutrients of nitrogen, phosphorus, and potassium, farmers turned to chemists who developed synthetic nitrogen fertilizer from petroleum. While it promotes rapid plant growth and makes plants appear to be healthy, this is an illusion. Rather, synthetic fertilization fails to replenish the soil with life-giving organic matter and the trace minerals plants and animals (including humans) that consume them need to thrive. Enter the organic and sustainable farming movement, which makes complete soil fertility its top priority—without the use of toxic and persistent organic-polluting pesticides (POPs), weed-killing herbicides, and synthetic fertilizers. To eat optimally, eat plants and animals that were fed from nutrient-rich soil. Eating locally makes it easier, because you can talk to the farmers who grew the fruits or vegetables you're eating, and the ranchers who raised animal foods you consume.

7. Choose wild-caught fish from the least-polluted waters. Documenting his experience traveling the world in the 1930s, visiting cultures that hadn't been influenced by the denatured Western diet, Weston Price summarized his optimal eating insights this way: "I have seldom found anywhere in the world such a high percentage of physical excellence with high immunity to our modern degenerative disease as among . . . people of the South Sea Islands. Their diet practically every day consisted of eating the proteins from the animal life of the sea with the carbohydrates of their land vegetables."[18] Today, with its recommendation to consume fresh fish at least twice weekly—and vegetables each day—the scientific community is confirming what Dr. Price observed more than seven decades ago: consume a diet rich in fish and vegetables for optimal health.

The suggestion seems simple enough, but recall what we discussed in "'Nourishment' Now," when we told you about the impact pollutants and toxicants have on genes and in turn, your health. Because of this, with today's polluted waters, this Green-Gene guideline may not be as simple as it sounds. Fish and shellfish do contain high-quality protein, other essential nutrients, and omega-3 fatty acids. Yet some have high levels of (for example) organic mercury (methylmercury) that fish absorb as they feed in waters affected by industrial pollution. And it is the methylmercury that may harm an unborn baby or the developing nervous system in a young child, or accumulate in an adult over time.

In selecting fish, the challenge is to find sustainable fish populations that are not polluted with heavy metals or organic pollutants. Use the internet to check fish advisories of fish caught from inland lakes and rivers in your area. Usually smaller, younger fish are less contaminated, and if they feed on plants rather than animals they will have less bio-accumulation of organic pollutants such as PCBs and dioxins. Common fish with less contamination include haddock, hake, flounder, pollock, wild Pacific salmon, speckled trout, white fish, wild Atlantic salmon, herring, smelt, sardines, anchovies, clams, shrimp, scallops, and lobster. Examples of fish to avoid are swordfish, Albacore white tuna, shark, king mackerel, and orange roughy. And avoid farmed fish, which, like their feedlot-raised cattle and poultry "relatives," are typically fed unnatural foods in crowded conditions that make them susceptible to sickness.

8. Select, store, and prepare food in ways that preserve its nutrients. This guideline about how to choose, keep, and prepare food is often overlooked in terms of optimal eating. But be assured: how you prepare your food has a big impact on its vitamin and mineral content, and in turn, on your health. The key concept to keep in mind is this: The more food is exposed to oxygen, the faster it deteriorates (oxidizes) and loses its nutrient value. To keep it fresh and nutrient-dense, follow these guidelines.

SELECTION. It's optimal to buy smaller quantities of highly perishable produce two to three times each week, than to buy a lot once a week. Choose only food that looks fresh and refrigerate it as soon as possible.

STORAGE. The longer food is stored in the refrigerator, the more likely it is to lose its nutrient value.

- To cut down on nutrient loss, place highly perishable vegetables in the proper bins and consume them within two, maximum three, days.
- Ideally, cook paper-wrapped fresh meat and poultry the same day you purchase it, and not more than one day afterward.
- If you've purchased fish, poultry, or meat sealed in plastic, cook it as soon as possible.
- If you're freezing food, freeze it at its freshest.
- To keep the oil in raw nuts and seeds from turning rancid, store them in airtight containers in the freezer section.
- If unprocessed bottled oil, such as olive, has been opened, keep it in the refrigerator until next usage. To protect freshness, also be sure to refrigerate PUFA-rich oils and seeds, such as flax.
- Store cooked food in airtight glass containers to preserve nutrients. However, do not store or heat food in plastic containers. Clear, hard plastic is made with bisphenol-A, which leaches into

your food. We told you about the toxic effects of bisphenol-A on genes in "Diet, DNA, and Health." It is the number one, most pervasive, and toxic chemical to avoid.

PREPARATION. Overcooking food at high temperatures not only influences vitamin content; it can damage food and actually make a healthy food unhealthy.

- Do not allow any oil or fat you heat to get so hot, it smokes. This is because heating oils to smoking levels means the chemical structure has changed, rendering it both unrecognizable and harmful to our genes.
- Avoid boiling vegetables in water, because their water-soluble vitamins and other nutrients are lost to the water. Lightly steam or sauté vegetables.
- Keep in mind that grilling or char-broiling meat at high temperatures creates heterocyclic amines, chemicals that can cause cancer. Instead, try baking or slow cooking methods.
- Prepare and serve fermented vegetables, such as sauerkraut. Not only does the fermentation process increase digestibility, it provides beneficial bacteria for the gut.
- Pre-soak beans and grains (such as brown rice) in water to reduce cooking time and preserve nutrients. Soaking legumes and grains has other benefits: it leeches out gas-forming oligo-saccharides, indigestible complex sugars in the outer coating of beans, while soaking grains reduces mineral-binding phytates, molecules that attach to minerals in the digestive tract, making them unavailable to the body.

9. Drink clean water. When you turn on your faucet for drinking water, what might be in your tap water . . . besides water? The answer to this question is pivotal both to gene health and for preventing disease. For decades, agencies have known that the quality of tap water varies, depending on where you live, the source of your tap water, and the effectiveness of local treatment plants. What has also been known is that hundreds of synthetic, industrial chemicals have found their way into Americans' drinking water. At any one time, an average of 200 industrial chemicals, pesticides, and more may be in your drinking water.

In 2008, the concern about pollutants in U.S. tap water was compounded with the discovery by the Environmental Working Group (EWG) that 41 million Americans are also exposed to low-level mixtures of pharmaceuticals in every glass of water they drink. How did medications, ranging from antibiotics and hormones in birth control pills to anti-depression medication, contribute to contaminated drinking water? Most are drug residues from pills we take. While the body absorbs most medication, what isn't absorbed is excreted in urine.[19] Add the undependable quality and contaminants found in most bottled water, and you have chemical cocktail that creates endocrine-disrupting compounds that not only can disrupt our epigenome but can be especially harmful to infants, pregnant women, or to those with chronic health conditions.

Here is EWG's guide to safe drinking water:

· Drink and cook with filtered tap water instead of bottled water.
· Learn what's in your tap water.
· Change water filters regularly, because they can harbor bacteria.
· When you're on the go, carry water in safe containers, such as stainless steel, glass, or other non-plastic bottles. Avoid hard plastic bottles (#7), which can leach bisphenol A (BPA, a harmful plastic chemical). While pregnant, stay hydrated with safe water.
· Use safe water for infant formulas.
· For extra protection, use a whole house water filter.

10. Give regard to every aspect of the meal. In "It's the Lifestyle, Stupid!" we introduced you to the ways in which not only diet but other lifestyle "ingredients," such as exercise, stress, and social support, can switch genes on and off and in turn influence health and healing. In the same way, not only what you eat but also how, why—even with whom—

The Dirty Dozen

Consume five servings a day of the following conventionally grown "dirty dozen" fruits and vegetables and, unless they're grown organically, you'll eat an average of ten pesticides a day. To avoid pesticide-laden produce: go organic. (Source: Environmental Working Group, www.foodnews.org/walletguide.php)

X peaches	X nectarines	X lettuce
X apples	X strawberries	X grapes
X bell peppers	X cherries	X carrots
X celery	X kale	X pears

The Clean 15

You can reduce your exposure to pesticides up to 80 percent by choosing fruits and vegetables from the "clean 15" conventionally grown options, below. You may want to pay special attention to the "clean 15," especially if it's hard for you to find, or pay for, organic produce. (Source: Environmental Working Group www. foodnews.org/walletguide.php)

√ onions	√ asparagus	√ papaya
√ avocado	√ sweet peas	√ watermelon
√ sweet corn	√ kiwi	√ broccoli
√ pineapple	√ cabbage	√ tomato
√ mango	√ eggplant	√ sweet potato

you eat influences how food is metabolized and in turn, your health. Co-authors Larry Scherwitz and Deborah Kesten have identified seven eating styles that can empower you to restyle your food life by re-discovering not only what, but also how to eat, so that you can metabolize food optimally. Here is a brief overview of the seven eating styles they discovered. Each is a compilation of their published research[20] on the eating styles, as well as *The Enlightened Diet*, [21] their book on the topic. As with the other guidelines, we are proposing the seven eating styles as a way of life and eating—not as a rigid, restricted regimen.

FRESH WHOLE FOODISM. Replace a mostly fast-food, processed, denatured diet, with organic fresh whole foods such as fruits, vegetables, whole grains, beans and peas, nuts and seeds; free-range poultry and eggs; and grass-fed beef and related dairy products.

APPETITE-BASED EATING. Most of us are familiar with emotional eating—eating to soothe frazzled, unpleasant feelings, such as anxiety, anger, or loneliness; or eating to celebrate positive happenings, such as finishing a particularly challenging project. Appetite-based eating means eating when you have a positive, comfortable, natural desire for food; you're neither famished nor full.

ENJOYING FOOD. Are you a "food fretter," who counts calories, lives with a "diet mentality," and worries a lot about the "best" way to eat? Such behaviors have become normal in our culture, but they're not. Replace food fretting with enjoying food and relating to the experience of eating as one of life's most pleasurable experiences.

MINDFULNESS EATING. If you're a "task snacker," you typically eat while doing other things, such as watching TV, driving, or working at your computer. Replace task snacking with mindfulness eating, by only eating when you eat. This doesn't have to be time-consuming. For instance, if you're eating while driving, why not pull over in a nearby park and eat while enjoying some greenery and calm surroundings?

APPETIZING ATMOSPHERE. Both the psychological and the aesthetic atmosphere in which you dine hold the power to influence your psyche and the way in which you metabolize meals. Surround yourself in a healing environment when you eat by being both people-wise and atmosphere-wise. Choose serene, soothing company and surroundings when you eat.

SOCIAL DINING. The guideline to share food-related experiences with others is seemingly simple. But though we evolved eating in groups and clans around a fire, today, "solo dining" in front of the TV, while driving, or at work, is more common than not. To turn this around, take a tea or lunch break with a co-worker; have family meals as often as possible; or if you live alone, invite friends or neighbors over for a potluck once a week.

SAVOR FLAVORS. If you've ever eaten without taking the time to truly taste your food; indeed, if you sometimes don't even quite recall you've eaten—possibly because you typically eat quickly—you're not savoring flavors. To turn this around, the next time you eat, focus your attention inside your mouth. Identify various flavors—such as salty, sweet, or sour—and the ones you most enjoy.

Each Green-Gene guideline tells us there are a lot of actions you can take to switch on genes that can set health and healing into motion. To reap the rewards, follow the guidelines as often as you realistically can.

4

Let's now turn to one more aspect of the Green-Gene Guidelines, which you'll need to know about to make the most of the guidelines and to optimize the food-gene-health equation: biochemical individuality. Throughout the book, we've seen that humans can adapt to a wide range of diets and be healthy. For instance, some of our Paleolithic ancestors thrived on relatively lean wild animals and plant foods, while others, such as those living in the Far North, fared well on a diet consisting of a lot of high-fat marine mammals and relatively low vegetable intake. Since the Neolithic era, many of us have adapted to grains and dairy, while others developed gluten sensitivity or lactose intolerance in response to these food groups, respectively.

The fact that we evolved on a host of different diets means there is no ideal diet for all individuals. Rather, our genetic and family histories have programmed how our genes respond to the food we eat, and because of this, human beings have a wide range of individual biochemical differences; in other words, biochemical individuality. For example, in addition to gluten sensitivity and lactose intolerance, some of us may need a higher intake of essential vitamins and minerals than others. Because of such biochemical differences, each of us must search for the ideal diet by considering personal genetic history, health, ethnic food preferences, how your body responds to certain foods when you eat them, and by how satisfied you feel when you eat different foods. Here are some other considerations to keep in mind as you create your own ideal diet:

- Adjust your caloric intake based on your current weight and activity level (energy expenditure). If you are very active, exercise a lot, and live in a cold climate, you will burn more calories than those who are sedentary and live in warmer climates.
- Health status and healing can influence dietary needs. For instance, after surgery, or during a fast-growth period such as during infancy and adolescence, energy needs and nutrient intake requirements go up.
- If you have a short history of exposure to grains and dairy, or if you've over-consumed these foods, you're more likely to be sensitive to gluten or be lactose or casein intolerant. If so, consume small amounts or avoid them altogether.
- There are large differences in how much nutrition each of us needs to be healthy. For instance, some of us may not absorb or metabolize certain nutrients and therefore might need to compensate by eating foods with more of these nutrients or by supplementation.

To reap the rewards now, here is an overview of the ten guidelines—the key principles—of the 10 Green-Gene Food Guidelines. Look them over carefully, and familiarize yourself with them. Having an intimate understanding of each one is pivotal to optimizing gene health.

The 10 Green-Gene Food Guidelines

Here are the ten elements of the Green-Gene Guidelines, the essential principles for activating the food-gene-health link we've discussed throughout this book.

1. Eat fresh whole food in its natural state as often as possible.
2. Eat a wide variety of foods.
3. Select organic, grass-fed, free-range, local and sustainable foods whenever possible.
4. Consume high-quality food with the proportion of protein, carbohydrates, and fats our genes adapted to over the millennia.
5. Choose ONLY minimally processed oils and fats that have retained their naturally occurring proportion of nutrients.
6. Choose plant and animal foods that have been grown or raised on sustainable and nutrient-rich soil.
7. Choose wild-caught fish from the least-polluted waters.
8. Select, store, and prepare food in ways that preserve its nutrients.
9. Drink clean water.
10. Give regard to every aspect of the meal.

Each time you eat or participate in any food-related activity, remember that all ten guidelines count and that optimal nourishment includes both the familiar nutrients in food, as well as the organic, grass-fed, free-range, and "enlightened eating" nutrients missing from the food charts. We created the elements of the Green-Gene Guidelines to make it easy for you to practice them daily. For only by actually doing them each day will you be empowered to nourish your genes in the ways they are meant to be nourished.

Also, be patient with yourself: making such sweeping changes in what you eat is a process. In other words, changing your relationship to food isn't likely to happen overnight: success takes ongoing nurturing, care, and regard . . . for yourself. To enhance your odds for success and food-gene-health self-care, the next chapter, "Taking Action: If Not Now, When?" gives you still more practical strategies to integrate the elements of the Green-Gene Food Guidelines into your everyday life.

Green-Gene Food Tips

Cook smart. Our hunter-gatherer ancestors didn't cook foods at high temperatures; rather, food was typically baked or consumed raw. This means that our genes—and health—pay a price when we eat foods that are either overcooked or cooked at high heat levels. For instance, overcooking vegetables reduces their nutrient content, while high temperatures change the chemical structure of proteins, fats, and even carbohydrates. For instance, overcook food such as pasta—even whole grain pasta—and you'll increase its sugar content, and in turn, its rank in the glycemic index. To preserve the nutrient balance of cooked foods avoid overcooking or cooking at a high temperature. Some suggestions: consider poaching eggs or serving them sunny-side up instead of scrambling them in hot oil, and steam or sauté vegetables over a low flame. The most healthful step you can take toward cooking smart is this: don't heat cooking oil so much that it smokes.

Get fresh. If you find that you don't eat all the vegetables and fruits you purchase within three or four days; that you forget about them; or they age and spoil in the refrigerator bin, consider shopping for fresh fruits and vegetables twice weekly, and purchase smaller amounts.

Figure in ferments. What do sourdough bread, sauerkraut, yogurt, and cheese have in common? They're all fermented, made by the ancient process of fermentation, which occurs when lactic acid bacteria convert starch and sugar into lactic acid and alcohol and in the process make milk, grains, and fiber more digestible. Supplementing your daily diet with fresh fermented foods, which contain living microbes, provides a plethora of health benefits—mostly through the probiotics they produce that protect the gut from harmful pathogens, and increases absorption of nutrients.

Get personal. Residing within your genes are the dietary requirements and food tolerances that fit you best, personally. In other words, the foods on which you're likely to thrive are based on the genetics you inherited from your ancient ancestors and the epigenetics that were passed on from more recent relatives (such as your great-grandparents, grandparents, and your parents) when you were conceived. Because of this, just as a pair of shoes fit each person differently, there isn't a single diet that's a right fit for everyone. To create your ideal diet, ask yourself:

- What foods were available to your ancestors?
- Do you have health concerns to consider, such as lactose intolerance or gluten sensitivity?
- What's your physical activity level? (If you're quite sedentary, for instance, you might want to cut back on carbohydrate- and calorie-dense foods, especially highly processed and sweetened cookies, cakes, ice cream, and so on.)
- Do you have any ethical or health beliefs about food that influence your food choices?
- And of course, ask yourself which foods make you feel best? Once you identify them, adjust your food choices accordingly.

Consider raw dairy. Clean raw milk from grass-fed, pastured cows and goats has been swathed in controversy for more than a decade. Is it healthful and safe? Lately, the debate has moved from fringe to mainstream as more and more consumers are letting government, industry, and politicians know they want the freedom to choose between health-giving dairy of their choice and processed, pasteurized milk. Indeed, raw milk is becoming so popular that "buying clubs" have been popping up in America. If milk and dairy are typically part of your diet—and you're not lactose intolerant or allergic—consider raw dairy as an alternative.

Chapter 10

Taking Action: If Not Now, When?

The message throughout *Pottenger's Prophecy* is clear: a change in our food choices—a shift in what we eat each day—holds the timeless genetic secret not only to your health status, but to the health of generations to come—indeed, our very evolution as humans. In other words, our food choices empower us to reprogram "health traits" we inherit through our genes so that they express themselves through good health and vibrant well-being. *And we have control over this.* In this chapter, we are making a call to personal and community action, a call for creating fundamental changes both in both what and how much we eat, as well as in how we raise, prepare, consume, and share our food. For if we don't take action now, we're choosing to stand by passively and watch as what passes for food today does nothing less than change both our health destiny and the arc of human evolution.

I

When considering how to eat to reset genes for health and healing, it might be tempting to return to the "old-think" of just pondering what and how much to eat. But because this reductionist view of food and eating is just a small piece of the gene-health pie, it doesn't even begin to touch on the deeper emotional, social—even spiritual (in that food contains the mystery of life, as do we human beings)—needs that food satisfies. Rather, such a limited view undermines the sublime experience that food and eating can offer.

How might you capture this sublime experience? Actually, chances are you've already had a numinous dining experience. To get in touch with it, think back to one of your most memorable meals. What was special that made it stand out in your memory? Was it an impromptu get-together with friends at a favorite restaurant with fantastic, fresh-made food and an appetizing atmosphere? Or did you conjure up memories of your mom's homemade meals during the holiday season when you were a child; a time when you dined with family surrounded by holiday lights; at the same time, the air crackled with promise and possibilities, because in place of routine, there was celebration, ceremony, and socializing?

Or perhaps you recalled the time you camped out with your spouse and children, and after a long afternoon hike, you brought a healthy appetite to the fresh fish you had just caught and cooked over a campfire?

What does each scenario have in common? Chances are, you were eating fresh fare; you took the time to taste and savor the food (meaning, you ate mindfully, sans TV); you shared meals with friends or family; and you dined in pleasant surroundings. In other words, you weren't eating-by-number, by yourself, in a car or in front of your computer; nor were you in a fast-food outlet, eating processed, polluted food, surrounded by formica, glaring lights, and plastic utensils. Rather, you were simply enjoying mostly homemade food and the experience of eating as a social, celebratory, delightful pleasure. What if your most-of-the-time way of eating were like this?

We're asking you to reframe your vision of optimal foods, and your very relationship to food and eating. This is because there's more . . . far more . . . to the diet-gene-health story than feeding our genes the *types* and *proportions* of foods they adapted to over the millennia. For throughout this book, we have revealed that in addition to the nutritional content in food, our behaviors, feelings, even the regard (consciousness) we bring to meals[1] are mirrored in genetic expression. By journeying into this neglected place, the "simple truth" that emerges is that there is more to food than the biological effects it has on our body and genes. Which brings us to the simple truth of optimal eating, and that truth is that food not only offers sustenance for our physical health, it also nourishes us emotionally, spiritually, and socially.

That these "invisible nutrients" are especially relevant to Pottenger's Prophecy first surfaced in "It's the Lifestyle, Stupid," when we disclosed state-of-the-art research not only about how food switches genes on and off, but also how emotions (specifically, feeling stressed vs. relaxed) and social support influence whether genes express themselves by being silenced or activated. Indeed, clinical psychologist Ernest Lawrence Rossi believes that "novelty" (such as new recipes, taste sensations, and so on) and "environmental enrichment" (for instance, eating with people you like in a pleasant atmosphere) send messages to our genes that, ultimately, modulate gene expression, which in turn, influences health and healing.[2-4]

Doesn't such state-of-the-art science suggest that *what* we eat matters a lot, but also that the emotions, sense of meaning and connection, and social milieu we bring to meals influence the diet-DNA-disease equation?[5-8] In other words, isn't it possible (indeed, likely) that not only what we eat, but also the emotional, spiritual, and social "ingredients" we bring to meals make a difference in how food is metabolized, how our genes express themselves, and in turn, whether we are healthy . . . or not? We think so, and in light of the multidimensional ways in which food heals—based on the consciousness you bring to food choices as well as to how you eat—we are asking you this: If you don't get intimately involved in the foods you choose and eat; if you don't care about what, how, even with whom you eat NOW, when, indeed, will the time be right to take charge of what you eat to reset your genes for health and healing and in turn, live up to your genetic and health potential?

2

We've been on quite an odyssey throughout this book. In the first chapter, we introduced you to Dr. Francis M. Pottenger, who predicted as early as the 1930s that the food we eat each day is a strong determinant of our health, which, in turn, reflects the health of the genes we pass on to our children. We met researchers in Överkalix, Sweden, who both explained and verified Pottenger's Prophecy 70 years later through the emerging science of nutritional epigenetics—the focus of this book. We shed still more light on the food-gene-health link in "Curtailing Cancer," when Dr. Dean Ornish put epigenetics into action by showing prostate cancer could be curtailed through diet and other lifestyle changes, which silence genes that express as prostate cancer. And then in "Food, Genes, and Health Over Time," we introduced you to the nutrients and foods our genes adapted to over hundreds of thousands of years; nutrients on which we thrived, while "'Nourishment' Now" revealed toxins that have made their way into our food supply—pollutants to which our genes have *not* adapted. To turn the tide in favor of our genes, our "10 Green-Gene Guidelines" provided valuable clues about what to eat and what not to eat to reset genes for health and healing.

If you want to reap the food-gene-health rewards, though, you need to do more than read this book; rather, you must put into action what you've been reading by engaging in food and eating on multiple levels: personally, with others, and through the larger community. In other words, this chapter is a call to action in response to the epigenetic and health damage we've been doing to ourselves and our offspring through the polluted, processed foods most of us have been consuming for decades. The good news: your body—including your genes—has a miraculous power to recover when given the nutrients it needs through what co-author Deborah Kesten describes as the "four facets of food": biological, psychological, spiritual, and social sustenance.[7] We've shown how get an idea of how to return to what has nourished humankind for millennia—and in the process, how to eat to reset your genes for health and healing. Each step is simply and briefly described, but together, they have the power to transform your relationship to food, and in turn, reset your genes for health and healing. The key concept: TAKE ACTION . . . NOW! To get started, act on the ideas you resonate with the most . . . for yourself, others, community; even globally.

Taking Action: Yourself Whether you use one, some, or all of the following suggestions to optimize your relationship with food, you'll be setting in motion the potential to heal. The key concept: Return to the multidimensional, quality nourishment that served humankind for millennia.

GET FRESH. Consuming fresh whole food in its natural state as often as possible is the key concept for optimizing your diet. How do you know if food is fresh? Food that's alive rots, spoils, or goes bad, and food with such "living properties" is better for you than "dead," processed, packaged foods. At the same time, consuming fresh food enables you to avoid antibiotics, growth hormones, pesticides, herbicides, and other unwanted additives in food that damage genes and health. For more fresh-food insights, please review our "10 Green-Gene Guidelines" chapter.

START COOKING. The most empowering step you can take to take control of your food—and what you, friends, and family eat—is to buy fresh, unadulterated foods and prepare dishes and meals from foods you choose and purchase yourself. As a contrast, when the processed food industry does your cooking for you (such as with microwave meals), it doesn't do a good job. Rather, Dr. David Kessler, former head of the Food and Drug Administration (FDA), says the desire to addict you to lots of added salt, sugar, health-harming, highly processed fats, and food additives is what motivates most of the food industry's meals and products.[9]

SPICE UP YOUR KITCHEN. Aesthetics count! Whether it's the color, cabinets, layout, or appliances, if you don't like your kitchen, it'll be hard (perhaps, even impossible) to enjoy cooking in it. As a first step toward turning your kitchen into a dream cooking space, decide which part of it bothers you the most. Then fix it to your liking.

SHOP THE PERIPHERY. On average, the American supermarket has about 47,000 packaged food products.[10] Most fresh food (fruit, vegetables, dairy, fish, poultry, etc.) is kept cool, and is therefore to be found on the outside border of the supermarket, where it's kept refrigerated. In comparison, you're likely to find highly processed, packaged food *products*, filled with dubious chemicals and sugar, on the inside isles.

MEET "100-MILE" DINING. Have you tried "100 mile" dining? More and more restaurants and caterers are creating locally-sourced dishes, with many meals made from ingredients sourced within 100 miles. Become more of a locavore by seeking out local food. One way to do this is to eschew, say, peaches that have traveled 2000 miles so that you can buy them in winter months when they're not locally grown.

FIND NEARBY FARMS AND FARMERS MARKETS. The periphery of your supermarket is likely to have limited options for finding real food grown in your area or state. Ask around to find out about nearby farms. Then buy produce from farmers you know. And take advantage of the growing number of farmers' markets in your community for yet another way to find fresh food. Though farmers' markets may be a new option for many Americans, they have been part of the worldwide food culture for centuries.

GROW YOUR OWN. You can start to make food changes in your own backyard by planting and growing your own fruits and vegetables. The more you put into growing your own food (attention, time, etc.), the more you'll get out of it (flavor-filled, nutrient-dense foods, plus personal satisfaction and gratification). If you don't have the time or grounds to create your own garden, consider sprouting grains and seeds indoors on your countertop, or fermenting your own food. Or find out if your town has a community garden you can join. If not, would you be interested in starting one? Other options: consider urban or rooftop gardens.

BECOME NUTRITION-SMART. Co-author Gray Graham founded the Nutritional Therapy Association (NTA) in 1998 to give health care practitioners the tools they need to provide optimal nutrition guidance for their patients and clients. In 2001, Graham expanded NTA by creating a new training program for health professionals, so that they can work alongside other health professionals as nutrition therapists. To find an NTA-trained holistic nutrition practitioner, or for more information about becoming a practitioner, go to www.nutritionaltherapy.com or call 800.918.9798.

Take Action: You, Others, Community Our "10 Green-Gene Guidelines" are templates not only for *what* to eat, but also for *how* to take action to eat to activate positive epigenetic changes. Here, some soothing suggestions for nourishing every aspect of your being each time you eat.

TAKE ACTION: YOU

Take a break from the busyness of everyday life with a calming cup of herbal tea. Play a soothing CD as you sip.

Treat yourself to a favorite food at a favorite restaurant or café. Eat slowly, and take the time to savor the flavor.

Turn casual, everyday meals into a special event by serving food on your best dinnerware. Set the table and light subtly scented candles.

TAKE ACTION: OTHERS The experience of food and eating is about more than what to eat, it also includes connection with self, family, friends, and neighbors—with food as the unifying flavor. Here are some suggestions for creating social sustenance each time you eat.

Ask a relative, spouse, or partner, for a time-honored recipe, then prepare it for her or him and other family members.

Invite your children to make their favorite snack with you. Enjoy the rewards of your "snack cook-in" while talking at the table. Afterward, watch a favorite movie together.

Finesse family fare. If you, your spouse, and your children have busy schedules, is it possible to commit to one or two mornings to having breakfast together?

Set a table for two—even if you're dining alone. Then "socialize" by placing a photograph of someone you love on the table. As you sit down to eat, conjure up favorite food memories you've shared.

Take a social nutrition break. Whether you're "brown-bagging" it with a tuna sandwich or dining on a simple mixed salad when you're at work, why not make it a point to have lunch with coworkers? Or, in the afternoon, take a break by enjoying a cup of yogurt or freshly popped popcorn with like-minded coworkers.

Take a moment to contemplate this insight from authors Manuela Dunn Mascetti and Arunima Borthwick: "Sitting together around a table for meals is far more than a practical necessity. In its sacral character the sharing of food and drink is probably the most ancient ritual of mankind."[13]

Take Action: Practice Whole Person Nutrition

Co-author Deborah Kesten's "Whole Person Nutrition" program (www.EnlightenedDiet.com) includes strategies for optimizing your physical, emotional, spiritual, and social well-being through food choices you make each day.[7, 11, 12] Here are her suggestions for integrating the "four facets of food" into your own life, so that you—and your genes—may benefit each time you eat:

Socializing. If you're dining alone, conjure up a favorite food memory that you enjoyed with others, such as a family picnic or romantic dinner. At the office, ask a coworker to join you for lunch. Or have a weekly potluck with special friends.

Feelings. Most of us overeat and gain weight because of "emotional eating"—turning to food (especially sugary food products) to soothe negative feelings, such as anger, anxiety, or depression. The solution is threefold: replace junk food with real food; eat because you have a healthy appetite, not because you want to "treat" unpleasant emotions with food; and find the source of your anxiety, then deal with it directly. In other words, develop awareness, then honor your needs by nourishing yourself in ways that have nothing to do with food.

Mindfulness. Commit to being in the present moment when you eat, shop for food or prepare it—even when cleaning up. Start with small steps by focusing on the appearance (such as color), aroma, and texture of the food.

Appreciation. Foster an attitude of gratitude by expressing appreciation for the food before you. If you're short on time, try the Native American Seneca greeting, "Thank you for being." Whether cooking, dining at a favorite restaurant, or selecting produce, flavor food with gratitude by holding regard in your heart.

Connection. Regardless of the setting, remain mindful of the gift of food. After all, all food has been passed to you by a chain of human hands—such as the farmer or rancher, trucker, and grocer.

Optimal foods. The key concept for eating optimally is to consume fresh, pesticide-free plant-based foods (fruits, vegetables, whole grains, legumes, and nuts and seeds), and pollution- and chemical-free dairy, fish, poultry, and meat. The bottom line: to eat *real food*—not processed food products that pass as food.

TAKE ACTION: COMMUNITY In addition to making proactive, green-gene food choices for yourself, family, and friends, consider community-oriented actions you can take to change the future of food. Here are some ways to get involved and become a food activist. As you look over the options, remember that even one change can make a big difference.

Pass legislation. In March 2004, voters in Mendocino County, CA passed a bill banning the planting of genetically modified crops in their county (please see "'Nourishment' Now" for more about GE crops). Since then, other counties in California have followed suit with their own initiatives. Might your town, city, or county benefit from similar actions?

Get the word out. From banning GMO crops to protecting organic standards—whatever you're passionate about, get the word out by starting a free online petition, sending email updates about your area of concern, or use the "e-mail this article" link to pass on information about a relevant article you just read.

Start with schools. Award-winning chef Alice Waters transferred her passion for fresh organic food to students at Berkeley's Martin Luther King, Jr. Middle School by partnering with parents to start the Edible Schoolyard project in Berkeley, CA. Now middle school students use their formerly useless school grounds to plan, plant, and cultivate fresh food; and of course, make big salads with their abundant choices of vegetables. At the same time, many campaigns to get soft drinks and unhealthful vending-machine snacks out of schools have been successful, and a start-up company called "Revolution Foods" delivers affordable, fresh-food meals to 235 public and private schools in California, Colorado, and the District of Columbia.

Create change with your purchasing power. So many consumers protested GE ingredients in some food items sold at Whole Foods, Trader Joe's, and Wild Oats markets that the chain stores now sell only GMO-free foods. If you want more additive-free food choices in your own local market, write a letter to your supermarket manager, and visit www.truefoodnow.org/supermarkets for more "take action" activities.

Send letters to legislators. The U.S. Department of Agriculture (USDA) subsidizes poor quality crops, such as corn, so that industrial farmers can grow and sell such crops cheaply; in turn, this enables you to buy cheap corn products, such as chips, or other food products with lots of high fructose corn syrup. Fresh fruits and vegetables aren't subsidized, so they're more costly than processed foods. Send letters to your state and local representatives, expressing your concerns about the abundance of processed food filled with GMOs, pesticides, and other pollutants that harm you, your children, and the genes you pass on to your offspring. Let them know you want chemical-free fruits, vegetables, grains, dairy, and meat to be affordable. You can find out the addresses of your state and federal representatives at www.congress.org.

Ultimately, the message in our personal, other-oriented, and community "take action" steps is simple: you can reset your genes for health and healing each time you eat by making conscious food choices on a personal level and by being community-wise. As a matter of fact, every time you shop for, prepare, and eat food, we are suggesting that you can empower yourself by experiencing food as the symphonic masterpiece that it is; one that plays the notes of fresh food, positive feelings, in-the-moment mindfulness, culinary delight, pleasing surrounds, savory flavors, and social connection. That is—if you don't put off making changes and you take action NOW.

3

"We need a food revolution," Oprah said. "Yes, we need a food revolution," food expert and author Michael Pollan agreed when he appeared on her show to discuss America's poor quality food and what to do about it.[10] "Cheap food is great," Pollan said, "but we also have to acknowledge the cost of it." To highlight his point, Pollan reflected on being a boy in 1960, when Americans spent 18 percent of their national income on food and 5 percent on health care. Today, though, there's been quite a flip-flop: 9 percent of our income goes to cheap, poor quality, highly processed, chemical-laden food that makes us sick; and 17 percent goes to health care—in large part, because of our diet. The equation is clear: If you spend less on cheap food, you'll spend more on health care. Given this, Pollan posits this rhetorical question: "Who would you rather pay?"[10]

Who indeed? In response, Pollan isn't the only one proposing a food revolution. Farmer Will Allen has founded Growing Power, with the slogan, "The Good Food Movement is now a Revolution."[14] At the same time, it seems that chef Jamie Oliver is leading the media movement with his book *Jamie's Food Revolution*[15] and his TV show on the topic. Consider this description:

> A revolution is about to start. Impassioned chef, TV personality, and best-selling author Jamie Oliver is ready. He's taking on the high sta-

tistics of obesity, heart disease and diabetes in this country, where our nation's children are the first generation not expected to live as long as their parents. In the thought provoking new series, "Jamie Oliver's Food Revolution," Oliver invites viewers to take a stand and change the way America eats, in our home kitchens, schools, and workplaces.[16]

One definition of "revolution" describes it as "a procedure or course, as if in a circuit, back to a starting point."[17] We especially like this definition, because, at its core, it describes our message throughout Pottenger's Prophecy—which is that we've veered so off course from the foods on which we—and our genes—thrived that it's time to have a food revolution and return to our "starting point," meaning, a way of eating that merges fresh food with ancient food wisdom and the latest science.

Food technology may have changed over the years, but our bodies' needs have not. Given this, what greater gifts can we give to ourselves and children—indeed, humankind—than to eat the kinds of foods that nourish us multidimensionally each time we eat? The visionary food pioneers we introduced you to earlier have already been leading the Food Revolution. For instance, recall the 100 percent grass-fed cattle ranch in Wyoming; chef Dan Barber who serves farm-to-table food; pediatrician Alan Greene, who includes organic food as part of his treatment plan; Ed, Malea, Jake, and Eliza Balmuth, who raise their own farm-fresh food; and a unique Organic Farming major offered at Washington State University.

At the heart of each pioneer's view of food is this: *You eat who you are* (in terms of values). For surely, the food they grow, eat, and recommend is motivated by an all-pervasive commitment and concern for healing ourselves—and the Earth. With the ideas in this chapter, we are inviting you join the Food Revolution; to become part of the swelling chorus of women and men who are passionate about a more profound and meaningful relationship with true food; people who care about the role food—and each of us—play in Pottenger's Prophecy. For by returning to our nutritional roots, we may access food's invisible power to sustain, rejuvenate, and heal—and in the process, find true nourishment.

References, Notes, and Links

Introduction: Pottenger's Prophecy

Note: The PMID (Pub Med Identifier) is a unique number assigned to each journal article, and listed after the journal references that appear in Pub Med. Entering this number in Pub Med search will provide the reader the abstract, and often the full text of the articles referenced in this bibliography.

1. Wikipedia, "Atchison, Topeka and Santa Fe Railway," www.en.wikipedia. org/wiki/Santa Fe Railroad. (Accessed June 7, 2009).

2. Price Pottenger Nutrition Foundation, "Biography of Francis M. Pottenger, Sr., MD," www.ppnf.org/catalog/ppnf/PottBio.htm. (Accessed June 7, 2009).

3. Price Pottenger Nutrition Foundation, "Biography of Francis M. Pottenger, Sr., MD," www.ppnf.org/catalog/ppnf/PottBio.htm. (Accessed June 7, 2009).

4. Telephone interview with Robert T. Pottenger, Jr., MD, by Deborah Kesten, MPH, May 12, 2009. Dr. Pottenger's father was the brother of Francis Marion Pottenger. He is a retired physician who practiced general medicine with an emphasis in allergies. He was eight years old when Francis M. Pottenger began his feeding experiments with cats and, at 82 years of age, has clear memories of the sanatorium. "The road from US Route 66 ended (at the sanatorium)," he recalls. "On the right was the old sanatorium, which sat on a hill. On the left was a driveway with a hill where my uncle lived. His house had five cottages, a tower for distillery extracts; on the top of the hill were the cat bins."

5. Pottenger married Teresa Elizabeth Saxour on June 17, 1925, the day both graduated from Otterbein College in Westerville, Ohio. They had four children: Francis Marion III; Margaret Elizabeth; Barbara Jane; and Samuel Slatter. Available from www.ppnf.org http://ppnf.org/catalog/ppnf/PottBio. htm. (Accessed on June 3, 2009).

6. The Pottenger Cat Studies, Introduction by David J. Getoff, Vice-President, Price-Pottenger Nutrition Foundation, TRT2830, 2006.

7. The cooked meat scraps included liver, tripe, sweetbread, brains, heart, and muscle. From Wikipedia, "Francis M. Pottenger, Jr." www/en.wikipedia. org/wiki/Francis Pottenger. (Accessed June 6, 2006).

8. Francis M. Pottenger, "The effect of heat-processed foods and metabolized Vitamin D milk on the dentofacial structures of experimental animals." American Journal of Orthodontics and Oral Surgery, Vol. 32, No. 8 (1946): 467–485.

9. Francis M. Pottenger, Pottenger's cats: A study in nutrition, 2nd ed. Edited by Elaine Pottenger with Robert T. Pottenger. La Mesa, CA: Price-Pottenger Nutrition Foundation, Inc., 1983.

10. Francis M. Pottenger, "Evidence of the protective influences of adrenal hormones against tuberculosis in guinea pigs." Endocrinology, Vol. 21, No. 4 (July 1937): 529–532.

11. Francis M. Pottenger, "Adrenal cortex in treating childhood asthma: Clinical evaluation of its use." California and Western Medicine, Vol. 49, No. 4 (October, 1938).

12. How could feeding heated meat and milk have such a rapid deleterious effect on cats? Were Pottenger's findings valid? If Pottenger had done the study today with funding, say, from the National Institutes of Health, he would have been able to acquire cats with similar genetic history, age, gender, and dietary history. He would have fed all cats the same pieces of meat with the only difference being whether it was cooked or raw. And he would have randomly assigned cats to each condition and used measures and statistics to assess the strength of his treatment effect. Given that these conditions were not in place when the research was done, we cannot rule out obvious biases in his research methods, such as the fact that when he examined his cats, he knew what they had been fed. His expectations or desires could have influenced his outcome measures of the cat's health, particularly his visual observations.

Nevertheless, the high quality photographs show contrasting differences, if representative of all the cats, which compel us to ask, "How could this be and how does it apply to humans?" In fact, Pottenger's studies do not apply to cats, which in the wild eat a varied diet including insects and plants to complete their nutrition. In contrast, Pottenger indicated feeding the cats only meat, milk, and cod liver oil, so cats that have access to a varied diet would probably fare better when being fed primarily a cooked meat and milk diet.

The results also show how cooking meat and milk destroys certain nutrients that the cats needed to thrive. Taurine is one of those proteins that is altered and could account for the poor health effects of the cooked food diet. It is most significant that Pottenger found that diet determines heritable differences in offspring. Diet can deteriorate (at least the cat) genome quickly and diet can help it to recover. If true for humans, diet is more important that we ever thought, for it determines not only our health but whether we survive or thrive as a species.

"At the time of Pottenger's Study the amino acid taurine had been discovered but had not yet been identified as an essential amino acid for cats. Today many cats thrive on a cooked meat diet where taurine has been added after cooking. The deficient diets lacked sufficient taurine to allow the cats to properly form protein structures and resulted in the health effects observed. Pottenger himself concluded that there was likely an 'as yet unknown' protein factor that may have been heat sensitive." Available from "Francis M. Pottenger, Jr." http://en.wikipedia.org/wiki/Francis. (Accessed June 6, 2009).

13. A.M. Branum and Susan L. Lukacs," Food allergy among U.S. children: trends in prevalence and hospitalizations," http://www.cdc.gov/nchs/data/databriefs/db10.pdf. (Accessed June 6, 2010).

14. QuickStats: "Prevalence of overweight among children and teenagers, by Age Group and Selected Period—United States, 1963–2002"; Available from: http://www.cdc.gov/mmwr/preview/mmwrhtml/mm5408a6.htm. (Accessed July 31, 2010).

15. Center for Disease Control and Prevention, "Crude and age-adjusted incidence of diagnosed diabetes per 1,000 population aged 18–79 years, United States, 1980–2007." 2009; Available from: http://www.cdc.gov/diabetes/statistics/incidence/fig2.htm. (Accessed June 6, 2009).

16. Child Trends Databank, "Adolescents who feel sad or hopeless, 2009." http://www.childtrendsdatabank.org/?q=node/321. (Accessed July 31, 2010).

17. D.S. Mandell, W.W. Thompson, E.S. Weintraub, F. Destefano, and M.B. Blank, "Trends in diagnosis rates for autism and ADHD at hospital discharge in the context of other psychiatric diagnoses." Psychiatric Services, 56, 1 (2005): 56–62. PMID 15637193.

18. E. Carlsen, A. Giwercman, N. Keiding, and N.E. Skakkebaek, "Evidence for decreasing quality of semen during past 50 years." British Medical Journal, 305, 6854 (1992): 609–613. PMID 1393072.

19. S.H. Swan, E.P. Elkin, and L. Fenster, "The question of declining sperm density revisited: An analysis of 101 studies published 1934–1996." Environmental Health Perspectives, 108, 10 (2000): 961–966. PMID 11049816.

20. Much to our delight and surprise we found intriguing evidence for transgenerational effects of diet from the grandmother and grandfather to their grandchildren. The best studies across three generations were done in the northern most province in Sweden. They provide evidence that access to higher levels of food availability during the slower developmental periods of children (8–12 years old) corresponded to increased mortality from diabetes and heart disease of their grandchildren. See references 21–23 below for access to this research.

21. G. Kaati, L.O. Bygren, and S. Edvinsson, "Cardiovascular and diabetes mortality determined by nutrition during parents' and grandparents' slow growth period." European Journal of Human Genetics, 10, 11 (2002): 682–628. PMID 12404098.

22. G. Kaati, L.O. Bygren, M. Pembrey, and M. Sjostrom, "Transgenerational response to nutrition, early life circumstances and longevity." European Journal of Human Genetics, 15, 7 (2007): 784-790. PMID 17457370.

23. M.E. Pembrey, L.O. Bygren, G. Kaati, S. Edvinsson, K. Northstone, M. Sjostrom, and J. Golding, "Sex-specific, male-line transgenerational responses in humans." European Journal of Human Genetics, 14, 2 (2006): 159–166. PMID 16391557.

24. D.K. Morgan and E. Whitelaw, "The case for transgenerational epigenetic inheritance in humans." Mammalian Genome, 19, 6 (2008): 394–397. PMID 18663528.

25. R.L. Jirtle and M.K. Skinner, "Environmental epigenomics and disease susceptibility." Nature Review of Genetics, 8, 4 (2007): 253–62. PMID 17363974.

CHAPTER 1: THE GENE-HEALTH PROMISE

1. Dr. Joseph Pizzorno and his colleagues have developed a sophisticated artificial intelligence, evidence-based tool to help health professionals and consumers create personalized recommendations for health care. The tool has provisions for entering personal data such as age, gender, weight, ethnic group, diagnoses, genomic testing, and medications. This data is then considered and probable underlying conditions are listed as well as a list of supplements, dietary recommendations, and botanicals to consider adding to one's treatment regimen.

2. Co-author Deborah Kesten interviewed Dr. Pizzorno by telephone on May 13, 2009. Co-authors Kesten and Larry Scherwitz conducted a second interview that focused on genetic testing and on genes as they relate to the future of medicine at Dr. Pizzorno's home in Seattle, Washington, on June 23, 2009.

3. Dr. Joseph Pizzorno is an educator, physician, researcher and a leading authority on natural medicine. Dr. Pizzorno is founding president of Bastyr University, which under his leadership became the first fully accredited, multidisciplinary university of natural medicine. He founded Salugenecist.com in 2002.

4. "Osteoporosis can lead to dowagers' humps." In advanced osteoporosis, a person sometimes develops vertebral fractures, and kyphosis or a spinal hump often occurs. Kyphosis and its resultant bent-over posture are often associated with older women (although men get them also). Kyphosis is a result of advanced osteoporosis. Spinal vertebrae become so porous that they weaken and often fracture spontaneously. Available from http://www.osteopenia3.com/dowagers-humps.html

5. The most common bone mineral density test is called DEXA or DXA, an x-ray that measures bone density. According to WebMD "DXA is relatively easy to perform and the amount of radiation exposure is low. A DXA scanner is a machine that produces 2 x-ray beams, each with different energy levels. One beam is high energy while the other is low energy. The amount of x-rays that pass through the bone is measured for each beam. This will vary depending on the thickness of the bone. Based on the difference between the 2 beams, the bone density can be measured. " Osteoporosis Guide. DEXA Scan (Dual X-ray Absorptiometry). Available from http://www.webmd.com/osteoporosis/guide/dexa-scan. (Accessed August 20, 2009).

6. Osteoporosis is a disorder whereby the bones become increasingly porous, brittle, and subject to fracture, because of a loss of calcium and other mineral components. Osteopenia is a condition where bone mineral density (BMD) is lower than normal peak BMD but not low enough to be considered osteoporosis. Bone mineral density is a measurement of the level of minerals in the bones, which indicates how dense and strong they are. If your BMD is low compared to normal peak BMD, you are said to have osteopenia. For more information check out National Osteoporosis Foundation at nof.org.

7. In addition, the National Osteoporosis Foundation recommends getting tested, as well as avoiding smoking and excessive alcohol intake. See http://www.nof.org/osteoporosis/index.htm (Accessed August 20, 2009). Commonly prescribed medications for osteoporosis include a class of drugs called bisphosphonates such as Fosamax, Actonel, and Boniva, which act to reduce or stop the natural process that dissolves bone tissue. There is good research to support their effectiveness. However, there have been recent reports that bisphosphonates cause bone death in the jaw. Most of these cases, however, have been with intravenous infusions with cancer patients to stop bone loss. For an impartial consideration of the risks of bisphosphonates see http://bisphosphonates.org/. (Accessed August 20, 2009).

8. "Kids Health"; "Genetic Testing," www.kidshealth.org/parent/system/medical/genetics.html. (Accessed July 2, 2009).

9. "Genetics Home Reference: Your Guide to Understanding Genetic Conditions." Available from http://ghr.nlm.nih.gov/. (Accessed July 11, 2009).

10. Genetic tests look at genotypes which includes the genetic structure of the DNA; genetic tests scan for mutations (a sudden departure from the parent type in one or more heritable characteristics, caused by a change in a gene). Genotypes are contrasted with phenotypes, which are the appearance of an organism resulting from the interaction of the genotype and the environment. Human cells contains 46 chromosomes, 23 from each parent. This set is contained in the nucleus of almost every cell in the body except for red blood cells.

11. Joseph Pizzorno knew such high levels wouldn't be harmful for Lara, because he reviewed the research literature, which more and more was revealing that the dosage required to achieve optimal levels of vitamin D ranges from a low of 400 IUs a day (which is the RDA) to a high of about 10,000 IUs a day. According to Pizzorno, the average person needs about 400 IUs a day. A study of sun-deprived women suggested they need between 600 and 1000 IUs per day. For a good review of dosage levels, toxicity levels, and the effects of too little vitamin D, you can get the full text, cited in the next reference.

12. R. Vieth, "Vitamin D supplementation, 25-hydroxyvitamin D Concentrations, and Safety." American Journal of Clinical Nutrition, 69, 5 (1999): 842–856.

13. Joseph Pizzorno said that "what's particularly relevant about Lara's story is that she grew up in southern Florida. As a teenager, it was typical for her to

lie on tin foil and sunbath with oil to get a deep tan. Because of this, today, she is prone to about 15–20 skin cancers a year. This meant that she went from being in the sun all the time and getting a lot of vitamin D to now, when she avoids the sun because she's so prone to skin cancer. So Lara has the combination of VDR deficit and avoiding the sun, which translates into low levels of vitamin D, and in turn, loss of bone mass."

14. "Jean Baptiste- Lamarck." Available from http://en.wikipedia.org/wiki/Jean-Baptiste_Lamarck. (Accessed August 20, 2009).

15. Seung Yon Rhee, "Gregor Mendel." Available from www.accessexcellenc.org/RC/AB/BC/Gregor_Mendel.php. (Accessed August 9, 2009).

16. Gregor Mendel, "Experiments on plant hybridization (1865)." Available from http://www.mendelweb.org/Mendel.html. (Accessed August 20, 2009).

17. One of the reasons that Mendel's work was such an outstanding contribution to genetics is the rigorous methodology he used. First he carefully selected a species suited to his experiments. The variety of self-pollinating peas he choose were, by their morphology, protected from cross-fertilization, allowing him less contamination by other plants. Another important aspect is that he conducted experiments rather than just observations. He removed the immature male part of the pea plants and then manually pollinated these plants from other plants while carefully documenting the characteristics of both plants. And he had large samples, as well as carrying on the studies as far as six generations. His paper (see previous reference) is a masterpiece of careful work.

18. "Gregor Mendel: 1822–1884," EMuseum@Minnesota State University, Mankato. Available from www.mnsu.edu/emuseum/information/biography/klmno/mendel_gregor.html. (Accessed August 10, 2009).

19. Two German botanists rediscovered Mendel's work in the early 1900s. Both Hugo De Vries and Carl Correns replicated the work with another plant model and they rediscovered Mendel's paper. "Hugo de Vries." Available from http://en.wikipedia.org/wiki/Hugo_de_Vries. (Accessed August 20, 2009); Carl Correns, from Wikipedia. Available from http://en.wikipedia.org/wiki/Carl_Correns. (Accessed August 20, 2009).

20. Definition of "Chromosome" from http://dictionary.reference.com/browse/chromosome. (Accessed August 20, 2009).

21. Thomas Hunt Morgan won the Nobel Prize in 1933 "for his discoveries concerning the role played by the chromosome in heredity." Available from http://nobelprize.org/nobel_prizes/medicine/laureates/1933/. (Accessed August 20, 2009).

22. Chris Evers, "The one gene/one enzyme hypothesis: Beadle and Tatum's 1941 breakthrough." Available from http://www.accessexcellence.org/RC/AB/BC/One_Gene_One_Enzyme.php. (Accessed July 31, 2010).

23. G. W. Beadle, E. L. Tatum (1941). "Genetic control of biochemical reactions in Neurospora." Proceedings of the National Academy of Sciences

of the United States of America 27, (11): 499–506. doi:VL -27. Available from http://www.pnas.org/content/27/11/499.short. (Accessed June 1, 2009).

24. Mark Hickman and John Cairns (2003). "The centenary of the one-gene one-enzyme hypothesis." Genetics, 163(3): 839–841. Available from http://www.genetics.org. (Accessed June 1, 2009).

25. N.H. Horowitz (1995–05). "One-gene-one-enzyme: Remembering biochemical genetics." Protein Science: A Publication of the Protein Society 4(5): 1017–1019. ISSN 0961-8368. Available from http://www.ncbi.nlm.nih.gov/pubmed/7663338. (Accessed June 1, 2009).

26. James Watson and Francis Crick, "Molecular structure of nucleic acids; a structure for deoxyribose nucleic acid." Nature, 171, 4356 (1953): 737–738.

27. ". . . on 28 February 1953, Francis Crick walked into the Eagle pub in Cambridge, UK, and announced something for which he would later share a Nobel Prize. 'We have found the secret of life,' his collaborator and subsequent fellow Nobel laureate James Watson later quoted him as saying." Available from http://news.bbc.co.uk/2/hi/science/nature/2804545.stm. (Accessed August 20, 2009).

28. "When do doctors recommend genetic testing?" Available from www.Kidshealth.org/parent/system/medical/genetics.html. (Accessed July 8, 2009).

29. Diane Allingham-Hawkins, "Successful genetic tests are predicated on clinical utility." Genetic Engineering & Biotechnology News, 28, 14: 6–9. Available from http://www.genengnews.com/articles/chitem.aspx?aid=2544. (Accessed August 20, 2009).

30. S.A. Lee, J.H. Fowke, W. Lu, C. Ye, Y. Zheng, Q. Cai, K. Gu, Y.T. Gao, X.O. Shu, and W. Zheng, "Cruciferous vegetables, the gstp1 ile105val genetic polymorphism, and breast cancer risk." American Journal of Clinical Nutrition, 87, 3 (2008): 753–760. PMID 18326615.

31. S.M. Getahun and F.L. Chung, "Conversion of glucosinolates to isothiocyanates in humans after ingestion of cooked watercress." Cancer Epidemiology Biomarkers Prevention, 8 (5) (1999): 447–451. PMID 10350441.

32. C.C. Conaway, S.M. Getahun, L.L. Liebes, D.J. Pusateri, D.K. Topham, M. Botero-Omary, and F.L. Chung, "Disposition of glucosinolates and sulforaphane in humans after ingestion of steamed and fresh broccoli." Nutrition and Cancer, 38, 2 (2000): 168–178. PMID 11525594.

33. J.W. Lampe and S. Peterson, "Brassica, biotransformation and cancer risk: Genetic polymorphisms alter the preventive effects of cruciferous vegetables." Journal of Nutrition, 132, 10 (2002): 2991–2994. PMID 12368383.

34. A.E. Guttmacher and F.S. Collins, "Genomic medicine—a primer." New England Journal of Medicine, 347, 19 (2002): 1512–1520. PMID 12421895.

35. Human Genome Project Information, "Fast forward to 2020: What to expect in molecular medicine." Available from www.ornl.gov/sci/techresources/Human_Genome/medicine/tnty.shtml. U.S. Department of Energy Office of Science, Office of Biological and Environmental Research, Human Genome

Program. (Last modified October 29, 2003; Accessed August 20, 2009).

36. "Moving genomic medicine into the doctor's office: W. Gregory Feero, M.D., Ph.D., joins NHGRI as Senior Advisor." Available from www.genome. gov/25520892. (Accessed July 9, 2009).

CHAPTER 2: EPIGENETICS: A FAMILY AFFAIR . . . AND FARE

1. Heart of Lapland website available from http://www.heartoflapland. com/. (Accessed September 22, 2009).

2. Heart of Lapland, featuring Överkalix, available from http://overkalix. heartoflapland.com/sv-SE/default.aspx. (Accessed September 22, 2009).

3. Marcus Pembrey, "Imprinting and transgenerational modulation of gene expression: Human growth as a model." Acta geneticae medicae et gemellologiae (Roma), 45, 1–2 (1996): 111–125. PMID 8872020.

4. "The ghost in your genes." BBC documentary (2006). XviD.avi video available at: http://video.google.com/videoplay?docid=112804583576167593. (Accessed September 22, 2009).

5. Conrad Waddington, "The epigenotype." Endeavour, 1 (1942): 18–20.

6. Linda Van Speybroeck, "From epigenesis to epigenetics: The case of C. H. Waddington." Annals of the New York Academy of Sciences, 981 (2002): 61–81. PMID 12547674.

7. D.J. Barker, J.G. Eriksson, T. Forsen, and C. Osmond, "Fetal origins of adult disease: strength of effects and biological basis." International Journal of Epidemiology, 31, 6 (2002): 1235–1239. PMID 12540728.

8. D. J. Barker, "The developmental origins of well-being." Philosophical Transactions of the Royal Society London B Biological Science, 359, 1449 (2004): 1359–1366. PMID 15347527.

9. D.J. Barker, "The origins of the developmental origins theory." Journal of Internal Medicine, 261, 5 (2007): 412–417. PMID 17444880.

10. L.O. Bygren, G. Kaati, and S. Edvinsson, "Longevity determined by paternal ancestors' nutrition during their slow growth period." Acta Biotheoretica, 49, 1 (2001): 53–59. PMID 11368478.

11. G. Kaati, L.O. Bygren, and S. Edvinsson, "Cardiovascular and diabetes mortality determined by nutrition during parents' and grandparents' slow growth period." European Journal of Human Genetics, 10, 11 (2002): 682–688. PMID 12404098.

12. G. Kaati, L.O. Bygren, M. Pembrey, and M. Sjostrom, "Transgenerational response to nutrition, early life circumstances and longevity." European Journal of Human Genetics, 15, 7 (2007): 784–790. PMID 17457370.

13. M.E. Pembrey, L.O. Bygren, G. Kaati, S. Edvinsson, K. Northstone, M. Sjostrom, and J. Golding, "Sex-specific, male-line transgenerational responses in humans." European Journal of Human Genetics, 14, 2 (2006): 159–166. PMID 16391557.

14. "The ghost in your genes." BBC documentary (2006). XviD.avi video available at: http://video.google.com/videoplay?docid=112804583576167593. (Accessed September 22, 2009).

15. "The ghost in your genes." BBC documentary (2006). XviD.avi video available at: http://video.google.com/videoplay?docid=112804583576167593. (Accessed September 22, 2009).

16. Harvey Angelman, "Children: A report of three cases." Developmental Medicine and Child Neurology, 7 (1965): 681–688.

17. Prada-Willi Syndrome, available from http://en.wikipedia.org/wiki/Prader-Willi_syndrome. (Accessed September 22, 2009).

18. M. Pembrey, S.J. Fennell, J. van den Berghe, M. Fitchett, D. Summers, L. Butler, C. Clarke, M. Griffiths, E. Thompson, and M. Super, "The association of Angelman's syndrome with deletions within 15q11-13." Journal of Medical Genetics, 26, 2 (1989): 73–77. PMID 2918545.

19. J.H. Knoll, R.D. Nicholls, R.E. Magenis, J.M. Graham, Jr., M. Lalande, and S.A. Latt, "Angelman and Prader-Willi Syndromes share a common chromosome 15 deletion but differ in parental origin of the deletion." American Journal of Medical Genetics, 32, 2 (1989): 285–290. PMID 2564739.

20. M. Bhatia, "Miasms: A new look through epigenetics." http://hpathy.com/homeopathy-scientific-research/miasms-a-new-look-through-epigenetics-i/ (17 December 2006).

21. Science & Nature: TV & Radio Follow-up, "The ghost in your genes" Available from www.bbc.co.uk/sn/tvradio/programmes/horizon/ghostgenes.shtml. (Accessed August 22, 2009).

22. "In vitro fertilization" http://en.wikipedia.org/wiki/In_vitro_fertilisation. (Accessed September 22, 2009).

23. E.R. Maher, L.A. Brueton, S.C. Bowdin, A. Luharia, W. Cooper, T.R. Cole, F. Macdonald, J.R. Sampson, C.L. Barratt, W. Reik, and M.M. Hawkins, "Beckwith-Wiedemann syndrome and assisted reproduction technology." Journal of Medical Genetics, 40, 1 (2003): 62–64. PMID 12525545.

24. "The ghost in your genes." BBC documentary (2006). XviD.avi video available at: http://video.google.com/videoplay?docid=112804583576167593. (Accessed September 22, 2009).

25. W. Reik and A. Lewis, "Co-evolution of X-chromosome inactivation and imprinting in mammals." Nature Reviews Genetics, 6, 5 (2005): 403–410. PMID 15818385.

26. W. Reik and J. Walter, "Genomic imprinting: parental influence on the genome." Nature Reviews Genetics, 2, 1 (2001): 21–32. PMID 11253064.

27. W. Reik, W. Dean, and J. Walter, "Epigenetic reprogramming in mammalian development." Science, 293, 5532 (2001): 1089–1093. PMID 11498579.

28. F. B. Churchill, "William Johannsen and the genotype concept." Journal of the History of Biology, 7, (1974): 5–30. PMID 11610096.

29. W. Johannsen, "The genotype conception of heredity." American Naturalist, 45, (1911): 129–159.

30. "The ghost in your genes." BBC documentary (2006). XviD.avi video available at: http://video.google.com/videoplay?docid=112804583576167593. (Accessed September 22, 2009).

31. "The ghost in your genes." BBC documentary (2006). XviD.avi video available at: http://video.google.com/videoplay?docid=112804583576167593. (Accessed September 22, 2009).

32. "The ghost in your genes." BBC documentary (2006). XviD.avi video available at: http://video.google.com/videoplay?docid=112804583576167593. (Accessed September 22, 2009).

33. Dawson Church, The genie in your genes. Santa Rosa, CA: Elite Books, 2007.

34. S. Henikoff and M.A. Matzke, "Exploring and explaining epigenetic effects." Trends in Genetics, 13, 8 (1997): 293–295. PMID 9260513.

35. B. Lewin, "The mystique of epigenetics." Cell, 93, 3 (1998): 301–303. PMID 9590160.

36. R.A. Waterland and R.L. Jirtle, "Transposable elements: Targets for early nutritional effects on epigenetic gene regulation." Molecular Cell Biology, 23, 15 (2003): 5293–5300. PMID 12861015.

37. A.P. Feinberg, "Epigenetics at the epicenter of modern medicine." Journal of the American Medical Association, 299, 11 (2008): 1345–1350. PMID 18349095.

38. G. Taubes, "RNA revolution," in Discover. New York: Discover Media LLC, 2009.

39. C.D. Davis and S.A. Ross, "Evidence for dietary regulation of microRNA expression in cancer cells." Nutritional Review, 66, 8 (2008): 477–482. PMID 18667010.

40. D.P. Bartel, "MicroRNAs: Genomics, biogenesis, mechanism, and function." Cell, 116, 2 (2004): 281–297. PMID 14744438.

41. "Science and reason," MicroRNA and Cancer. Posted March 14, 2007, www.scienceandreason.blogspot.com/2007/03/microrna.html. (Accessed October 7, 2009).

42. M.F. Fraga, E. Ballestar, M.F. Paz, S. Ropero, F. Setien, M.L. Ballestar, D. Heine-Suner, J.C. Cigudosa, M. Urioste, J. Benitez, M. Boix-Chornet, A. Sanchez-Aguilera, C. Ling, E. Carlsson, P. Poulsen, A. Vaag, Z. Stephan, T.D. Spector, Y.Z. Wu, C. Plass, and M. Esteller, "Epigenetic differences arise during the lifetime of monozygotic twins." Proceedings of the National Academy of Science U.S.A., 102, 30 (2005): 10604–10609. PMID 16009939.

43. Ethan Watters, "DNA is not destiny." Discover, 27, 11, November 2006. www.discover.com/printer-friendly-discover/?pid=106585.

44. M.E. Pembrey, "Time to take epigenetic inheritance seriously." European Journal of Human Genetics, 10, 11 (2002): 669–671. PMID 12404095.

45. R. Lamb, "What is the human epigenome project?" Available from: http:/science.howstuffworks.com/genetic-science/human-epigenome-project. htm/printable. (Accessed September 23, 2009).

46. H.T. Bjornsson, M.D. Fallin, and A.P. Feinberg, "An integrated epigenetic and genetic approach to common human disease." Trends in Genetics, 20, 8 (2004): 350–358. PMID 15262407.

SIDEBAR: PERSPECTIVE: A TRANSGENERATIONAL VIEW

1. G. Kaati, L.O. Bygren, M. Pembrey, M. Sjostrom, "Transgenerational response to nutrition, early life circumstances and longevity." European Journal of Human Genetics, vol. 15, No. 7 (2007): 784–790. PMID 17457370.

2. C. Matyn, D. Barker C. and Osmond, "Mothers' pelvic size, fetal growth, and death from stroke and coronary heart disease in men in the UK." Lancet, 348 (1996): 1264–1268. PMID 8909378.

3. M.E. Pembrey, L.O. Bygren, G. Kaati, S. Edvinsson, K. Northstone M. Sjostrom, "Sex-specific, male-line transgenerational responses in humans." European Journal of Human Genetics, 14, 2 (2006): 159–166. PMID 16391557.

4. L.H. Lumey, and A.D. Stein, "Offspring birth weights after maternal intrauterine undernutrition: a comparison within sibships." American Journal of Epidemiology, 146, 10 (1997): 810–819. PMID 9384201.

5. J. Allen, "U.S. kids even fatter than believed," Available from www.today. msnbc.msn.com/id/35938575/ns/health-kids_and_parenting/. (Accessed May 17, 2010).

CHAPTER 3: DIET, DNA AND DISEASE

1. D. Engelhardt, "Children getting fat younger. 2003." Available from: www.smh.com.au/articles/2003/05/16/1052885392617.html. (Accessed February 25, 2010).

2. J.B. Meigs, "Epidemiology of the metabolic syndrome." American Journal of Managed Care, 8, 11 Suppl (2002): S283–292; quiz S293–296; PMID 12240700.

3. R.A. Waterland, M. Travisano, K.G. Tahiliani, M.T. Rached, and S. Mirza, "Methyl donor supplementation prevents transgenerational amplification of obesity." International Journal of Obesity, (London) 32, 9 (2008): 1373–1379. PMID 18626486.

4. D.C. Dolinoy, J.R. Weidman, R.A. Waterland, and R.L. Jirtle, "Maternal genistein alters coat color and protects AVY mouse offspring from obesity by modifying the fetal epigenome." Environmental Health Perspectives, 114, 4 (2006): 567–572. PMID 16581547.

5. Deborah Kesten and Larry Scherwitz interviewed Dana Delinoy, MPH, PhD, on September 3, 2009.

6. M.B. Schwartz and K.D. Brownell, "Actions necessary to prevent child-

hood obesity: Creating the climate for change." Journal of Law and Medical Ethics, 35, 1 (2007): 78–89. PMID 17341218.

7. E. Schlosser, Fast food nation: The dark side of the all-American meal. New York: HarperCollins, 2002.

8. Safer States, "Tests find BPA in 'microwave safe' plastics." Available from www.saferstates.com/2008/11/tests-find-bpa.html. Posted November 17, 2008, based on tests conducted by the Milwaukee Journal Sentinel, reported by investigative journalists Susanne Rust and Meg Kissinger. (Accessed February 25, 2010).

9. D.C. Dolinoy, D. Huang, and R.L. Jirtle, "Maternal nutrient supplementation counteracts bisphenol a-induced DNA hypomethylation in early development." Proceedings of the National Academy of Sciences U.S. A, 104, 32 (2007): 13056–13061. PMID 17670942.

10. T. Colborn, J. Myers, and D. Dumanoski, "The partnership call: Endocrine disruption and environmental health: Ten years after our stolen future" (2006). Collaborative on Health and the Environment. Available from http://www.healthandenvironment.org/articles/call_resources/420. (Accessed August 1, 2010).

11. D. Melzer, N.E. Rice, C. Lewis, W.E. Henley, and T.S. Galloway, "Association of urinary bisphenol a concentration with heart disease: Evidence from NHANES." PLoS One, 5, 1, (2003): e8673. PMID 20084273.

12. National Diabetes Factsheet 2007. Department of Health and Human Services, Center for Disease Control and Prevention. Available from http://www.cdc.gov/diabetes/pubs/pdf/ndfs_2007.pdf. (Accessed February 28, 2010).

13. American Diabetes Association (ADA). "Standards of medical care in diabetes." Diabetes Care, 32 (2009): S13–S61. PMID 19118286.

14. B.M. Jucker, G.W. Cline, N. Barucci, and G.I. Shulman, "Differential effects of safflower oil versus fish oil feeding on insulin-stimulated glycogen synthesis, glycolysis, and pyruvate dehydrogenase flux in skeletal muscle: A 13c, nuclear magnetic resonance study. " Diabetes, 48, 1 (1999): 134–140. PMID 9892234.

15. D.H. Han, P.A. Hansen, H.H. Host, and J.O. Holloszy, "Insulin resistance of muscle glucose transport in rats fed a high-fat diet: A reevaluation." Diabetes, 46, 11 (1997): 1761–1767. PMID 9356023.

16. A.H. Harding, L.A. Sargeant, A. Welch, S. Oakes, R.N. Luben, S. Bingham, N.E. Day, K.T. Khaw, and N.J. Wareham, "Fat consumption and HBA(1c) levels: The EPIC-Norfolk study." Diabetes Care, 24, 11 (2001): 1911–1916. PMID 11679456.

17. N.D. Oakes, K.S. Bell, S.M. Furler, S. Camilleri, A.K. Saha, N.B. Ruderman, D.J. Chisholm, and E.W. Kraegen, "Diet-induced muscle insulin resistance in rats is ameliorated by acute dietary lipid withdrawal or a single bout of exercise: Parallel relationship between insulin stimulation of glucose

uptake and suppression of long-chain fatty acyl-CoA." Diabetes, 46, 12 (1997): 2022–2028. PMID 9392490.

18. Two studies referenced above show that a high fat diet increases the insulin resistance in rats (reference 15 and 17) while a high fat diet is associated with higher HA1c levels in humans (reference 16).

19. J.A. Marshall, D.H. Bessesen, and R.F. Hamman, "High saturated fat and low starch and fibre are associated with hyperinsulinaemia in a non-diabetic population: The San Luis Valley diabetes study." Diabetologia, 40, 4 (1997): 430–438. PMID 9112020.

20. E.J. Feskens, S.M. Virtanen, L. Rasanen, J. Tuomilehto, J. Stengard, J. Pekkanen, A. Nissinen, and D. Kromhout, "Dietary factors determining diabetes and impaired glucose tolerance. A 20-year follow-up of the Finnish and Dutch cohorts of the seven countries study." Diabetes Care 18, 8 (1995): 1104–1112; PMID 7587845.

21. E.J. Mayer-Davis, J.H. Monaco, H.M. Hoen, S. Carmichael, M.Z. Vitolins, M.J. Rewers, S.M. Haffner, M.F. Ayad, R.N. Bergman, and A.J. Karter, "Dietary fat and insulin sensitivity in a triethnic population: The role of obesity. The insulin resistance atherosclerosis study (IRAS)." American Journal of Clinical Nutrition, 65, 1 (1997): 79–87. PMID 8988917.

22. S. Jacob, J. Machann, K. Rett, K. Brechtel, A. Volk, W. Renn, E. Maerker, S. Matthaei, F. Schick, C.D. Claussen, and H.U. Haring, "Association of increased intramyocellular lipid content with insulin resistance in lean nondiabetic offspring of type 2 diabetic subjects." Diabetes, 48, 5 (1999): 1113–1119. PMID 10331418.

23. N.D. Oakes, G.J. Cooney, S. Camilleri, D.J. Chisholm, and E.W. Kraegen, "Mechanisms of liver and muscle insulin resistance induced by chronic high-fat feeding." Diabetes, 46, 11 (1997): 1768–1774. PMID 9356024.

24. R. Barres, M.E. Osler, J. Yan, A. Rune, T. Fritz, K. Caidahl, A. Krook, and J.R. Zierath, "Non-cpg methylation of the pgc-1alpha promoter through dnmt3b controls mitochondrial density." Cell Metabolism, 10, 3, (2009): 189–198. PMID 19723495.

25. M. Haag and N.G. Dippenaar, "Dietary fats, fatty acids and insulin resistance: Short review of a multifaceted connection." Medical Science Monitoring, 11, 12 (2005): RA359–367. PMID 16319806.

26. "Dynamic changes in DNA linked to human diabetes," available from www.scienceblog.com/cms/dynamic-changes-dna-linked-human-diabetes-24684.html. (Accessed February 17, 2010)

27. "Don't blame your genes," The Economist, Sept. 3, 2009, Science and Technology section: 86

28. H.M. Roche, C. Phillips, and M.J. Gibney, "The metabolic syndrome: The crossroads of diet and genetics." Proceedings of the Nutrition Society, 64, 3 (2005): 371–377. PMID 16048671.

29. E.S. Ford, W.H. Giles, and A.H. Mokdad, "Increasing prevalence of

the metabolic syndrome among U.S. Adults. Diabetes Care, 27, 10 (2004): 2444–2449. PMID 15451914.

30. C. Gallou-Kabani and C. Junien, "Nutritional epigenomics of metabolic syndrome: New perspective against the epidemic." Diabetes, 54, 7 (2005): 1899–1906. PMID 15983188.

31. P.D. Gluckman, M.A. Hanson, and H.G. Spencer, eds. "Predictive adaptive responses and human evolution." Trends in Ecology and Evolution, 20 (2005): 527–533.

SIDEBAR: PERSPECTIVE: ANOTHER FAT-DIABETES VIEW

1. Cordain, L., et al., "Plant-animal subsistence ratios and macronutrient energy estimations in worldwide hunter-gatherer diets." American Journal of Clinical Nutrition, 71, 3, (2000): 682–692. PMID 10702160.

2. Agriculture Fact Book 2000–2001, "Chapter 2: Profiling Food Consumption in America," 14. Available from http://www.usda.gov/factbook/chapter2.htm. (Accessed August 2, 2010).

3. Sugar consumption. Available from: http://www.healingdaily.com/detoxification-diet/sugar.htm. (Accessed August 2, 2010).

4. F.B. Hu, J.E. Manson, and W.C. Willett, "Types of dietary fat and risk of coronary heart disease: A critical review." Journal of the American College of Nutrition, 20, 1 (2001): 5–19. PMID 11293467.

5. "National diabetes statistics, 2007: Prevalence of diagnosed and undiagnosed diabetes in the United States, all ages, 2007." Available from: www.diabetes.niddk.nih.gov/dm/pubs/statistics/index.htm. (Accessed May 17, 2010).

6. National Diabetes Information Clearinghouse, "National diabetes statistics, 2007: Incidence of diagnosed diabetes in people younger than 20 years of age, United States, 2002 to 2003." (Accessed May 17, 2010).

CHAPTER 4: CURTAILING CANCER: EPIGENETICS IN ACTION

1. National Cancer Institute "SEER stat fact sheets" Lifetime Risk, http://seer.cancer.gov/statfacts/html/prost.html. (Accessed August 3, 2009).

2. Deborah Kesten interviewed Robert Caldwell (a pseudonym is being used at the request of the interviewee) during a telephone interview at his home and office on May 6, 2009. All quotations, experiences, and opinions from and about Caldwell were derived from the interview.

3. Caldwell's prostate specific antigen scores before diagnosis were low and normal; on successive readings they were 1.5 and 1.5 before the diagnosis of prostate cancer. At the time of diagnosis, his Gleason score was 3+3, with tumor tissue involving less than 5 percent of the sampled tissue (based on one of twelve core samples). Follow-up readings after the biopsy were 1.6, 1.8, and 2.9, respectively. After following and implementing the Ornish lifestyle intervention, a second biopsy showed no evidence of cancerous tissue in any of 16

core samples. The PSA values that followed this second biopsy were 1.9, 10.2, 3.6, and 1.9 respectively. These results show that PSA values may not necessarily indicate evidence of cancer in an early stage, and that PSA values can spike when there is no evidence of cancer.

4. Dean Ornish, L.W. Scherwitz, R.S. Doody, D. Kesten, S.M. McLanahan, S.E. Brown, E. DePuey, R. Sonnemaker, C. Haynes, J. Lester, G.K. McAllister, R.J. Hall, J.A. Burdine, and A.M. Gotto, Jr., "Effects of stress management training and dietary changes in treating ischemic heart disease." Journal of the American Medical Association, 249, 1 (1983): 54–59. PMID 6336794.

5. Ornish and his team had conducted an earlier pilot study with nine patients with heart disease (1977). To implement the intervention, for 30 days the nine research participants lived in a residential retreat environment in Houston, Texas. After following the program for one month, the participants showed substantial weight loss and the frequency and duration of chest pain diminished, as did serum cholesterol levels. Perhaps most interesting is that two of the research participants had an exercise thallium scan prior to starting the program and one month later and they both showed improved blood flow to the heart muscle during exercise. Ornish and his team designed a second study that would build upon the success of the pilot project.

Co-author Dr. Larry Scherwitz was an assistant professor at Baylor College of Medicine in Houston, Texas, when he met Ornish, who was a medical student at the time. Scherwitz became Ornish's Co-Principal Investigator and research collaborator. In this capacity, Ornish and Scherwitz planned, implemented, and evaluated the first randomized controlled clinical trial cited in this chapter, the results of which were published in the Journal of the American Medical Association in 1983; co-author Deborah Kesten was the nutritionist on Ornish's first clinical trial for reversing heart disease. To conduct the intervention, Ornish and his team of investigators lived with the 24 research participants for 24 days at a lakeside residential resort. During this time, Ornish repeated all four components of his lifestyle intervention.

Post-intervention tests revealed that the research participants had a 55 percent mean increase in total work performed; a 20.5 percent decrease in plasma cholesterol levels; and a 91.0 percent mean reduction in frequency of angina episodes. Most interestingly, the ability of their heart to pump blood during exercise had significantly improved when compared with those in the usual care group. We still needed to demonstrate whether RPs could make lifestyle changes for the long term.

After Ornish completed his internal medicine residency at Massachusetts General Hospital in 1984, he moved to San Francisco where Ornish, Scherwitz, and eight other colleagues conducted a comprehensive study, which demonstrated that lifestyle changes can reverse coronary heart disease without drugs or surgery. To do this, they studied 48 participants for five years and then published the results in The Lancet (1990); a five year follow-up on the intervention was published in the Journal of the American Medical Association (1998).

The study was the first to show that combining diet, exercise, stress management, and social support results in better blood flow through coronary arteries (determined by angiographies) and better blood flow to the heart muscle (demonstrated with Positive Emission Tomography [PET] scans) compared to those in the usual-care control group whose heart disease worsened during this interval. For more information, visit the Ornish website at www.PMRI.org.

6. D. Ornish, G. Weidner, W.R. Fair, R. Marlin, E.B. Pettengill, C.J. Raisin, S. Dunn-Emke, L. Crutchfield, F.N. Jacobs, R.J. Barnard, W.J. Aronson, P. McCormac, D.J. McKnight, J.D. Fein, A.M. Dnistrian, J. Weinstein, T.H. Ngo, N.R. Mendell, and P.R. Carroll, "Intensive lifestyle changes may affect the progression of prostate cancer." Journal of Urology, 174, 3 (2005): 1065–1070. PMID 16094059.

7. Dean Ornish, J. Lin, J. Daubenmier, G. Weidner, E. Epel, C. Kemp, M.J. Magbanua, R. Marlin, L. Yglecias, P.R. Carroll, and E.H. Blackburn, "Increased telomerase activity and comprehensive lifestyle changes: A pilot study." Lancet Oncology, 9, 11 (2008): 1048–1057. PMID 18799354.

8. Dean Ornish, M.J. Magbanua, G. Weidner, V. Weinberg, C. Kemp, C. Green, M.D. Mattie, R. Marlin, J. Simko, K. Shinohara, C.M. Haqq, and P.R. Carroll, "Changes in prostate gene expression in men undergoing an intensive nutrition and lifestyle intervention." Proceedings of the National Academy of Sciences U S A, 105, 24 (2008): 8369–8374. PMID 18559852.

9. D. Ornish, L.W. Scherwitz, J.H. Billings, S.E. Brown, K.L. Gould, T.A. Merritt, S. Sparler, W.T. Armstrong, T.A. Ports, R.L. Kirkeeide, C. Hogeboom, and R.J. Brand, "Intensive lifestyle changes for reversal of coronary heart disease." Journal of the American Medical Association, 280, 23 (1998): 2001–2007. PMID 9863851.

10. Dean Ornish, "Avoiding revascularization with lifestyle changes: The multicenter lifestyle demonstration project." American Journal of Cardiology, 82, 10B (1998): 72T–76T. PMID 9860380.

11. Ornish et al., "Intensive lifestyle changes." (1998).

12. K.L. Gould, D. Ornish, L. Scherwitz, S. Brown, R.P. Edens, M.J. Hess, N. Mullani, L. Bolomey, F. Dobbs, W.T. Armstrong, et al., "Changes in myocardial perfusion abnormalities by positron emission tomography after long-term, intense risk factor modification." Journal of the American Medical Association, 274, 11 (1995): 894–901. PMID 7674504.

13. G.A. Sonn, W. Aronson, and M.S. Litwin, "Impact of diet on prostate cancer: A review." Prostate Cancer Prostatic Disease, 8, 4 (2005): 304–310. PMID 16130015.

14. C. L. Van Patten, J.G. de Boer, and E.S. Tomlinson Guns, "Diet and dietary supplement intervention trials for the prevention of prostate cancer recurrence: A review of the randomized controlled trial evidence." Journal of Urology, 180, 6 (2008): 2314–2322. PMID 18930254.

15. J.M. Chan, C.N. Holick, M.F. Leitzmann, E.B. Rimm, W.C. Willett, M.J. Stampfer, and E.L. Giovannucci, "Diet after diagnosis and the risk of prostate cancer progression, recurrence, and death (United States)." Cancer Causes Control, 17, 2 (2006): 199–208. PMID 16425098.

16. M.F. Leitzmann, M.J. Stampfer, D.S. Michaud, K. Augustsson, G.C. Colditz, W.C. Willett, and E.L. Giovannucci, "Dietary intake of n-3 and n-6 fatty acids and the risk of prostate cancer." American Journal of Clinical Nutrition, 80, 1 (2004): 204–216. PMID 15213050.

17. E. Giovannucci, E.B. Rimm, Y. Liu, M.J. Stampfer, and W.C. Willett, "A prospective study of tomato products, lycopene, and prostate cancer risk." Journal of the National Cancer Institute, 94, 5 (2002): 391–398. PMID 11880478.

18. H.S. Kim, P. Bowen, L. Chen, C. Duncan, L. Ghosh, R. Sharifi, and K. Christov, "Effects of tomato sauce consumption on apoptotic cell death in prostate benign hyperplasia and carcinoma." Nutrition and Cancer, 47, 1 (2003): 40–47. PMID 14769536.

19. S. Rohrmann, E.A. Platz, C.J. Kavanaugh, L. Thuita, S.C. Hoffman, and K.J. Helzlsouer, "Meat and dairy consumption and subsequent risk of prostate cancer in a U.S. cohort study." Cancer Causes & Control, 18, 1 (2007): 41–50. PMID 17315319.

20. S. Koutros, A.J. Cross, D.P. Sandler, J.A. Hoppin, X. Ma, T. Zheng, M.C. Alavanja, and R. Sinha, "Meat and meat mutagens and risk of prostate cancer in the agricultural health study." Cancer Epidemiology Biomarkers and Prevention, 17, 1 (2008): 80–87. PMID 18199713.

21. Cancer has traditionally been more resistant to all but the most radical conventional therapies. Because of this, Ornish set the standards of his lifestyle-change recommendations higher to avoid missing the treatment effect, if it existed. He reasoned that if he could piece together the various associations among diet, stress, exercise, and social support to build a case for his comprehensive approach, he could justify asking the research participants to make more extreme changes. The study successfully achieved great dietary-, exercise-, and social-support adherence, likely, in large part, because the research participants faced the possibility of impotence and incontinence if they had to opt for surgery. The low-fat, plant-based diet is not designed for the general public. See Dean Ornish, The Spectrum, New York, Ballantine Books (2007) for an overview of his lifestyle approach.

22. Recruiting individuals who were willing to participate in the study was a major undertaking. First, it involved finding patients who were willing to participate and not seek conventional treatment and whose physicians were willing to forego providing conventional treatment for their patients. The research team also needed to convince the research participants to make a lifestyle change so extreme that it had never been done before. And finally participation in the intervention also meant getting a second biopsy for research purposes. Visit www.pmri.org for more information.

23. The weekly support group meetings, with their emphasis upon disclosure and reflection on feelings, made the program's intervention and its aims a truly tribal effort. This component of the program helped to encourage adhering to intensive lifestyle changes, it bonded the research participants, and it had the added benefit of providing social support to spouses and other family members.

24. Research participants were prescribed a vegan diet supplemented with soy (1 daily serving of tofu plus 58 grams of a fortified soy protein powdered beverage), fish oil (3 grams daily), vitamin E (400 IU daily), selenium (200 mcg daily) and vitamin C (2 grams daily), moderate aerobic exercise (walking 60 minutes, six days weekly), stress management techniques (gentle yoga-based stretching, breathing, meditation, imagery and progressive relaxation for a total of 60 minutes daily), and participation in a one-hour support group once weekly to enhance adherence to the intervention.

25. The rationale for the diet was based on avoiding foods that may be a risk factor and to include foods that were believed to be beneficial. The basic diet consisted mostly of fresh, whole, plant-based food in its natural state as often as possible. The diet was predominantly fruits, vegetables, whole grains (complex carbohydrates), legumes, and soy products. Additionally, it was designed to be low in simple carbohydrates, with approximately 10 percent of calories from fat (see Ornish 2005, note 5, above). The diet was also designed to replace higher calorie foods, e.g., meat, nuts and seeds, and dairy products with more nutrient-dense foods, e.g., fresh vegetables such as broccoli, leafy greens and tomatoes. This diet resulted in weight loss for the research participants, while providing a higher level (per calorie) of the macro- and micronutrients we need for our bodies to function optimally.

Another strong contributor to the dietary guidelines was based on the dietary recommendations and results from Dr. Ornish and team's San Francisco Lifestyle Heart Trial. During the trial, research participants completed three-day diet diaries at baseline and following two follow-up angiograms. When the results were analyzed, it became apparent that the level of fat and cholesterol intake was significantly correlated with regression or progression of disease, as was weight gain. Put another way, those who had the lowest intake of fat and cholesterol had a better chance of reversing their blocked coronary arteries than those who consumed even a little more dietary fat and cholesterol. Conversely, those in the control group who gained the most weight had the most progression of heart disease. Ornish and his team reasoned that if a low-fat, plant-based diet was an effective component of the heart disease reversal program, that it would be good to be consistent and try a comparable diet (with modifications) for men with prostate cancer.

26. Also, soy-based foods and soy-protein beverages were included to replace casein, which has been found to correspond to increased prostate tumor growth in rats. See Hakkak, R., et al., "Soy protein isolate consumption pro-

tects against azoxymethane-induced colon tumors in male rats," Cancer Letter, 166, 1 (2001): 27–32. PMID 11295283.

In addition, Ornish may have known about the study conducted at the University of California, Los Angeles, in 1998 in which a low-fat + soy protein + isoflavone extract diet reduced the growth rates of human prostate cancer cells in vivo. See W.J. Aronson, C.N. Tymchuk, R.M. Elashoff, W.H. McBride, C. McLean, H. Wang, D. Heber, "Decreased growth of human prostate LNCaP tumors in SCID mice fed a low-fat, soy protein diet with isoflavones," Nutrition and Cancer, 35, 2 (1999): 130–136. PMID 10693166.

27. L.Q. Qin, J.Y. Xu, P.Y. Wang, T. Kaneko, K. Hoshi, and A. Sato, "Milk consumption is a risk factor for prostate cancer: Meta-analysis of case-control studies." Nutrition and Cancer, 48, 1 (2004): 22–27. PMID 15203374.

28. Several cohort and case-control studies associate milk, yogurt, and cheese consumption with prostate cancer. For a review see Ganmaa, D. and A. Sato, "The possible role of female sex hormones in milk from pregnant cows in the development of breast, ovarian and corpus uteri cancers." Medical Hypotheses, 65(6) 2005: 1028–1037. PMID 16125328.

29. W.B. Grant, "An ecologic study of dietary links to prostate cancer." Alternative Medicine Review, 4(3) 1999: 162–169. PMID 10383480.

30. J.M. Hamilton-Reeves, S.A. Rebello, W. Thomas, M.S. Kurzer, and J.W. Slaton, "Effects of soy protein isolate consumption on prostate cancer biomarkers in men with HGPIN, ASAP, and low-grade prostate cancer." Nutrition and Cancer, 60, 1 (2008): 7–13. PMID 18444130.

31. E. Kesse, S. Bertrais, P. Astorg, A. Jaouen, N. Arnault, P. Galan, and S. Hercberg, "Dairy products, calcium and phosphorus intake, and the risk of prostate cancer: Results of the French prospective su.Vi.Max (supplementation en vitamines et mineraux antioxydants) study." British Journal of Nutrition, 95, 3 (2006): 539–545. PMID 16512941.

32. S. Torniainen, M. Hedelin, V. Autio, H. Rasinpera, K.A. Balter, A. Klint, R. Bellocco, F. Wiklund, P. Stattin, T. Ikonen, T.L. Tammela, J. Schleutker, H. Gronberg, and I. Jarvela, "Lactase persistence, dietary intake of milk, and the risk for prostate cancer in Sweden and Finland." Cancer Epidemiology Biomarkers and Prevention, 16, 5 (2007): 956–961. PMID 17507622.

33. Zhang, J. and H. Kesteloot, "Milk consumption in relation to incidence of prostate, breast, colon, and rectal cancers: Is there an independent effect?" Nutrition and Cancer, 53, 1, (2005): 65–72. PMID 16351508.

34. S.I. Berndt, H.B. Carter, P.K. Landis, K.L. Tucker, L.J. Hsieh, E.J. Metter, and E.A. Platz, "Calcium intake and prostate cancer risk in a long-term aging study: The Baltimore longitudinal study of aging." Urology, 60, 6 (2002): 1118–1123. PMID 12475694.

35. One possible mechanism by which milk could increase the chances of prostate cancer is through the xenoestrogens in much of the modern milk supply. Modern dairies milk pregnant cows and this raises the estrogen levels in

milk. In turn, high estrogen levels in milk have been linked to growth of prostate cancer cells.

36. L.Q. Qin, P.Y. Wang, T. Kaneko, K. Hoshi, and A. Sato, "Estrogen: One of the risk factors in milk for prostate cancer." Medical Hypotheses, 62, 1 (2004): 133–142. PMID 1472901937. For a closer look at the clinical and epidemiological studies examining processed meats such as bacon and salami, see D. S. Michaud, K. Augustsson, E.B. Rimm, M.J. Stampfer, W. C. Willet, E. Giovannucci, "A prospective study on intake of animal products and risk of prostate cancer." Cancer Causes Control, 12, 6 (2001): 557–567 PMID 11519764; see also S. Rohrmann, E.A. Platz, C.J. Kavanaugh, L. Thuita, S. Hoffman, K.J. Helzlsouer, "Meat and dairy consumption and subsequent risk of prostate cancer in a U.S. cohort study," Cancer Causes and Control, 18, 1, (2007): 41–50. PMID 17315319.

37. Well-grilled and processed red meat is more strongly related to prostate cancer than fresh and unprocessed red meat. See A. J. Cross, U. Peters, V. A. Kirsh, G.L. Andriole, D. Reding, R. B. Hayes, R. Sinha, "A prospective study of meat and meat mutagens and prostate cancer risk," Cancer Research, 65, 24, (2005): 11779–11784. PMID16357191. See also D. Tang, J.J. Liu, A. Rundle, C. Neslund-Dudas, A. T. Savera, C. H. Bock, N. L. Nock, J.J. Yang, B. A. Rybicki, "Grilled meat consumption and PhIP-DNA adducts in prostate carcinogenesis." Cancer Epidemiology Biomarkers and Prevention, 16, 4 (2007): 803–808. PMID 17416774.

Not all studies are negative for meat; however, two laboratory studies show tallow and other components of meat to promote prostate cancer cell growth in animals. J. A. Mobley, I. Leav, P. Zielie, C. Wotkowitz, J. Evans, Y.W. Lam, B.S. L'Esperance, Z. Jiang, S.M. Ho, "Branched fatty acids in dairy and beef products markedly enhance alpha-methylacyl-CoA racemase expression in prostate cancer cells in vitro." Cancer Epidemiology Biomarkers and Prevention, 12,8 (2003): 775–783. PMID 12917210. See also T. Mori, K. Imaida, S. Tamano, M. Sano, S. Takahashi, M. Asamoto, M. Takeshita, H. Ueda, T. Shirai, "Beef tallow, but not perilla or corn oil, promotion of rat prostate and intestinal carcinogenesis by 3,2'-dimethyl-4-aminobiphenyl." Japanese Journal of Cancer Research, 92, 10 (2001): 1026–1033. PMID 11676852.

38. M. Hedelin, E.T. Chang, F. Wiklund, R. Bellocco, A. Klint, J. Adolfsson, K. Shahedi, J. Xu, H.O. Adami, H. Gronberg, and K.A. Balter, "Association of frequent consumption of fatty fish with prostate cancer risk is modified by cox-2 polymorphism." International Journal of Cancer, 120, 2 (2007): 398–405. PMID 17066444.

39. P. Terry, P. Lichtenstein, M. Feychting, A. Ahlbom, and A. Wolk, "Fatty fish consumption and risk of prostate cancer." Lancet, 357, 9270 (2001): 1764–1766. PMID 11403817.

40. K. Augustsson, D.S. Michaud, E.B. Rimm, M.F. Leitzmann, M.J. Stampfer, W.C. Willett, and E. Giovannucci, "A prospective study of intake of fish

and marine fatty acids and prostate cancer." Cancer Epidemiology Biomarkers and Prevention, 12, 1 (2003): 64–67. PMID 12540506.

41. The statistical analysis correlated self-reported adherence to diet, exercise, and stress management with percent diameter stenosis, a measure of the blockage of the coronary arteries. Consistently, practicing stress management was more highly correlated with reversal of blockage than either diet or exercise after one year and again after the five-year angiogram. These results however should be considered tentative because all three components are correlated with one another (to some degree) and stress management was related to reversal of disease in those who were doing the recommended exercise and following the diet.

42. Billings J, Scherwitz L, Ornish D, Sullivan M, "Group Support Therapy in the Lifestyle Heart Trial." in R. Allan and S. Scheidt (Eds.) Heart and mind: The practice of cardiac psychology (Washington D.C.: American Psychological Association, 1996).

43. D. Spiegel, J.R. Bloom, H.C. Kraemer, and E. Gottheil, "Effect of psychosocial treatment on survival of patients with metastatic breast cancer." Lancet, 2, 8668 (1989): 888–891. PMID 2571815.

44. The down-regulated pathways were involved in protein metabolism and modification, intracellular protein traffic, and protein phosphorylation; see Ornish et al., 2008. "Changes in prostate gene expression in men."

45. S. Gonzalez, "Change your lifestyle, Change your genes," Ornish explains surprising new research (2009) at http://www.naturalnews.com/024015. html. (Accessed August 2, 2010).

46. One significant facet of this study is the degree of extreme change in lifestyle it took to achieve such results. During the three-month program, the average fat intake of the RPs was 11.6 percent of total calories (to give you some perspective, 30 percent is generally recommended in non-therapeutic diets); the research participants practiced stress management for an average of 4.5 hours each week; exercise averaged 3.6 hours weekly; and an additional one hour was dedicated to social support gatherings.

47. The improvement with the research participants diagnosed with prostate cancer may have been greater if they had done more than 45 minutes stress management. For example, most of the reversal achieved by the heart patients in the San Francisco Lifestyle Heart Trial was among those who did more than an hour a day. Eighty percent of participants got reversal if they did an hour and a half or more of stretching, deep relaxation, breathing techniques, meditation, and visualization. The practice of these stress management techniques in terms of minutes per week was better correlated with reversal of coronary artery blockages than either diet or exercise.

48. In other words, success requires a commitment of both time and dedication to "being in the world" in a new and different way. Make the commitment, though, and you're likely to reap still more rewards: the research participants

lost a substantial amount of weight; they lowered their blood pressure and cholesterol levels; and their psychological distress and mental health measures also improved.

49. The research participants' body mass index (BMI) went from 26.5 to 23.9 [waist circumference decreased by 7.7 centimeters), they lowered their blood pressure (from 129/68 to 120/63) and cholesterol (192 to 147) levels; and their psychological distress and mental health improved. Total PSA did not change significantly (from 4.8 to 4.6), although percent free PSA was improved. Free PSA means that the PSA molecule is not attached to other blood proteins and levels of free PSA are lower in men with prostate cancer compared with men with benign conditions.

50. Text from Dr. Ornish's keynote presentation at the Summit on Integrative Medicine and the Health of the Public, Institute of Medicine of the National Academies, Washington, D.C., February 26, 2009.

51. The GEMINAL study on gene expression was a pilot project done with one group of participants. Before it can be validated and verified as an approach for treating prostate cancer, the study needs to be replicated with a control group.

SIDEBAR PERSPECTIVE: A RE-VISIONING OF THE HIGH-FAT, LOW-FAT VIEW

1. F.B. Hu, J.E. Manson, and W.C. Willett, "Types of dietary fat and risk of coronary heart disease: A critical review." Journal of the American College of Nutrition, 20, 1 (2001): 5–19. PMID 11293467.

2. A. Esmaillzadeh, P. Mirmiran, and F. Azizi, "Whole grain consumption and the metabolic syndrome: A favorable association in Tehranian adults." European Journal of Clinical Nutrition, 59 (2005): 353–362, PMID 15536473.

3. A Simopoulos, A. and J. Robinson, The omega diet: The life saving nutritional program based on the diet of the island of Crete. New York: Harper, 1999.

4. A. Esmaillzadeh, and L. Azadbakht, "Consumption of hydrogenated versus nonhydrogenated vegetable oils and risk of insulin resistance and the metabolic syndrome among Iranian adult women." Diabetes Care, 31, 2 (2007): 223–226. PMID 18000178.

CHAPTER 5: IT'S THE LIFESTYLE, STUPID!

1. M.J. Reeves and A.P. Rafferty, "Healthy lifestyle characteristics among adults in the United States, 2000." Archives of Internal Medicine, 165, 8 (2005): 854–857. PMID 15851634.

2. "Healing Quest"; Wednesday, April 22, 2009; channel 3, KBTC; 10–10:30am PST; 30 minutes

3. DrGreene Content: Special Feature, "Breast Cancer—A Story of Sur-

vival," Available from www.drgreene.com/21_625.html. (Accessed August 21, 2009).

4. Jessica Tripp, "Information on the Fountain of Youth" eHow Contributing Writer, www.ehow.com/about_5135620_information-fountain-youth. html. (Accessed August 27, 2009).

5. Stibich, Mark, "The Fountain of Youth: Myth or Fact?" www.longevity. about.com/od/longevitylegends/p/fountain.htm. Updated: August 18, 2008. (Accessed August 26, 2009).

6. L Scherwitz L and R. Rugulies, "Lifestyle and hostility." Hostility, coping and health. Ed. H. Friedman. Washington, D.C., American Psychological Association, 1992.

7. D. Ornish, L.W. Scherwitz, R.S. Doody, D. Kesten, S.M. McLanahan, S.E. Brown, E. DePuey, R. Sonnemaker, C. Haynes, J. Lester, G.K. McAllister, R.J. Hall, J.A. Burdine, and A.M. Gotto, Jr., "Effects of stress management training and dietary changes in treating ischemic heart disease." Journal of the American Medical Association, 249, 1 (1983): 54–59. PMID 6336794.

8. D. Ornish, L.W. Scherwitz, J.H. Billings, S.E. Brown, K.L. Gould, T.A. Merritt, S. Sparler, W.T. Armstrong, T.A. Ports, R.L. Kirkeeide, C. Hogeboom, and R.J. Brand, "Intensive lifestyle changes for reversal of coronary heart disease." Journal of the American Medical Association, 280, 23 (1998): 2001–2007. PMID 9863851.

9. D. Ornish, G. Weidner, W.R. Fair, R. Marlin, E.B. Pettengill, C.J. Raisin, S. Dunn-Emke, L. Crutchfield, F.N. Jacobs, R.J. Barnard, W.J. Aronson, P. McCormac, D.J. McKnight, J.D. Fein, A.M. Dnistrian, J. Weinstein, T.H. Ngo, N.R. Mendell, and P.R. Carroll, "Intensive lifestyle changes may affect the progression of prostate cancer." Journal of Urology, 174, 3 (2005): 1065–1069; discussion 1069–70. PMID 16094059.

10. D. Ornish, M.J. Magbanua, G. Weidner, V. Weinberg, C. Kemp, C. Green, M.D. Mattie, R. Marlin, J. Simko, K. Shinohara, C.M. Haqq, and P.R. Carroll, "Changes in prostate gene expression in men undergoing an intensive nutrition and lifestyle intervention." Proceedings of the National Academy of Science U.S.A, 105, 24 (2008): 8369–8374. PMID 18559852.

11. Larry King Live, August 12, 2009, 12m, CNN, discussion on health care, moderated by Wolf Blitzer.

12. A.P. Feinberg, "Epigenetics at the epicenter of modern medicine." Journal of the American Medical Association, 299, 11 (2008): 1345–1350. PMID 18349095.

13. Z. Attias, H. Werner, and N. Vaisman, "Folic acid and its metabolites modulate IGFI-I receptor gene expression in colon cancer cells in a p53-dependent manner." Endocrine Related Cancer, 13, 2 (2006): 571–581. PMID 16728583.

14. T.S. Church, C.K. Martin, A.M. Thompson, C.P. Earnest, C.R. Mikus, and S.N. Blair, "Changes in weight, waist circumference and compensatory

responses with different doses of exercise among sedentary, overweight post-menopausal women." PLoS One, 4, 2 (2009): e4515. PMID 19223984.

15. K. Brownell, "Yale Rudd Center for Food Policy and obesity." 2009; Available from: http://www.yaleruddcenter.org (cited 2009; accessed September 3, 2009).

16. John Cloud, "Why exercise won't make you thin," Time, August 17, 2009, 43.

17. D. Kesten, Feeding the body, nourishing the soul. Amherst, MA: White River Press, 2008.

18. L. Scherwitz and D. Kesten, "Seven eating styles linked to overeating, overweight, and obesity." Explore (NY), 1, 5 (2005): 342–359. PMID 16781565.

19. D. Kesten and L. Scherwitz, The enlightened diet: 7 weight-loss solutions that nourish body, mind, and soul. Berkeley, CA: Ten Speed Press, 2007.

20. H. Benson and W.M. Klipper, The relaxation response. New York: Harper Collins, 1975.

21. J.A. Dusek and H. Benson, "Mind-body medicine: A model of the comparative clinical impact of the acute stress and relaxation responses." Minnesota Medicine, 92, 5 (2009): 47–50. PMID 19552264.

22. E.M. Sternberg, "Emotions and disease: From balance of humors to balance of molecules." Nature Medicine, 3 (2008): 264–267. PMID 9055845.

23. H. Benson, I.L. Goodale. "The relaxation response: Your inborn capacity to counteract the harmful effects of stress." Journal of Florida Medical Association, 68 (1981): 265–267. PMID 7014762.

24. J.E. Platt , X. He, D. Tang, J. Slater, and M. Goldstein, "C-fos expression in vivo in human lymphocytes in response to stress." Progress in Neuro-Psychopharmacology and Biological Psychiatry, 19, (1995): 65–74. PMID 7708933.

25. R. Glaser, S. Kennedy, W.P. Lafuse, R.H. Bonneau, and C. Speicher, J. Hillhouse, J.K. Kiecolt-Glaser, "Psychological stress-induced modulation of interleukin 2 receptor gene expression and interleukin 2 production in peripheral blood leukocytes." Archives of General Psychiatry, 47 (1990): 707–712. PMID 2378541.

26. R. Glaser, W.P. Lafuse, R.H. Bonneau, C. Atkinson, and J.K. Kiecolt-Glaser, "Stress-associated modulation of proto-oncogene expression in human peripheral blood leukocytes." Behavioral Neuroscience, 107 (1993): 525–529. PMID 8329139.

27. J.A. Dusek, H.H. Otu, A.L. Wohlhueter, M. Bhasin, L.F. Zerbini, M.G. Joseph, H. Benson, and T.A. Libermann, "Genomic counter-stress changes induced by the relaxation response." PLoS One, 3, 7 (2008): e2576. PMID 18596974.

28. C.W. Christian, N.J. Blum, Nelson's essentials of pediatrics (Section V, Chapter 21) Philadelphia: Elsevier, 2005.

29. D. Schwartz, "Failure to thrive: An old nemesis in a new millenium." Pediatrics in Review, 21 (2000): 257–264. PMID 10922022.

30. D. Spiegel, J.R. Bloom, H.C. Kraemer, and E. Gottheil, "Effect of psychosocial treatment on survival of patients with metastatic breast cancer." Lancet, 2, 8668 (1989): 888–891. PMID 2571815.

31. R.M. Nerem, M.J. Levesque, and J.F. Cornhill, "Social environment as a factor in diet-induced atherosclerosis." Science, 208, 4451 (1980): 1475–1476. PMID 7384790.

32. D. Ornish, Love and survival: The scientific basis for the healing power of intimacy. New York: HarperCollins, 1998.

33. J. Cassel, "The contribution of the social environment to host resistance: The fourth Wade Hampton Frost lecture." American Journal of Epidemiology, 104, 2 (1976): 107–123. PMID 782233.

34. K. Kendler, J. Myers, and C. Prescott, "Sex differences in the relationship between social support and risk for major depression: A longitudinal study of opposite-sex twin pairs." American Journal of Psychiatry, 162, 2 (2005): 250–256. PMID 15677587.

35. P.O. McGowan, M.J. Meaney, and M. Szyf, "Diet and the epigenetic (re)programming of phenotypic differences in behavior." Brain Research, 1237 (2008): 12–24. PMID 18694740.

36. P.O. McGowan, A. Sasaki, A.C. D'Alessio, S. Dymov, B. Labonte, M. Szyf, G. Turecki, and M.J. Meaney, "Epigenetic regulation of the glucocorticoid receptor in human brain associates with childhood abuse." Nature Neuroscience, 12, 3 (2009): 342–348. PMID 19234457.

37. S. Hyman, "How adversity gets under the skin." Nature Neuroscience, 12, 3 (2009): 241–243. PMID 19238182.

38. Price, Rhonda, "Mariel Hemingway believes that extraordinary health starts in the kitchen." Extraordinary Health, 7 (2009): 12.

39. Samueli Institute, "A wellness initiative for the nation," PDF available from http://www.siib.org/news/611-IIB/version/default/part/AttachmentData/data/WIN%20Summary%2020Apr09.pdf. (Accessed September 5, 2009).

40. "The Take Back Your Health Act of 2009" by U.S. Senator Ron Wyden (D-Oregon) Available from http://webferret.search.com/click?wf6,take+back+your+health+act+2009,,wyden.senate.gov%2Fnewsroom%2Frecord.cfm%3Fid%3D316933,,aol,l. (Accessed September 5, 2009).

Chapter 6: Food, Genes, and Health Over Time

1. "History of the Aborigines." Available from http://library.thinkquest.org/CR0215290/history.htm. (Accessed December 28, 2009).

2. "Australian Aborigines." Available from www.factmonster.com/ce6/society/A0805377.html. (Accessed December 28, 2009).

3. D. Nathan, "Aboriginal Languages of Australia." Aboriginal Languag-

es of Australia Virtual Library, http://www.dnathan.com/VL/austLang.htm, 2007. (Accessed December 28, 2009).

4. K. O'Dea, P.A. Jewell, A. Whiten, S.A. Altmann, S.S. Strickland, and O.T. Oftedal, "Traditional diet and food preferences of Australian aboriginal hunter-gatherers." Philosophical Transactions: Biological Sciences, 334, (1991): 233–241 PMID 1685581.

5. "History of the Aborigines." Available from http://library.thinkquest. org/CR0215290/history.htm. (Accessed December 28, 2009).

6. G. Burenhult, ed. Traditional peoples today: Continuity and change in the modern world. Vol. 5 of Illustrated history of humankind. New York: Harper Collins, 1994.

7. L. Cordain, J.B. Miller, S.B. Eaton, N. Mann, S.H. Holt, and J.D. Speth, "Plant-animal subsistence ratios and macronutrient energy estimations in worldwide hunter-gatherer diets." American Journal of Clinical Nutrition, 71, 3 (2000): 682–692; PMID 10702160.

8. L.E. Cordain, B Sebastian, A. Mann, N. Lindebery, S. Watkins, B. O'Keefe, J. Brand-Miller J, "Origins and evolution of the western diet: Health implications for the 21st century." American Journal of Clinical Nutrition, 81 (2004): 341–354. PMID 15699220.

9. R. Lee and I. DeVore, eds. What hunters do for a living, or how to make out on scarce resources. Man the hunter. Chicago: Aldine, 1968: 30–48.

10. J.D. Speth, K.A. Spielmann KA, "Energy source, protein metabolism, and hunter-gatherer subsistence strategies." Journal of Anthropological Archaeology, 2, (1983): 1–31.

11. J.D. Speth, K.A. Spielmann KA, "Energy source, protein metabolism, and hunter-gatherer subsistence strategies." Journal of Anthropological Archaeology, 2 (1983): 1–31.

12. L. Cordain, "The hunter-gatherer diet," letter to the editor. Mayo Clinic Proceedings, 79, (2004): 703–704.

13. The two fatty acids considered "essential" are linoleic fatty acid (omega-6) and alpha-linolenic acid (omega-3). Both omega-6 and omega-3 produce three derivatives each, which are conditionally essential. We refer to them in the text as essential fatty acids (EFAs).

14. A. Simopoulos and J. Robinson, The omega diet: The life-saving nutritional program based on the diet of the island of Crete. New York: HarperPerennial, 1999.

15. A. Simopoulos and J. Robinson, The omega diet: The life-saving nutritional program based on the diet of the island of Crete. New York: HarperPerennial, 1999: 25.

16. A. Simopoulos and J. Robinson, The omega diet: The life-saving nutritional program based on the diet of the island of Crete. New York: HarperPerennial, 1999: 25.

17. A.P. Simopoulos, "Evolutionary aspects of omega-3 fatty acids in the

food supply." Center for Genetics, Nutrition and Health, Washington, DC 20009, USA, 60, 5–6 (1999): 421–429.

18. Gagné, Steve, "The origin of agriculture." Available from www.gold-enageproject.org.uk/965.html. (Accessed December 29, 2009).

19. L. Cordain, The paleo diet: Lose weight and get healthy by eating the food you were designed to eat. New York: Wiley, 2002.

20. D. Kesten, The healing secrets of food. Novato, CA: New World Library, 2001.

21. Food Science/Nutrition Updates, "Origins and evolution of the Western diet: Health implications for the 21st century," August 12, 2006, Available from: www.my-healthscience.blogspot.com/2006/08origins-and-evolution-of-western-diet.html. (Accessed January 2, 2010).

22. D. Mozaffarian and W.C. Willett, "Trans fatty acids and cardiovascular risk: A unique cardiometabolic imprint?" Current Atherosclerosis Reports, 9, 6 (2007): 486–93. PMID 18377789.

23. Daniel DeNoon, "Eat Trans Fat, Get Big Belly: Trans Fats Add—and Move—Weight to Belly," Available from www.webmd,com/diet/news/20060612/eat-trans-fat-get-big-belly. (Accessed, January 8, 2010).

24. S.B. Eaton, "The ancestral human diet: What was it and should it be a paradigm for contemporary nutrition?" Proceedings of the Nutritional Society, 65, 1 (2006): 1–6. PMID 16441938.

25. S.B. Eaton, M. Shostak, and M. Konner, The paleolithic prescription: A program of diet and exercise and a design for living. New York: Harper and Row, 1988.

26. Michael F. Roizen and Mehmet C. Oz, "Food Fight: The Ghrelin versus Leptin Grudge Match," You: On a Diet. New York: Free Press, 2006.

27. W.A. Price, Nutrition and physical degeneration. San Diego, CA: Price-Pottenger Nutrition Foundation, 2008.

28. D. Nathan, "Aboriginal languages of Australia." Aboriginal Languages of Australia Virtual Library. Available from http://www.dnathan.com/VL/austLang.htm 2007. (Accessed January 10, 2010).

29. P.D. Gluckman and M.A. Hanson, The fetal matrix: Evolution, development and disease. West Nyack, NY: Cambridge University Press, 2005.

30. P.D. Gluckman, M.A. Hanson, H.G. Spencer, P. Bateson, "Environmental influences during development and their later consequences for health and disease: Implications for the interpretation of empirical studies." Proceedings of Biological Science, 1564, (2002): 671–577. PMID 15870029.

31. P.D. Gluckman and M.A. Hanson, "Adult disease: Echoes of the past." European Journal of Endocrinology, 155, (2006): S47–S50.

32. P.D. Gluckman, M.A. Hanson, and H.G. Spencer, "Predictive adaptive responses and human evolution." Trends in Ecology and Evolution, 20 (2005): 527–533. PMID 16701430.

33. C.E. Ramsden, K.R. Faurot, P. Carrera-Bastos, L. Cordain, M.D. Lorg-

eril, and L.S. Sperling, "Dietary fat quality and coronary heart disease prevention: A unified theory based on evolutionary, historical, global, and modern perspectives." Current Treatment Options in Cardiovascular Medicine, 11 (2009): 289–301. PMID 19627662.

34. N. Saravanan, A. Haseeb, N.Z. Ehtesham, and Ghafoorunissa, "Differential effects of dietary saturated and trans-fatty acids on expression of genes associated with insulin sensitivity in rat adipose tissue." European Journal of Endocrinology, 153, 1 (2005): 159–65. PMID 15998628.

35. F.B. Hu, J.E. Manson, and W.C. Willett, "Types of dietary fat and risk of coronary heart disease: A critical review." Journal of the American College of Nutrition, 20, 1 (2001): 5–19. PMID 11293467.

36. L.H. Storlien, A.B. Jenkins, D.J. Chisholm, W.S. Pascoe, S. Khouri, and E.W. Kraegen, "Influence of dietary fat composition on development of insulin resistance in rats. Relationship to muscle triglyceride and omega-3 fatty acids in muscle phospholipid." Diabetes, 40, 2 (1991): 280–289. PMID 1991575.

37. A. Ibrahim, S. Natrajan, and R. Ghafoorunissa, "Dietary trans-fatty acids alter adipocyte plasma membrane fatty acid composition and insulin sensitivity in rats." Metabolism 54, 2 (2005): 240–246. PMID 15789505.

38. A.H. Lichtenstein and U.S. Schwab, "Relationship of dietary fat to glucose metabolism." Atherosclerosis, 150, 2 (2000): 227–43. PMID 10856515.

39. G.P. Nabhan, Some like it hot: Food, genes, and cultural diversity. Washington, D.C.: Island Press, 2004.

40. "Prevalence, age & genetics of lactose intolerance." Available from ww.foodreactions.org/intolerance/lactose/prevalence.html. (Accessed January 16, 2010).

41. M. Pollan, In defense of food: An eater's manifesto. New York: Penguin, 2008.

CHAPTER 7: "NOURISHMENT" NOW

1. A.P. Simopoulos, "The importance of the omega-6/omega-3 fatty acid ratio in cardiovascular disease and other chronic diseases." Experimental Biology and Medicine, 233, 6 (2008): 674–688. PMID 18408140.

2. A.P. Simopoulos, "Evolutionary aspects of diet, the omega-6/omega-3 ratio and genetic variation: Nutritional implications for chronic diseases." Biomedicine and Pharmacotherapy, 60, 9 (2006): 502–507. PMID 17045449.

3. A.P. Simopoulos, "Omega-3 fatty acids in health and disease and in growth and development." American Journal of Clinical Nutrition, 54, 3 (1991): 438–463. PMID 1908631.

4. S.D. Hursting, M. Thornquist, and M.M. Henderson, "Types of dietary fat and the incidence of cancer at five sites." Preventive Medicine, 19, 3 (1990): 242–253. PMID 2377587.

5. U.P. Kelavkar, J. Hutzley, R. Dhir, P. Kim, K.G. Allen, and K. McHugh, "Prostate tumor growth and recurrence can be modulated by the omega-

6:omega-3 ratio in diet: Athymic mouse xenograft model simulating radical prostatectomy." Neoplasia, 8, 2 (2006): 112–124. PMID 16611404.

6. J. Nair, C.E. Vaca, I. Velic, M. Mutanen, L.M. Valsta, and H. Bartsch, "High dietary omega-6 polyunsaturated fatty acids drastically increase the formation of etheno-DNA base adducts in white blood cells of female subjects." Cancer Epidemiology Biomarkers and Prevention, 6, 8 (1997): 597–601. PMID 9264272.

7. M.Y. Wang and J.G. Liehr, "Induction by estrogens of lipid peroxidation and lipid peroxide-derived malonaldehyde-DNA adducts in male Syrian hamsters: Role of lipid peroxidation in estrogen-induced kidney carcinogenesis." Carcinogenesis, 16, 8 (1995): 1941–1945. PMID 7634425.

8. X. Han, J.G. Liehr, and M.C. Bosland, "Induction of a DNA adduct detectable by 32p-postlabeling in the dorsolateral prostate of nbl/cr rats treated with estradiol-17 beta and testosterone." Carcinogenesis, 16, 4 (1995): 951–954. PMID 7728979.

9. A. Ascherio and W.C. Willett, "Health effects of trans fatty acids." American Journal of Clinical Nutrition, 66, 4 Suppl (1997): 1006S–1010S. PMID 9322581.

10. N. Bakker, P. Van't Veer, and P.L. Zock, "Adipose fatty acids and cancers of the breast, prostate and colon: An ecological study. Euramic study group." International Journal of Cancer, 72, 4 (1997): 587–591. PMID 9259395.

11. J.E. Chavarro, J.W. Rich-Edwards, B.A. Rosner, and W.C. Willett, "Dietary fatty acid intakes and the risk of ovulatory infertility." American Journal of Clinical Nutrition, 85, 1 (2007): 231–237. PMID 17209201.

12. A.T. Merchant, L.E. Kelemen, L. de Koning, E. Lonn, V. Vuksan, R. Jacobs, B. Davis, K.K. Teo, S. Yusuf, and S.S. Anand, "Interrelation of saturated fat, trans fat, alcohol intake, and subclinical atherosclerosis." American Journal of Clinical Nutrition, 87, 1 (2008): 168–174. PMID 18175752.

13. A.P. Simopoulos,"Is insulin resistance influenced by dietary linoleic acid and trans fatty acids?" Free Radical Biology and Medicine, 17, 4 (1994): 367–372. PMID 8001841.

14. N. Saravanan, A. Haseeb, and N.Z. Ehtesham, "Differential effects of dietary saturated and trans-fatty acids on expression of genes associated with insulin sensitivity in rat adipose tissue." European Journal of Endocrinology, 153, 1 (2005): 159–165. PMID 15998628.

15. I.M. Jazet, H. Pijl, and A.E. Meinders, "Adipose tissue as an endocrine organ: Impact on insulin resistance." Netherlands Journal of Medicine, 61, (2003): 194–212. PMID 12948164.

16. T.M. Willson, M.H. Lambert, and S.A. Kliewer, "Peroxisome proliferator activated receptor gamma and metabolic disease." Annual Review of Biochemistry, 70, (2001): 341–367. PMID 11395411.

17. I.J. Goldberg, "Lipoprotein lipase and lipolysis: Central roles in lipoprotein metabolism and atherogenesis." Journal of Lipid Research, 37, (1996):

693–707. PMID 8732771.

18. J.K. Kim, J.J. Fillmore, Y. Chen, C. Yu, I.K. Moore, M. Pypaert, E.P. Lutz, Y. Kako, W. Velez-Carrasco, I.J. Goldberg, J.L. Breslow, and G.I. Shulman, "Tissue-specific overexpression of lipoprotein lipase causes tissue-specific insulin resistance." Proceedings of the National Academy of Sciences, 98, (2001): 7522–7527.

19. L. Giovannelli, C. Saieva, G. Masala, G. Testa, S. Salvini, V. Pitozzi, E. Riboli, P. Dolara, and D. Palli, "Nutritional and lifestyle determinants of DNA oxidative damage: A study in a Mediterranean population." Carcinogenesis, 23, 9 (2002): 1483–1489. PMID 12189191.

20. K. Shimoi, A. Okitsu, M.H. Green, J.E. Lowe, T. Ohta, K. Kaji, H. Terato, H. Ide, and N. Kinae, "Oxidative DNA damage induced by high glucose and its suppression in human umbilical vein endothelial cells." Mutation Research, 480 (2001): 371–378. PMID 11506829.

21. Adams, Mike "High fructose corn syrup produces chemical 'HMF' when heated." From NaturalNews.com. Available from http://www.naturalnews.com/027286_HFCS_food_honey.html. (Accessed December 7, 2009).

22. B.W. Leblanc, G. Eggleston, D. Sammataro, C. Cornett, R. Dufault, T. Deeby, and E. St Cyr, "Formation of hydroxymethylfurfural in domestic high-fructose corn syrup and its toxicity to the honey bee (Apis mellifera)." Journal of Agriculture and Food Chemistry, 57, 16 (2009): 7369–7376. PMID 19645504.

23. L.J. Durling, L. Busk, and B.E. Hellman, "Evaluation of the DNA damaging effect of the heat-induced food toxicant 5-hydroxymethylfurfural (HMF) in various cell lines with different activities of sulfotransferases." Food Chemistry Toxicology, 47, 4 (2009): 880–884. PMID 19271322.

24. "Nunavik: Adventure awaits!" Québec: Official tourist site of the government of Québec, available from www.bonjourquebec.com/qc-en/nunavik0.html. (Accessed November 11, 2009.)

25. "Nunavik: The place to live." Available from www.nunavik-travelguide.com. (Accessed November 10, 2009).

26. Statistics Canada (2006). "2006 census, Aboriginal population profiles". Available from http://www12.statcan.ca/english/census06/data/profiles/aboriginal/Details/Page.cfm?Lang=E&Geo1=PR&Code1=62&Geo2=PR&Code2=01&Data=Count&SearchText=Nunavut&SearchType=Begins&SearchPR=01&B1=All&GeoLevel=&GeoCode=62. (Accessed December 7, 2009).

27. Searles, Edmund. "Food and the making of modern Inuit identities."Food & Foodways: History & Culture of Human Nourishment, 10 (2002): 55–78.

28. H. Kuhnlein and N. Turner, "Traditional plant foods of Canadian indigenous people: Nutrition, botany and use." Amsterdam: Overseas Publishers Association, 1991.

29. Inuit Tapiriit Kanatami. "Arctic Wildlife." Available from http://www.itk.ca/publications/arctic-wildlife 2007-11-20. "Not included are the myriad of

other species of plants and animals that Inuit use, such as geese, ducks, rabbits, ptarmigan, swans, halibut, clams, mussels, cod, berries and seaweed." (Accessed December 8, 2009).

30. J. Bennett and S. Rowley, "Chapter 5. Gathering." Uqalurait: An oral history of Nunavut. Kingston and Montreal: McGill-Queen's University Press, 2004: 84–85. http://books.google.com/books?id=6cjGnMRRrcEC&pg=PA8 4&dq=inuit+seaweed&sig=zIqIahWu8leC3FoRhzMnufW_QsU#PPR9,M1. "On the tidal flats and rocky shorelines, Inuit gathered seaweed and shellfish. For some, these foods were a treat; for others their consumption was a sign that the men were out hunting and there was no meat in camp."

31. J. Bennett and S. Rowley, "Chapter 5. Gathering." Uqalurait: An oral history of Nunavut. Kingston and Montreal: McGill-Queen's University Press, 2004: 78–85. Available from: http://books.google.com.books?id=6cjGnMRRr cEC&pg=PA78&lpg=PA78&dq=%22in+the+land+where+it+was+flat%22&s ource=web&ots=sQbLTAucNS&sig=QU5LmIueYJ2fBqtFsx8Zzzpzepg. (Accessed December 8, 2009).

32. P. Gadsby, "Health and medicine nutrition. The Inuit paradox." Available from http://discovermagazine.com/2004/oct/inuit-paradox/article print. Published October 1, 2004. (Accessed November 11, 2009).

33. E. Searles, "Food and the making of modern Inuit identities." Food & Foodways: History & Culture of Human Nourishment, 10 (2002): 55–78.

34. J. Dyerberg, H.O. Bang, and N. Hjorne, "Fatty acid composition of the plasma lipids in Greenland Eskimos." American Journal of Clinical Nutrition, 28, 9 (1975): 958–966. PMID 1163480.

35. H.O. Bang, J. Dyerberg, and H.M. Sinclair, "The composition of the Eskimo food in Northwestern Greenland." American Journal of Clinical Nutrition, 33, 12 (1980): 2657–2661. PMID 7435433.

36. P. Bjerregaard, T.K. Young, E. Dewailly, and S.O. Ebbesson, "Indigenous health in the Arctic: An overview of the circumpolar Inuit population." Scandanavian Journal of Public Health, 32, 5 (2004): 390–395. PMID 15513673.

37. S. Iverson, K. Frost, and S.Y. Lang, "Fat content and fatty acid composition of forage fish and invertebrates in Prince William Sound, Alaska: Factors contributing to among and within species variability." Marine Ecology Progress Series, 241 (2002): 161–181.

38. Maria Cone, "Pollutants drift north, making Inuits' traditional diet toxic," Los Angeles Times, January 18, 2004.

39. Daly, Gay, "A special report: Bad chemistry," On Earth Magazine, Natural Resources Defense Council, www.nrdc.org/OnEarth/06win/chem1.asp. (Accessed November 12, 2009).

40. L.D. Berkson, Hormone deception. New York, New York: Contemporary Books, 2000.

41. W.G. McBride, "Studies of the etiology of thalidomide dysmorphogenesis." Teratology, 14, 1 (1976): 71–87. PMID 960013.

42. "Thalidomide." For a historical account of the discovery of thalidomide see http://www.vaccinetruth.org/thalidomide.htm. (Accessed December 8, 2009).

43. "Thalidomide horrors show up in the children of victims," Gold Coast Bulletin, Australia, April 26, 1995.

44. R.A. Hatcher and C.C. Conrad, "Adenocarcinoma of the vagina and stilbestrol as a 'morning-after' pill." New England Journal of Medicine, 285, 22 (1971): 1264–1265. PMID 5113718.

45. H. Ulfelder, D. Poskanzer, and A.L. Herbst, "Stilbestrol-adenosis-carcinoma syndrome: Geographic distribution." New England Journal of Medicine, 285, 12 (1971): 691. PMID 5563489.

46. J. Folkman, "Transplacental carcinogenesis by stilbestrol." New England Journal of Medicine, 285, 7 (1971): 404–405. PMID 5556579.

47. ITVS, "A healthy baby girl: A brief history of DES," www.itvs.org/external/babyg/timeline.html. (Accessed November 14, 2009).

48. R.R. Newbold, E. Padilla-Banks, and W.N. Jefferson, "Adverse effects of the model environmental estrogen diethylstilbestrol are transmitted to subsequent generations." Endocrinology, 147, 6 Suppl (2006): S11–S17 PMID 16690809.

49. T. Colborn, D. Dumanoski, and J. Peterson, Our stolen future. New York: Penguin, 1997.

50. "CHE partnership call: Endocrine disruption and environmental Health: Ten years after our stolen future," www.healthandenvironment.org/articles/partnership_calls/346. (Accessed November 12, 2009).

51. "CHE partnership call: Endocrine disruption and environmental Health: Ten years after our stolen future," www.healthandenvironment.org/articles/partnership_calls/346. (Accessed November 12, 2009).

52. J.L. Jacobson and S.W. Jacobson, "Intellectual impairment in children exposed to polychlorinate biphenyls in utero." New England Journal of Medicine, 335, 11 (1996): 783–789. PMID 8703183.

53. J.L. Jacobson, S.W. Jacobson, and H.E. Humphrey, "Effects of in utero exposure to polychlorinated biphenyls and related contaminants on cognitive functioning in young children." Journal of Pediatrics, 116, 1 (1990): 38–45 PMID 2104928.

54. J.L. Jacobson, S.W. Jacobson, and H.E. Humphrey, "Effects of exposure to PCBs and related compounds on growth and activity in children." Neurotoxicology and Teratology, 12, 4 (1990): 319–326. PMID 2118230.

55. Consumer Reports, June 1998, "Hormone mimics (endocrine disruptors): They're in our food, should we worry?" www.mindfully.org/Pesticide/Hormone-Mimics-In-Food.htm . (Accessed November 18, 2009).

56. F.S. vom Saal, B.G. Timms, M.M. Montano, P. Palanza, K.A. Thayer, S.C. Nagel, M.D. Dhar, V.K. Ganjam, S. Parmigiani, and W.V. Welshons, "Prostate enlargement in mice due to fetal exposure to low doses of estradiol

or diethylstilbestrol and opposite effects at high doses." Proceedings of the National Academy of Science U.S.A., 94, 5 (1997): 2056–2061.

57. Riverkeeper NY's Leading Clean Water Advocate is "an independent, member-supported environmental organization founded on the premise that citizens themselves must roll up their sleeves to defend our waterways." Available from: http://www.riverkeeper.org/about-us/our-story/. (Accessed December 8, 2009).

58. Moving Stars and Earth for Water define themselves as "an artistic happening broadcast online, organized on the occasion of the Poetic Social Mission seeking to raise everyone's awareness of water-related issues." Available from: http://www.onedrop.org/en/mission_space/world_event/About_Event. aspx. (Accessed December 8, 2009).

59. AMAP Symposium on Human Health and Arctic Environmental Contaminants. Iqaluit, Nunavut, Canada, June 10–12, 2009, Available from www. uarctic.org/singleNewsArticle.aspx?m=83&amid=7143. (Accessed November 11, 2009).

60. The Agency for Toxic Substances and Disease Registry is a U.S. Department of Health and Human Services agency. On the website displayed here is a lists of common organic and other pollutants. http://www.atsdr.cdc.gov/toxprofiles/tp35.pdf. (Accessed December 8, 2009).

61. E.D. Magnuson, J.M. Nash, P. Stoler, "The poisoning of America," Time, September 23, 1980, available from www.time.com/time/magazine/article/0,9171,952748,00.html. (Accessed October 26, 2009).

62. Authored by www.SixWise.com, "Organophosphates: What you don't know can indeed hurt you." Available from http://www.sixwise.com/newsletters/05/06/15/organophosphates_what_you_dont_know_can_indeed_hurt_you.htm. (Accessed November 20, 2009).

63. "Our stolen future: Body burden studies document wide exposures." Web article by Centers for Disease Control and Prevention. Second National Report on Human Exposure to Environmental Chemicals, 2003. NCEH Pub. No. 02-0716. Available from http://www.ourstolenfuture.org/NEWSCIENCE/oncompounds/bodyburden/2003-0131-CDC-bodyburden.htm. (Accessed December 8, 2009).

64. Deborah Kesten and Larry Scherwitz interviewed David Granatstein, M.S., at his office in Wenatchee, Washington, on July 29, 2009. With a master's degree in soil science, Granatstein is an extension agent and sustainable agriculture specialist with the Center for Sustaining Agriculture and Natural Resources in Washington.

65. "Better Living Through Chemistry" is a variation of the advertising slogan, "Better Things for Better Living...Through Chemistry," which was DuPont's slogan between 1935 and 1982, when it dropped the "Through Chemistry" part. Since 1999, their slogan has been "The miracles of science."

66. Trif Alatzas, "DuPont touts 'miracles'." News Journal (Wilmington,

DE), "We need to get away from the word 'things" [DuPont Chairman and Chief Executive Charles O.] Holliday said. "Because we're also about providing knowledge'." Available at: http://en.academic.ru/dic.nsf/enwiki/197574. (Accessed August 3, 2010).

67. Mark Lytle, The Gentle Subversive: Rachel Carson, Silent Spring, and the rise of the environmental movement. New York: Oxford University Press, 2007: 166–167.

68. L. Lear, Rachael Carson: Witness for Nature. New York: Henry Hoyten, 1997.

69. DDT was banned for agricultural use worldwide under the Stockholm Convention. Source: Malaria Foundation International. Available from http://www.malaria.org/DDTpage.html. (Accessed December 8, 2009).

70. U.S. Department of Health and Human Services. Toxicological Profile: for DDT, DDE, and DDE. Agency for Toxic Substances and Disease Registry, September 2002. Available from http://www.atsdr.cdc.gov/toxprofiles/tp35-p.pdf. (Accessed December 10, 2009).

71. R. Carson, Silent Spring. New York, New York: Houghton Mifflin, 1962.

72. M.D. Anway, A.S. Cupp, M. Uzumcu, and M.K. Skinner, "Epigenetic transgenerational actions of endocrine disruptors and male fertility." Science, 308, 5727 (2005): 1466–1469. PMID 15933200.

73. M.D. Anway, C. Leathers, and M.K. Skinner, "Endocrine disruptor vinclozolin induced epigenetic transgenerational adult-onset disease." Endocrinology, 147, 12 (2006): 5515–5523. PMID 16973726.

74. S. Schneider, W. Kaufmann, R. Buesen, and B. van Ravenzwaay, "Vinclozolin—the lack of a transgenerational effect after oral maternal exposure during organogenesis." Toxicology, 25 (2008): 352–360. PMID 18485663.

75. K. Inawaka, M. Kawabe, S. Takahashi, Y. Doi, Y. Tomigahara, H. Tarui, J. Abe, S. Kawamura, and T. Shirai, "Maternal exposure to anti-androgenic compounds, vinclozolin, flutamide and procymidone, has no effects on spermatogenesis and DNA methylation in male rats of subsequent generations." Toxicology and Applied Pharmacology, 237, 2 (2009): 178–187.

76. E. Carlsen, A. Giwercman, N. Keiding, and N.E. Skakkebaek, "Evidence for decreasing quality of semen during past 50 years." British Medical Journal, 305, 6854 (1992): 609–613. PMID 1393072.

77. N.H. Aneck-Hahn, G.W. Schulenburg, M.S. Bornman, P. Farias, and C. de Jager, "Impaired semen quality associated with environmental DDT exposure in young men living in a malaria area in the Limpopo Province, South Africa." Journal of Andrology, 28, 3 (2007): 423–434.

78. C. de Jager, N.H. Aneck-Hahn, M.S. Bornman, P. Farias, G. Leter, P. Eleuteri, M. Rescia, and M. Spano, "Sperm chromatin integrity in DDT-exposed young men living in a malaria area in the Limpopo Province, South Africa. " Human Reproduction, 24, 10 (2009): 2429–2438.

79. "Toxic pesticides above "safe" levels in many U.S. residents." Pesticide Action Network Updates Service (PANUP), Available from http://www.panna.org/legacy/panups/panup_20040511.dv.html. (Accessed August 3, 2010.)

80. Ivan Noble, "Mexican study raises GM concern, Genetic diversity is at stake, say campaigners," 2001. Available from http://news.bbc.co.uk/2/hi/science/nature/1680848.stm. (Accessed December 9, 2009).

81. Carmelo Ruiz-Marrero, "Genetic pollution: Biotech corn invades Mexico." Available from http://www.corpwatch.org/article.php?id=2088. (Accessed December 9, 2009).

82. Tom Abate, "Engineered food rules proposed." Available from http://www.sfgate.com/cgi-bin/article.cgi?f=/c/a/2001/01/18/BU80932.DTL&type=printable. (Accessed December 9, 2009).

83. Dan Glickman, "Opinion," Los Angeles Times, April 2, 2001.

84. Johannes Wirz, "The case of Mexican maize." The Nature Institute, Available from http://www.natureinstitute.org/pub/ic/ic9/maize.htm. (Accessed August 3, 2010).

85. Barbara Boster, "Issues of genetically modified crops as reported in the press." Available from http://www.berkeley.edu/news/berkeleyan/1999/0915/crop_report.html. (Accessed December 9, 2009).

86. David Barboza, "As biotech crops multiply, consumers get little choice." Available from http://www.nytimes.com/2001/06/10/business/10GENE.html. (Accessed December 9, 2009).

87. "History of horticulture" acknowledgment of Joseph Gottlieb 1733–1806, the first plant hybridizer. Available from http://www.hcs.ohio-state.edu/hort/history/110.html. (Accessed December 9, 2009).

88. Dan Barker, "The forgotten story of Luther Burbank." Available from http://www.ffrf.org/fttoday/back/burbankbio.html. (Accessed December 9, 2009).

89. Rozella Kennedy, "An interview with John Fagan." Available from http://mothering.com/genetically-engineered-foods-too-many-unknowns. (Accessed December 9, 2009).

90. Lucette Lagnado, "Genetically-altered baby foods are being rejected—by adults." Available from http://www.gene.ch/gentech/1999/Jul-Aug/msg00111.html. (Accessed December 2009).

91. I.F. Pryme and R. Lembcke, "In vivo studies on possible health consequences of genetically modified food and feed—with particular regard to ingredients consisting of genetically modified plant materials." Nutrition and Health, 17, 1 (2003): 1–8.

92. Martha Herbert, "Genetically modifed food:Unsafe until further notice." Available from http://www.rense.com/general9/gmm.htm. (Accessed December 9, 2009).

93. A. Kimbrell, Your right to know: Genetic engineering and the secret changes in your food. San Rafael, CA: Earth Aware Editions, 2007.

94. Nutrient balance is yet another dynamic that may be affected when a food is modified by GE. When a health-policy researcher analyzed the nutrient content in GM soybeans, he discovered that they had much lower levels of isoflavones, naturally occurring substances that lower cholesterol levels and the odds of cancer. ("Researcher questions nutritional value of genetically altered crops," San Francisco Chronicle, July 28, 1999; www.berkeley.edu/news) Allergic reactions, too—most often due to the creation of new proteins—are a key health concern that has been linked to consuming GM organisms. (Michael Jacobson, FDA "Meeting on the safety and labeling of GMOs, November 18, 1999, www.lumenfds.com/jacobson.htm).

95. William Engdahl, "Bird flu and chicken factory farms: Profit bonanza for US agribusiness," available from www.globalresearch.ca. (Accessed November 29, 2009).

96. Business Timeline: 1960s. Perdue Farms. 2008. Available from http://www.perdue.com/company/history/index.html. (Accessed August 3, 2010).

97. Debbie Weinhold, "The briefing room: National hog farmer business update, NutriDense® Grain and Perdue AgriBusiness announce contracting opportunity," November 18, 2009, http://blog.nationalhogfarmer.com/briefingroom/2009/11/18/nutridense-grain-and-perdue-agribusiness-announce-contracting-opportunity/. (Accessed August 3, 2010).

98. D.M. Henricks, S.L. Gray, and J.L. Hoover, "Residue levels of endogenous estrogens in beef tissues." Journal of Animal Science, 57, 1 (1983): 247–255. PMID 6885662.

99. D.M. Henricks, S.L. Gray, J.J. Owenby, and B.R. Lackey, "Residues from anabolic preparations after good veterinary practice." Acta Pathologica, Microbiologica et Immunologica Scandinavica, 109, 4 (2001): 273–283. PMID 11469498.

100. S.H. Swan, "Semen quality in relation to pesticide exposure in Missouri males." Missouri Medicine, 100, 6 (2003): 554. PMID 14699813.

101. S.H. Swan, R.L. Kruse, F. Liu, D.B. Barr, E.Z. Drobnis, J.B. Redmon, C. Wang, C. Brazil, and J.W. "Overstreet, Semen quality in relation to biomarkers of pesticide exposure." Environmental Health Perspectives, 111, 12 (2003): 1478–1484.

102. K. Brownell and K. Horgen, Food fight: The inside story of the food industry: America's obesity crisis, and what we can do about it. New York: McGraw-Hill, 2004.

103. "Don't blame your genes," The Economist, September 5, 2009: 86.

CHAPTER 8: FOOD PIONEER

1. "Panorama organic grass-fed meats: Rancher profile," available at www.panoramameats.com/panorama/our-story/rancher-profile/arapaho-ranch/. (Accessed October 5, 2009).

2. "Panorama: Organic grass-fed meats, Panorama meats exclusively sup-

plies organic grass-fed Angus beef from northern Arapaho Indian Tribe to Whole Foods Market Rocky Mountain Region," available at www.panorama-meats.com/panorama/news/press-releases/20090519-arapaho-ranch. (Accessed October 5, 2009).

3. Catherine Tsal, "Tribe secures deal to sell organic beef," Denver Post, www.denverpost.com. (Accessed October 5, 2009).

4. D. Brown, and C. McCrimmon, C; "An organic journey: One steer's transformation into dinner," Denver Post, Food, Section D, September 30, 2009. The website version called "Grass-fed beef: One steer's organic journey from ranch to dinner" is available from www.denverpost.com/food. (Accessed October 5, 2009).

5. Bryan Walsh, "Getting real about the high price of cheap food." Time, August 21, 2009. available from www.time.com/time/printout/0,8816,1917458,00.html. (Accessed September 22, 2009).

6. R. Sinha, A.J. Cross, B.I. Graubard, M.F. Leitzmann, and A. Schatzkin, "Meat intake and mortality: A prospective study of over half a million people." Archives of Internal Medicine, 169, 6 (2009): 562–571. PMID 19307518.

7. "The Northern Arapaho Tribe," available from http://www.windriver-country.com/windriverres/arapahofront.html. (Accessed October 5, 2009).

8. "Arapaho Ranch" available from www.arapahoranch.com . (Accessed October 15, 2009).

9. Dan Barber, "Ripe for the eating," Martha Stewart Living, August 2009, available from http://www.bluehillfarm.com/food/dans-musings. (Accessed October 15, 2009).

10. "Blue Hill Dan Barber wins James Beard Award for nation's top chef." Available from http://www.nydailynews.com/lifestyle/food/2009/05/05/2009-05-05 blue_hill_new_york_chef_dan_barber_wins_james_beard_award_for_nations_top_chef.html. (Accessed October 15, 2009).

11. Dan Barber, "Passions: Clean plate club," Food&Wine, available from www.foodandwine.com/articles/passions-clean-plate-club. (Accessed October 1, 2009).

12. Rubenstein, Hal, "Top of the Hill," June 19, 2000, available from http://nymag.com/nymetro/food/reviews/restaurant/3397/. (Accessed October 4, 2009).

13. Dan Barber, "Ripe for the eating," Martha Stewart Living, August 2009. (Accessed October 1, 2009).

14. Adam Platt, "Up on the Farm," New York Magazine, restaurant review, May 21, 2005, available from: http://nymag.com/nymetro/food/reviews/restaurant/9477/. (Accessed October 4, 2009).

15. Stone Barns Center for Food & Agriculture, "The Farm," available from www.stonebarnscenter.org/sb_about/farm.aspx. (Accessed October 4, 2009).

16. Frank Bruni, "Food You'd almost rather hug than eat," New York Times, Dining & Wine section, August 2, 2006, available from http://events.nytimes.

com/2006/08/02/dining/reviews/02rest.html. (Accessed October 16, 2006).

17. Dan Barber, "Back on the Farm," Gourmet, July 2004, available from: www.gourmet.com/magazine/2000s/2004/07/back_on_the_farm. (Accessed October 16, 2009).

18. "About Us: About DrGreene.com," mission statement, available from: www.drgreene.com/127.html. (Accessed October 7, 2009).

19. K.J. Baines, L.G. Wood, and P.G. Gibson, "The nutrigenomics of asthma: Molecular mechanisms of airway neutrophilia following dietary anti-oxidant withdrawal." OMICS: A Journal of Integrative Biology, 13, 5 (2009): 355–365. PMID 19715394.

20. B.S. Levine, M.M. Wigren, D.S. Chapman, J.F. Kerner, R.L. Bergman, and R.S. Rivlin, "A national survey of attitudes and practices of primary-care physicians relating to nutrition: Strategies for enhancing the use of clinical nutrition in medical practice." American Journal of Clinical Nutrition, 57, 2 (1993): 115–119. PMID 8424377.

21. "From the Centers for Disease Control and Prevention. Missed opportunities in preventive counseling for cardiovascular disease—United States, 1995." Journal of the American Medical Association, 279, 10 (1998): 741–742. PMID 9508138.

22. DrGreene Content, "Dr. Greene's Organic Journey," special feature, available from: www.drgreene.com/21_2072.html. (Accessed October 9, 2009).

23. DrGreene Content, "Dr. Greene's Organic Rx," video viewed at: http://www.drgreene.com/555560.html. (Accessed October 16, 2009).

24. Environmental Working Group,"Shoppers guide to pesticides," available from http://www.foodnews.org/. (Accessed October 16, 2009).

25. DrGreene Content, "Organic Rx: Dr. Greene's Organix RX," available from www.drgreene.com/21_2154.html. (Accessed October 8, 2009).

26. DrGreene Content, "Dr. Greene's Organic Prescription: What You Need to Know." Available from: www.drgreene.org/body.cfm?id=555560. (Accessed October 10, 2009).

27. DrGreene Content, "Press Room, 'Dr. Greene's Housecalls' voted 'Best Pediatric Site' by Yahoo Internet Life," and "Dr. Greene selected as one of the most influential forces in healthcare IT," available from www.drgreene.com/26.html. (Accessed October 7, 2009).

28. "The Mission," available from: www.organic-center.org/newmission/theMission.htm. (Accessed October 10, 2009).

29. DrGreene Content, "Feeding baby green: 5 ways to buy organic on a budget." Available from: www.drgreene.com. (Accessed October 10, 2009).

30. A. Greene, A. Chensheng , C. Benbrook, and P. Landrigan,"Successes and lost opportunities to reduce children's exposure to pesticides since the mid-1990s." Critical Issue Report, 1 (2006): Available from: www.organic-center.org/science.pest.php?action=view&report_id=55. (Accessed October 10, 2009).

31. In February 2006 The Organic Center sponsored a symposium at the

2006 annual meeting of the American Association for the Advancement of Science (AAAS). Four scientists spoke about steps taken in the last decade to reduce children's pesticide exposures and compared and contrasted progress made as a result of innovation in pesticide chemistry and integrated pest management systems, through ecolabel programs (including organic certification), and by regulation. While some progress has been made in reducing pesticide risks, the report presents the science supporting the need for stronger action and outlines constructive steps required to accelerate progress.

32. Deborah Kesten interviewed Malea Balmuth on September 27, 2009 at the Balmuth farm in Granbury, Texas.

33. Courtney Easton, "Look at 'em grow," Hood County News, Life section, 1B, July 4, 2009.

34. Steve Diver. "Biodynamic farming and compost preparation." National Sustainable Agriculture Information Service. Available from http://attra.ncat. org/attra-pub/biodynamic.html. (Accessed October 16, 2009).

35. Washington State University, College of Agricultural, Human, and Natural Resource Sciences, "Major in Organic Agriculture Systems." Available from www.afs.wsu.edu/majors/organic.htm. (Accessed October 13, 2009).

36. Educated Nation/Higher Education Blog, "Washington State University Offers Organic Farming Degree," June 28, 2006. Available from: http:// www.educatednation.com/2006/06/28/washington-state-university-offers-organic-farming-degree. (Accessed October 14, 2009).

37. "The organic industry market trends 2008." Organic Trade Association. Available from: http://www.ota.com/pics/documents/Mini%20fact%20 1-08%20confirming.pdf. (Accessed October 14, 2009).

38. Organic Center, "The Mission." Available from: www.organic center. org/newmission/theMission.htm. (Accessed October 10, 2009).

39. Organic Center, "The Mission." Available from: www.organic center. org/newmission/theMission.htm. (Accessed October 10, 2009).

40. Bob Condor, "Living Well: WSU's organic agriculture major takes root." Seattlepi: Health & Fitness. Available from: www.seattlepi.com/health/280983_ condor14.html. (Accessed October 16, 2009).

41. Paul Clarke, "Green degrees." Alaska Airlines Magazine, (February 2009): 47–57.

42. D. Davis, "Declining fruit and vegetable nutrient composition: What is the evidence." HortScience, 44, 1 (2009): 15–19.

43. A.M. Mayer, "Historical changes in the mineral content of fruits and vegetables." British Food Journal, 99 (1997): 207–211.

44. W.M. Jarrell and R.B. Beverly, "The dilution effect in plant nutrition studies." Advances in Agronomy, 34 (1981): 197–224.

45. Organic Center, "New evidence confirms the nutritional superiority of plant-based organic foods." Available from: www.organic-center.org/report-files/5367_Nutrient_Content_SSR_FINAL_V2.pdf. (Accessed October 16,

2009).

46. Brian Halwell, "Still no free lunch: Nutrient levels in U.S.. food supply eroded in pursuit of higher yields." Available from: www.organic-center.org/science.nutriphp?action=view&report_id=115. (Accessed October 16, 2009).

47. C.M. Williams, "Nutritional quality of organic food: Shades of grey or shades of green?" Proceedings of the Nutritional Society, 61, 1 (2002): 19–24. PMID 12002790.

48. V. Worthington, "Nutritional quality of organic versus conventional fruits, vegetables, and grains." J Alternative and Complementary Medicine, 7, 2 (2001): 161–173. PMID 11327522.

49. Hannah Hathaway, "The Daily Evergreen," April 25, 2008. Available from: www.dailyeverygreen.com/pages/print_story?storyId=25612. (Accessed October 12, 2009).

50. K. Clancy, Greener pastures: How grass fed beef and milk contribute to healthy eating, Cambridge, MA: Union of Scientists, 2006.

51. C.A. Daley, K. Harrison, P. Doyle, A. Abbott, G. Nader, and S. Larson, "A review of fatty acid profiles and antioxidant content in grass-fed and grain-fed beef." Nutrition Journal, 9 (2010): 10. PMID 20219103.

52. D.C. Rule, K.S. Broughton, S.M. Shellito, and G. Maiorano, "Comparison of muscle fatty acid profiles and cholesterol concentrations of bison, beef cattle, elk, and chicken." Journal of Animal Science, 80, 5 (2002): 1202–1211. PMID 12019607.

CHAPTER 9: 10 GREEN-GENE FOOD GUIDELINES

1. J. Cloud, "Why DNA isn't your destiny," Time, Jan. 6, 2010.

2. A.P. Feinberg, "Epigenetics at the epicenter of modern medicine." Journal of the American Medical Association, 299, 11 (2008): 1345–1350. PMID18349095.

3. S.J. Olshansky, D.J. Passaro, R.C. Hershow, J. Layden, B.A. Carnes, J. Brody, L. Hayflick, R.N. Butler, D.B. Allison, and D.S. Ludwig, "A potential decline in life expectancy in the United States in the 21st century." New England Journal of Medicine, 352, 11 (2005): 1138–1145. PMID 15784668.

4. K. O'Dea, "Marked improvement in carbohydrate and lipid metabolism in diabetic Australian aborigines after temporary reversion to traditional lifestyle." Diabetes, 33, 6 (1984): 596–603. PMID 6373464.

5. S.B. Eaton, M. Shostak, and M. Konner, The paleolithic prescription: A program of diet and exercise and a design for living. New York: Harper Row, 1988.

6. Miranda Hitti, WebMD Health News, "Americans eating fewer vegetables." Available from http://www.webmd.com/food-recipes/news/20070319/americans-eating-fewer-vegetables. (Accessed February 3, 2010).

7. "Quick overview: Organic agriculture and production," Organic Trade Association. Available from www.ota.com/definition/quickoverview.html. (Ac-

cessed February 3, 2010).

8. J. Weinstein, The ethical gourmet: How to enjoy great food that is humanely raised, sustainable, nonendangered, and replenishes the earth. New York: Crown Publishing, 2006.

9. Deborah Kesten and Larry Scherwitz interviewed David Granatstein at his office in Wenatchee, Washington, on July 29, 2009. With a master's degree in Soil Science, Granatstein is an Extension Agent and Sustainable Agriculture Specialist with the Center for Sustaining Agriculture and Natural Resources in Washington.

10. S.K. Searles and J.G. Armstrong, "Vitamin E, vitamin A, and carotene contents of Alberta butter." Journal of Dairy Science, 53, 2 (1970): 150–154. PMID 5413655.

11. G.C. Gast, N.M. de Roos, I. Sluijs, M.L. Bots, J.W. Beulens, J.M. Geleijnse, J.C. Witteman, D.E. Grobbee, P.H. Peeters, and Y.T. van der Schouw, "A high menaquinone intake reduces the incidence of coronary heart disease." Nutrition Metabolism and Cardiovascular Disease, 19, 7 (2009): 504–510. PMID 19179058.

12. J. Iwamoto, Y. Sato, T. Takeda, and H. Matsumoto, "High-dose vitamin K supplementation reduces fracture incidence in postmenopausal women: A review of the literature." Nutrition Research, 29, 4 (2009): 221–228. PMID 19410972.

13. Cocofeed, "What is pastured poultry?" Available from www.cocofeed. com/pastured_poultry.htm. (Accessed February 3, 2010).

14. Sustainable Table, "What is local?" Available from www.sustainabletable.org/issues/eatlocal/. (Accessed February 3, 2010).

15. M.C. Craig-Schmidt and B.M. Holzer, Fatty acid isomers in foods. Fatty acids in foods and their health implications, New York: Marcel Dekker, 2000: 307–356.

16. Omega-6, in the presence of high insulin, is shunted into the arachidonic acid (AA) cycle, so instead of progressing to prostaglandin 1, which is anti-inflammatory, it is shunted to AA, which becomes pro-inflammatory prostaglandin 2. In turn, this imbalance of omega 6: omega 3 becomes even more detrimental to health in the presence of a high glycemic diet and insulin resistance. In other words, excess omega-6 becomes inflammatory in the presence of too much insulin from processed carbohydrates.

17. R. Farzaneh-Far, J. Lin, E.S. Epel, W.S. Harris, E.H. Blackburn, and M.A. Whooley, "Association of marine omega-3 fatty acid levels with telomeric aging in patients with coronary heart disease." Journal of the American Medical Association, 303, 3 (2010): 250–257. PMID 20085953.

18. W.A. Price, "Nutrition and physical degeneration." San Diego: Price-Pottenger Nutrition Foundation, Inc., 2008.

19. Environmental Working Group, "Pharmaceuticals pollute U.S. tap water," Press Release: March 10, 2008; Available from www.ewg.org/node/26128.

(Accessed February 9, 2010).

20. L. Scherwitz and D. Kesten, "Seven eating styles linked to overeating, overweight, and obesity." Explore (NY), 1, 5 (2005): 342–359. PMID 16781565.

21. D. Kesten and L. Scherwitz, The enlightened diet: 7 weight-loss solutions that nourish body, mind, and soul. Berkeley, CA: Ten Speed Press, 2007.

CHAPTER 10: TAKING ACTION: IF NOT NOW, WHEN?

1. D. Kesten, Feeding the body, nourishing the soul. Berkeley, CA: Conari Press, 1997.

2. E. Rossi, The psychobiology of gene expression. New York: Norton, 2002.

3. E.L. Rossi, "The bioinformatics of psychosocial genomics in alternative and complementary medicine." Research in Complementary and Classical Natural Medicine, 10, (2003): 143–150. PMID 12853721.

4. E.L. Rossi, "Gene expression, neurogenesis, and healing: Psychosocial genomics of therapeutic hypnosis." American Journal of Clinical Hypnosis, 45, 3 (2003): 197–216. PMID 12570091.

5. D. Kesten, Feeding the body, nourishing the soul. Amherst, MA: White River Press, 2008.

6. Kesten's book is about the "spiritual ingredient" in food; the ways in which wisdom traditions (i.e., Judaism, Christianity, Islam, Hinduism, Buddhism, Native American food beliefs, African-American soul food, etc.) throughout the centuries have infused meals with meaning and tradition. Kesten supports time-tested food and nutrition guidelines from the wisdom traditions with state-of-the-art science, which suggests that infusing meals with love and meaning does, indeed, influence both food and the dining experience.

7. D. Kesten, The health secrets of food. Novato, CA: New World Library, 2001.

8. In this book, Kesten proposes an Integrative Nutrition model, which is about the effect food has not only on physical health but also on emotional, spiritual, and social well-being. Her Integrative Nutrition model is based not only on these four facets of food (i.e., the biological, psychological, spiritual, and social elements), but also on three worldviews about nutrition: 1) Western nutritional science; 2) Eastern healing systems that include nutrition (i.e., traditional Chinese medicine, Ayurveda, Tibetan Medicine, etc.); and 3) the world's wisdom traditions (i.e., world religions and cultural traditions).

9. D. Kessler, The end of overeating: Taking control of the insatiable American appetite. New York: Rodale, 2009.

10. O. Winfrey, Before you grocery shop again . . . Food 101, in The Oprah Show. (Channel 5 KING: USA, 2010, 60 minutes).

11. D. Kesten and L. Scherwitz, The enlightened diet: 7 weight-loss solutions that nourish body, mind, and soul. Berkeley, CA: Ten Speed Press, 2007.

12. D. Kesten, Website for the Enlightened diet, Available from www.En-lightened-Diet.com. (Accessed March 8, 2010).

13. D. Kesten, The healing secrets of food. Novato, CA: New World Library, p. 29, 2001.

14. Will Allen, "Let's grow the good food revolution," December 23, 2009, www.facebook.com/note.php?note_id=248460885489. (Accessed February 28, 2010).

15. J. Oliver, Jamie's food revolution: Rediscover how to cook simple, delicious, affordable meals. New York: Hyperion, 2009.

16. WSOCTV.com, ""America's Food Revolution Begins," posted January 13, 2010; updated February 24, 2010, www.wsoctv.com/print/22230261/detail.html. (Accessed February 28, 2010).

17. On-line Dictionary Available from www.dictionary.com. (Accessed March 3, 2010).

INDEX

About the Authors

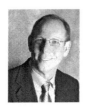

GRAY GRAHAM, NTP, has been an international consultant and teacher in the field of clinical nutrition for almost twenty years. During his career, he has taught hundreds of seminars on nutritional therapy to thousands of physicians and other healthcare practitioners worldwide. He is the founder of the Nutritional Therapy Association (NTA), and in 2001, started the Nutritional Therapy Training Program. Since then, NTA has certified more than a thousand Nutritional Therapist Practitioners (NTPs) throughout the United States. Website: www.nutritionaltherapy.com.

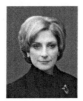

DEBORAH KESTEN, MPH, is an international nutrition researcher, educator, author, and lecturer. She was Director of Nutrition on research showing heart disease can be reversed through lifestyle changes. Her books, which have been featured in magazines, include the award-winning *Feeding the Body, Nourishing the Soul*, *The Healing Secrets of Food*, and *The Enlightened Diet*, which is based on her original published research. She has presented at national conferences, and been a guest speaker on television and radio shows. Website: www.EnlightenedDiet.com

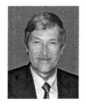

LARRY SCHERWITZ, PhD, is an international research scientist, with a specialty in mind-body medicine, lifestyle and its link to preventing and reversing both heart disease and obesity, and evidence-based Complementary and Alternative Medicine (CAM) research. His innovative research has been published in prestigious medical journals, ranging from *The Lancet* to the *American Journal of Cardiology* and the *Journal of the American Medical Association*. His more recent original research reveals seven newly discovered eating styles linked to overeating, overweight, and obesity. Website: www.EnlightenedDiet.com